Shunn
D0732814

Shunned: Discrimination against People with Mental Illness

Graham Thornicroft

Head, Health Service Research
Department, Institute of Psychiatry, London,
and Consultant Psychiatrist,
South London and Maudsley
NHS Trust

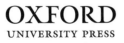

OXFORD
UNIVERSITY PRESS

OXFORD
UNIVERSITY PRESS

Great Clarendon Street, Oxford OX2 6DP

Oxford University Press is a department of the University of Oxford.
It furthers the University's objective of excellence in research, scholarship,
and education by publishing worldwide in

Oxford New York

Auckland Cape Town Dar es Salaam Hong Kong Karachi
Kuala Lumpur Madrid Melbourne Mexico City Nairobi
New Delhi Shanghai Taipei Toronto

With offices in

Argentina Austria Brazil Chile Czech Republic France Greece
Guatemala Hungary Italy Japan Poland Portugal Singapore
South Korea Switzerland Thailand Turkey Ukraine Vietnam

Oxford is a registered trade mark of Oxford University Press
in the UK and in certain other countries

Published in the United States
by Oxford University Press Inc., New York

© Graham Thornicroft 2006

The moral rights of the author have been asserted
Database right Oxford University Press (maker)

First published 2006
Reprinted 2007 (with corrections)

A catalogue record for this title is available from the British Library
Library of Congress Cataloging in Publication Data
Thornicroft, Graham.
Shunned : discrimination against people with mental illness/Graham Thornicroft.
Includes index.
ISBN-13: 978-0-19-857097-4 (hardback)
ISBN-13: 978-0-19-857098-1 (paperback)
1. Mental illness–Public opinion. 2. Discrimination against the mentally ill.
3. Stigma (Social psychology) I. Title.
[DNLM: 1. Mentally Ill Persons. 2. Prejudice. WM 29.5 T512s 2006]
RC454. T4556 2006   305.9'084–dc22   2006010942

Typeset by SPI Publisher Services, Pondicherry, India
Printed in Great Britain
on acid-free paper by
Biddles Ltd., King's Lynn.

10 9 8 7 6 5 4 3 2

Contents

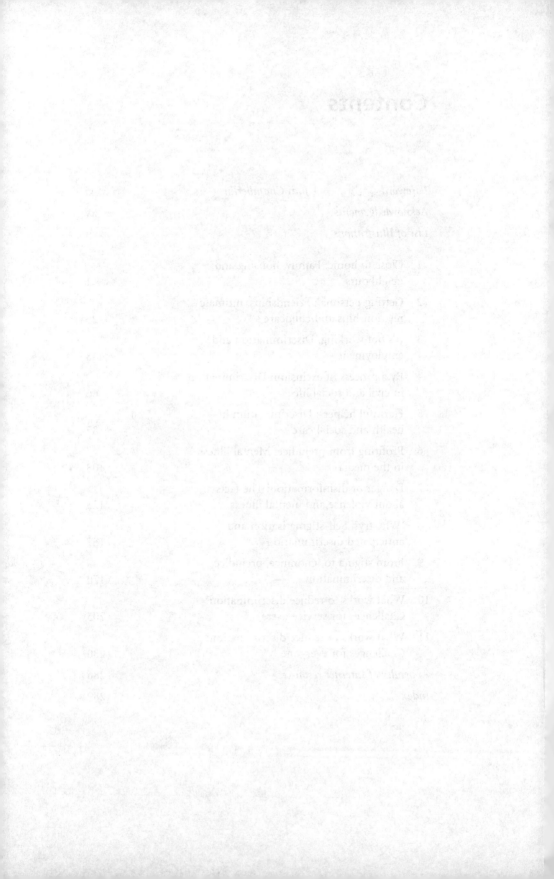

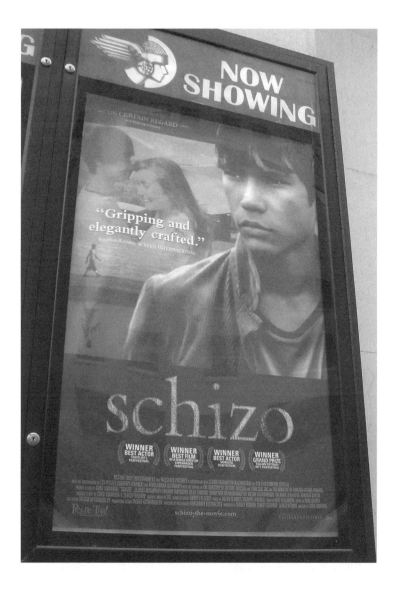

Billboard advertising film called 'Schizo', New York, 2005.

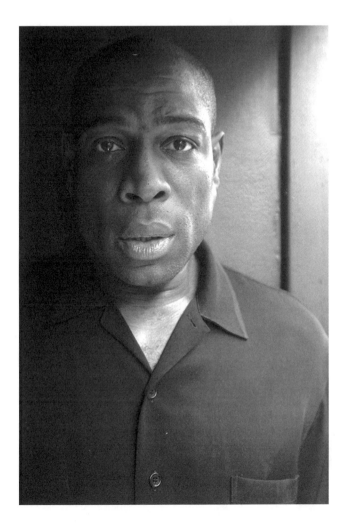

Frank Bruno – The battle to be happy.
Copyright Martin Godwin 2005. Courtesy of Guardian Newspapers
Limited.

Foreword

In the 1960s, I found out first-hand about the problems of prejudice, stigma, and discrimination in the mental health system, by becoming a victim of involuntary commitment and forced treatment. That experience had the unintended consequence of giving my life purpose and direction, and in the 1970s I became part of what was then called the 'mental patients' liberation movement'. Those of us who had experienced the system first-hand saw clearly that our basic rights as human beings and citizens had been violated by the very process of psychiatric diagnosis, labelling and treatment, and we worked to change those conditions. It is important to note that our campaign was *not* one against 'stigma', but instead was part of the broad-based anti-discrimination movement that insisted on basic rights for ethnic, gender and sexual identity groups that were marginalized within the dominant culture. These groups were run and controlled by the people who had experienced discrimination first-hand, starting with the black civil rights movement of the 1950s and 60s, on which other groups were modelled.

To fight against stigma is to engage in a side skirmish rather than to take on the basic problem – that once a person is labelled 'mentally ill', he or she loses fundamental rights that everyone else takes for granted. In fact, most so-called anti-stigma campaigns are run by the very people and organizations that control and support the process of diagnosis and treatment. It is not, therefore, surprising that the subtext of many such campaigns is to encourage *more* people to enter treatment, ignoring the fact that once they do so, they, too, will find themselves lacking both basic rights and the status to protest against them. Once a person has been defined as mentally ill, his or her own decision-making ability is called into question, and therefore, his or her protests are often discredited or, even worse, labelled one more 'symptom' of his or her illness.

In recent years, what is now usually called the psychiatric survivor or user movement *has* engaged with the question of stigma, but, significantly, only by linking it with discrimination. The solution is seen *not* as lessening stigma, but, instead, of ensuring that people labelled mentally ill retain their basic citizenship rights, particularly the right to challenge both the label and the treatment, and to retain basic control over one's own life.

It is important that the linked problems of stigma, prejudice, and discrimination against people labelled as mentally ill are now also being addressed by a mental health professional, as Graham Thornicroft has done in this book. By linking stigma to discrimination, he has joined those of us who have been labelled, who have always known that what others have defined as the 'stigma problem' lies at the root of the difficulties we face as we attempt to improve the conditions of our lives and to insure that we obtain the same legal and social status as people without psychiatric labels.

The very word stigma is problematic, locating the problem as *within the individual*. For this reason we have, in recent years, tried to replace the term stigma with two words that more accurately describe our situation:

- *Prejudice:* the unwarranted negative attitudes people hold toward us based on their own beliefs and preconceptions, rather than on our specific, individual attributes
- *Discrimination:* the societal codification of such attitudes, as expressed in laws and customs that result in us having a lower social status and fewer rights than non-labelled people.

The words that we choose to address this problem are important, because the activities that result are very much dependent upon the lens through which we view it. When the problem is framed as being stigma, the result is often so-called anti-stigma campaigns that do little or nothing to involve the very people who supposedly are the beneficiaries of these campaigns or to challenge their lesser legal status. In fact, in the language and images they choose to use, these campaigns often reinforce the very stigma they are supposedly designed to combat. This can be seen particularly in the embrace of the biologically based model of mental illnesses, despite the fact that there is *no* biologically based test that can distinguish a person diagnosed with a mental illness from one who has no such diagnosis. The mental health industry has been notably successful in convincing the public that people with psychiatric diagnoses are biologically distinguishable from so-called 'normal' people, yet there exists *no* blood test, x-ray, or any other biologically based marker that serves a diagnostic purpose. Psychiatric diagnosis continues to be, as it has been throughout its history, a matter of clinical impression in which a person's own protestations of *not* being mentally ill are taken as one of the strongest pieces of evidence that he or she in fact is.

Another problem is that many campaigns that purport to be about stigma are really about encouraging more people to enter mental health treatment, which is quite a different matter. Those of us who have experienced diagnosis and treatment, and who have become active in user/survivor[1] organizations, hold a wide variety of opinions about the value of treatment, including many who believe that treatment itself is part of the problem. Therefore, we are extremely sceptical about justifications for anti-stigma as 'removing barriers to treatment'. For example, the US Substance Abuse and Mental Health Services Administration states on its Website, under the headline, 'Anti-Stigma: Do You Know the Facts?,' 'Fear of stigma, and the resulting discrimination, discourages individuals and their families from getting the help they need.'[2] The National Mental Health Awareness Campaign, similarly, states its goals as to 'encourage people to identify, discuss, and seek help for mental health problems; and create a more accepting environment for them to do so,' and identifies stigma as a 'primary reason that people do not seek the mental health services they need'.[3]

When people labelled mentally ill are discriminated against, what makes more sense – to work against stigma, or to utilize the resources that other groups use when they face discrimination? While 'changing attitudes' may have a warm, fuzzy appeal, changing discriminating *behaviour* is, I believe far more important. A prospective landlord or employer needs to know that when he or she decides not to rent an apartment or offer a job to an otherwise qualified person because that person is perceived as being mentally ill, he or she is breaking the law, not just some vaguely defined social norm. Laws like the Americans with Disabilities Act in the US, or the Disability Discrimination Act in the UK, exist because people with disabilities worked hard to ensure that discrimination against them be recognized as just as real, and just as harmful, as discrimination based on race, ethnicity, religion, gender, or sexual orientation.

The attitudes that most people hold toward those labelled with mental illness are, as Graham Thornicroft illustrates here, major barriers to their being able to lead the lives they want – to hold down jobs they are qualified for, to live in ordinary housing, to engage in social relations and to enjoy their basic rights as citizens. Listen carefully to the personal accounts quoted from so liberally – they tell the tale of lives diminished not merely by stigmatization, but by outright prejudice and discrimination that is just as real, and as disabling, as those faced by other devalued groups. Until that discrimination is challenged, and becomes just as socially unacceptable as other forms of discrimination, there will continue to be the so-called 'stigma of mental illness'. Those of us who have devoted our lives to obtaining equal rights for people who have experienced the mental health system much prefer to put our energy into rights protection and advocacy, as a matter of basic social justice.

Judi Chamberlin
Arlington, Massachusetts, USA
February, 2006

Notes

1. The terms user and survivor are among the preferred terms by people who have been diagnosed with mental health difficulties. Other terms, such as consumer, may also be used. No single term has been found satisfactory to everyone.
2. Substance Abuse and Mental Health Services Administration, www.mentalhealth.samhsa.gov/publications/allpubs/OEL99-0004
3. National Mental Health Awareness Campaign, www.nostigma.org

Acknowledgements

My conviction that many people with mental illness are systematically discriminated against has come from discussions that I've had with service users and their family members, as I have worked as a psychiatrist over the last 20 years in Camberwell and Croydon in South London. I am grateful for their candour in telling me about their experiences. The focus here is upon adults of working age, as this reflects most of the relevant research and the testimonies available to me as a psychiatrist working in community mental heath services. This book stands upon these two foundations: evidence and experience.

The opportunity to undertake this work came because of the understanding and generosity of Stuart Bell, Chief Executive of the South London and Maudsley NHS Trust, and Dr George Szmukler, Dean of the Institute of Psychiatry, King's College London, who allowed me to take a period of study leave during which I wrote this book.

At present there is an active international debate on the appropriate words to use in the mental health field – in effect a terminological power struggle. This book reflects such diverse and conflicting views and uses a range of terms to refer to mental illnesses and to people who experience these conditions and their consequences. Where possible I have illustrated key points with direct quotations from people with mental illness, anonymized unless the individuals have specifically asked me to give their names. The stories which introduce Chapters 1–5 are anonymized composite accounts based upon what people with mental illness have told me of their experiences, while their quotations are reported verbatim.

The ideas presented here come from many sources, and I would like to give full credit to the contributions of many friends and colleagues who have helped me including: Matthias Angermeyer, Tania Burchardt, Peter Byrne, Cathy Carter, Judi Chamberlin, Richard Church, Pat Corrigan, Paul Corry, David Crepaz-Keays, Fiona Crowley, Bob Drake, Marina Economou, Paul Farmer, Ivan Fiser, Nick Glozier, Bob Grove, Sheilagh Hodgins, Gary Hogman, Kim Hopper, Louise Howard, John Illman, Jason, Nikos Kakavoulis, Aliya Kassam, Mike King, Jeremy Laurence, Ann Law, Sandra Lawman, Heidi Lempp, Oliver Lewis, Bruce Link, Jo Loughran, Sean Love, Tania Luhrmann, Jose Lumerman, Andrew McCulloch, William McKnight, Kirstin McLellan, Dave McDade,

Dave McDaid, Liz Main, David Morris, Paul Mullen, Jill Peay, Jo Phelan, Vanessa Pinfold, Diana Rose, Nik Rose, Norman Sartorius, Liz Sayce, Geoff Shepherd, Ezra Susser, Jeff Swanson, James Tighe, Alp Ucok, Norma Ware, Amy Watson, John Weinman, Til Wykes and Larry Yang.

List of Illustrations

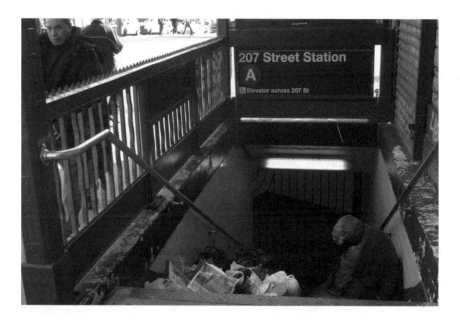

Homeless Person, 207th Street Subway Station, New York, 2005.
© Paul Treacy

Chapter 1 Close to home
Family, housing
and neighbours

Jasmine was 19 when her life changed. The British-born daughter of Pakistani parents, her life had been mostly straightforward until then. She had a large circle of friends, mostly Asian-British like herself, several young men actively interested in going out with her, and a full-time job as a clerk in a local bank. Then she began to suspect that her work colleagues were talking about her behind her back. Her suspicions gradually hardened into convictions until she felt that they were actively plotting to hurt her. On the day when all this came to a head she was sure that their glances meant that she was in imminent danger: she dashed out of her office in an attack of blind desperation, ran into a busy road, and was very nearly run over by a passing truck. To keep her safe, while they called her family, her workmates locked her in a side room, so confirming her worst fears.

Her parents had also noticed some changes. Jasmine, never before actively religious, began to pray up to five times a day. Their approval pleased her, 'they started liking me!' but for her own safety, after the episode at work, her family arranged for her to be continuously in the company of one of her relatives. 'My parents didn't let me go out or let me be alone on my own, because I might do something.' At that time Jasmine couldn't even make basic decisions about her day-to-day life, 'People around me helped me a lot, choosing clothes, choosing food, going out; there would always be somebody with me.' When her work manager called to ask about her health, her father said that she had resigned from her job, without discussing this with Jasmine.

Next her father brought in the Muslim priest. 'So they called the priest in to check me out, as they thought it was some sort of black magic.' He performed traditional rites, and her father gave her a special necklace containing extracts from the Koran to wear as protection against evil influences. Although she believed she was suffering from 'anxiety', she was prescribed antipsychotic medication at a local community mental health centre, and quickly felt better after taking it. Her father was strongly against her using this medication, but her mother quietly encouraged her to continue with the tablets, avoiding any open disagreement within the family.

Her parents then told Jasmine that her main problem was that she was not yet married, and so they began to make inquiries in their hometown in

Pakistan to find an eligible suitor. They told Jasmine that she was not particularly attractive or intelligent, and so she should not set her expectations too high. She is now looking at the details of some of the applicants, and feels that because she has a British passport she is likely to be seen as 'quite a catch'. Recently Jasmine began a part-time computing course, and she is just beginning to feel that she has regained enough confidence to start looking for a part-time job. She still retains her hope to train as a nursery nurse one day.

Reactions by family members

The reactions of Jasmine's family are not wholly typical. When features of mental illness first begin, relatives will often start by taking a common-sense view and recommend, for example, ways to avoid stress, or to adopt a more healthy lifestyle.

> I thought that if I had her at home for a while, with proper food and proper sleep and encouragement I thought I could pull her around and I thought she would get better, but she didn't get better she got worse. She was totally walled off in her own private world.
>
> Elizabeth, mother of Tania

When common sense is not effective, a second ordinary reaction is to see signs of unusual talk or actions as thoughtless or 'bad' behaviour, and to adopt a blaming or nagging attitude.

> At 16, in 1996, I suffered a bad mental breakdown where I was hospitalized for five years. It was very traumatic. There I was, the eldest son suffering a sudden deep depression, crying and unable to work. Often threatened by my confused Dad as being 'weak', 'a fuck-up', and a 'nutter'. No-one else in the family going back generations had gone 'mad like that'. I was told not to tell any of the neighbours what was happening - to stop the gossip. But I was far too ill to socialize until I was admitted as a day patient at a local mental hospital – formerly a workhouse – where I was to spend the next three years. Or was it four? Being with other 'nutters' and having a certain amount of freedom I soon became institutionalized.
>
> Paul

As members of the general population, until family members have direct experience of someone in the family with mental illness, they are likely to have the same background knowledge about mental illnesses as anyone else. As we shall see later in Chapter 9, this amounts in many cases to a profound level of ignorance mixed with prejudiced disinformation. Many surveys have found that most members of the general public do not have a clear understanding of the difference between, for example, mental illnesses and learning disability (mental retardation).[1] In this case it is understandable the family members will simply not know what to say for the best.

While family members can have some personal sense of what severe depression feels like, by imagining an exaggeration of times when they have themselves felt emotionally low, they usually struggle in particular to understand what is happening if someone in their family develops psychotic symptoms:

> I find it hard to understand it myself, actually, when I go to hospital I see people who are in the midst of their illness and I find it quite hard to reach them and I sort of think to myself - well if I've been there and I find it difficult how on earth do family and professional carers manage?
>
> Peter

> He thinks he's the second coming. He's here to salvage the world, he communicates with the television and alters world events in that way. What I hadn't realized at the time was that I couldn't argue with these ideas, so in the early stages we would argue and days later we would still be arguing about it, until it suddenly dawned on me that these were a solid fixation within his own illness that wouldn't budge, that you couldn't do anything with.
>
> Sarah, wife of Peter

Another reaction in the early stages of the condition is for family members to react to unusual behaviour with puzzled amusement, especially to people experiencing periods of mania, when their extravagance may be seen as highly entertaining.

> At university she behaved in a peculiar way ... she decided to camp out in the graveyard and this kind of thing was regarded as a great laugh by her friends of course ... she then began to experience delusions of being followed by the CIA.
>
> Greg, father of Tania.

Feeling at a loss about how to understand what is happening to their relative, and not able to connect it to their own direct experience, family members may also react with either withdrawal or attack.

> As far as friends and family were concerned, most people literally 'didn't know what to say'. This was in relation to the psychotic side of things. However, most of them understood depression. I think because they are all of a similar age and had experienced a crisis in their lives, I was lucky in a way, that I had an older age group to talk to who were full of common sense. The worst two examples were from my brother and a friend. My brother pronounced that 'I was off my rocker and completely mad', and the friend rested the phone receiver on a chair and I heard her doing the washing up while I was trying to speak to her. When I later asked her what happened she said 'I knew there was no point.' Both people are self-centred and are now off my Christmas card list. I think what is important is that none of these people knew what well thought-out, correct

medication can do for mental illness. All of them were surprised how much better I got and how quickly the medication kicked in and helped me return to a normal life. How could they know? So it can be treated. The most help were people who encouraged me to do normal things and rang up next day to see if I had done chores or been out.

Sonia

From the point of view of family members, their reluctance to talk directly about features of mental illness, which are increasingly plain to everyone in the family, can be very understandable. For example, they may feel that talking about the problems will make the situation worse. Commonly, for example, people believe that talking about suicide to a person who may be suicidal can trigger an act of self-harm, even though there is no evidence for this. In fact, the reverse is usually true. Someone so desperate that they are actively considering taking their own life first of all needs someone else to recognize their distress, and then to help them find treatment and care.

Another reason for family members to choose silence rather than discussing emerging mental health problems has to do with their understanding of the causes of mental illness. If, for example, relatives believe that mental illness is inherited, then guilt or shame can make it hard for them to talk openly about these problems. Alternatively, if the family believe that mental illness is infectious or contagious, then they may keep their distance as a consequence.

However, I have also had problems with members of my family. Some members of my family, such as my mother and some friends, don't know how to react after a crisis. They seem scared to talk about it, almost as if they might be 'infected' by my problems or fearful that anything they might say might spark off another crisis. They avoid the subject altogether and instead talk of trivialities.

Nadia

In fact it is common for people to react to the difficulties of others according to their understanding of the cause of the problems. Typically, for example, conditions which are thought to be under the voluntary control of the other person, such as obesity (assumed to be from deliberate overeating), produce unsympathetic reactions of blame and rejection. On the other hand, if the condition is understood to have developed 'through no fault of their own', for which the unwell person bears no personal responsibility, then reactions tend to be sympathetic and practically helpful. In other words a key early process for many family members is a search for meaning: why has this happened to us? What is the cause of all these problems? Is someone to blame? Psychologists have described these tendencies in relation to 'attribution theory'.[2,3]

One example of such attributions was described in a study in Wisconsin, which asked the brothers and sisters of people with 'serious mental illness' (which usually means a diagnosis of a psychotic disorder) about their experiences. Those relatives who viewed the unwell sib's behaviour as outside his or her own control felt less personal impact than did the family members who saw the symptoms as somehow brought on voluntarily, for example through 'laziness'.[4]

> I'm 40 on the 1st May, and I have had these phobias etc, since I was about 17. My main phobia is emetophobia (fear of vomiting), which I have quite severely. This has led to a social phobia, and depression, which then led to a kind of nervous breakdown, and I was referred to the women's service. Family? I gave up talking to them about this two years ago. They don't know half of what I'm going through. When I did try and talk to them, they told me not to be so stupid, and it's mind over matter. No-one in our family is allowed to have a mental health problem. They wouldn't admit that I have. They were worried about what people would think. As far as they are concerned, people with mental health problems, that makes them talk to themselves and do odd things, are on drugs.
>
> Eve

Another important issue which influences how families react to a relative with mental illness is whether they expect the person to recover. This is mainly influenced, to begin with, by the information which is available in the public domain, particularly from the print and broadcast media (this is discussed in more detail in Chapter 6). Since news stories and features overwhelmingly portray mental illness in its most negative aspects, families may genuinely know very little about the fact that most people with mental illness are able to make a full or partial recovery with treatment. If they believe that cure is impossible, then they are more likely to abandon their relatives, which was the fate of many of the long-term patients consigned to psychiatric institutions in the past.[5,6]

> From my family if I had a physical illness and was hospitalized because of it I got visits and get well cards, but when hospitalized because of my mental illness the visits were few and far between. And forget get well cards. You are not expected to get well from a mental illness.
>
> Maria

> People have got this idea that schizophrenia is incurable and a total disaster and you're not going anywhere, but that's not true and a lot can be done.
>
> Greg, father of Tania

On the other hand, it is important to recognize that many people with mental illness receive continuous, and unconditional support from their families.[7–9]

> I feel lucky to have a supportive family … and a loving husband who looks after us. He is also my carer. If he wasn't around I wouldn't be able to cope. Just before I met him I was going downhill, surviving on one meal a day and

depressed, and no one noticed. Then I met my husband and together we look after our one year old.

Barbara

Some of the theories developed by psychiatrists, psychologists and anthropologists in the past have made matters worse. Not only are popular ideas of mental disorder often profoundly damaging to mentally ill people: some professional theories have also had seriously negative consequences. One example of such stigmatizing ideas is that of the 'schizophrenogenic mother'.

In the 1950s,[10] the idea of the 'schizophrenogenic mother' began.[11] The notion is that harmful types of mother–child interaction can increase the likelihood that the child will later be given a diagnosis of schizophrenia. In particular, overprotective and nagging maternal behaviour was thought to be most harmful.[12–14] By the 1960s the concept had become discredited: 'None of the theories which have been put forward to explain the genesis of abnormal family relationships seems to have sufficient empirical foundation to be useful in planning services'.[15] In fact later research went on to show that unusual patterns of behaviour between a person with a diagnosis of schizophrenia and their family do not cause the condition, but can affect how the condition develops, and how often relapses occur.[16,17] This understanding led to valuable insights which were the basis for new types of family psycho-educational therapy which were later shown to reduce the risk of relapse.[17–20]

Nevertheless, ideas can survive in the popular imagination long after they have been scientifically undermined, and this was the case for the 'schizophrenogenic mother' theory.[21] So in addition to the difficulties experienced by parents of people with schizophrenia, according to this theory they were also asked to bear guilt and blame for the cause of the condition itself.[22] The uptake of these ideas in the wider community has contributed to the reluctance of some parents to disclose details about their relative's mental disorder to other people.[23,24] Even today it is still fairly common for family members of people with schizophrenia to say that they have the distinct impression from staff that they have in some way contributed to the cause of the condition.[25,26] The theory of the 'schizophrenogenic mother' therefore provides an example of an idea which has been positively harmful in increasing stigmatization.[25–27]

Reactions to family members

During the last 20 years it has been increasingly recognised that not only are people with mental illness themselves the butt of limited understanding, prejudiced attitudes and discriminatory behaviour, but so are their family members. In 1989 almost 500 members of the National Alliance for the Mentally Ill (NAMI) in 20 of the United States were surveyed about their experiences. They expressed very clear and consistent views. Almost all identified stigma as a key problem for their mentally ill relatives. They said that the most common effects of stigma on their unwell relatives were damage to self-esteem, difficulty making and keeping friends, difficulty finding a job and reluctance to admit mental illness. In terms of the worst effects that they experienced themselves, the most serious problems were lowered self-esteem and damaged family relationships. They gave mental health professionals mixed reviews. While not generally viewed as contributing to stigma, professionals were seen as generally unhelpful in dealing with stigma.[28]

This knock-on effect of negative attitudes towards the family members of people with mental illness has been described as 'stigma by association'. An interesting Swedish study interviewed the relatives of people admitted to acute psychiatric wards.[29] They found dramatic and disturbing results: 18 per cent of the relatives had at times thought that the patient would be better off dead, and among the family members 10 per cent had themselves experienced suicidal thoughts. This is reinforced by the findings of a similar study of family members in Germany. Going well beyond their expectations, the researchers found what they described as 'structural discrimination' (discussed in more detail in Chapter 9), including, for example, many ways that people with mental illness feel they receive a second-class service compared with care for people with physical disorders. They also reported that the common public images of mental illness, and some of the impressions left by psychiatrists, give a negative view of relatives.[30]

> We do feel strongly, both of us, that the image is all wrong, that more should be done to explain that most schizophrenics are frightened of people rather than frightening, that they are gentle, that they're not likely to hurt anybody.
>
> Gemma, wife of Mark

Such negativity can be expressed in different ways. For example, most of what has been written about the effects of living with someone with a severe mental illness has described this as a 'burden'.[31–33] Indeed it is common for family members to have a range of reactions to their situation. They will sometimes describe living with a relative with chronic difficulties as a type of bereavement. Worry is also a common feature, along with high rates of sleep disturbance, anxiety and depression, and they will often be troubled about what will happen when they are old and frail and can no longer actively care for their relative.[34]

> Tom has tried to commit suicide. Twice. I've never forgotten that and I've never stopped worrying since. What will happen when I die? That I think about everyday, I get up with that, and I go to bed with that.
>
> Margaret, mother of Tom

> I hope that he will go on getting better, but I do hope that I won't die first. Yes I do hope that.
>
> Sarah, wife of Peter

Nevertheless it is profoundly prejudiced to simply see the role of family members as having to shoulder a burden, as a type of dead weight. This is to over-simplify complex and varying relationships, and to deny the love and companionship that usually remains a part of these relations.

> You might go through the difficult times, but there will be good times when it's easy.
>
> Susan, wife of Harry
>
> However ill they are they're still worth it because it's your son or daughter, that's what it means. Mind you, sometimes it's so hard you almost have to give up. You think to yourself well maybe I've had enough. Maybe I'll give up, but you never do. But I said it is not a punishment is a pleasure. I really mean that, it's true.
>
> Margaret, mother of Tom

For these reasons what was previously called 'burden' is often referred to now by more neutral terms such as 'experience of care-giving'.[35,36] Just as it may be misleading to assume that most of the impact upon family members is negative, so relatives may chose not to see themselves as 'carers'. A large study of people with a diagnosis of psychosis in South London, for example, found that half of their family members were satisfied with their role,[37] and asked for no extra help. Even so it is clear that the situation can be very difficult for those looking after relatives who have long-term or severely disabling conditions. A study in Alberta in Canada, for example, found that many relatives did report significant distress from their care-giving role, and that this was worse the longer their relative was unwell.[38]

One way that some family members find of coping with their situation is to draw a clear distinction between the person they love and the harmful effects of the condition. In doing this they recognize that their relative bears no responsibility for the onset of the condition.

> I think it had a very deep and profound effect on me, really, and it's not the type of marriage I'd anticipated. But I mean we're still together, still trundling on, but there have been low moments from me and I'd gone into a depression, and usually by that stage he goes in hospital and I pick up because I start to get a rest. I love Peter as a person, but I hate the illness he has, because I think it's really destroying him in a lot of ways. It's just finding different ways of handling it.
>
> Sarah, wife of Peter

How does stigma affect families? One study in the USA examined this among 156 parents and spouses of people admitted to psychiatric hospital for the first time. While most family members did not see themselves as being shunned by others, half did say that they tried to hide the fact of hospital admission. Family members with more education, or whose relative had been unwell recently, reported more avoidance by others.[39]

> All my neighbours know that Tom is mentally ill. What I do not tell them is that he is schizophrenic, because a lot of nasty things are said about schizophrenic people.
>
> Margaret, mother of Tom

Interestingly most of the reports on the effects on family members refer to families with a person diagnosed as having schizophrenia (like most of the literature on stigma). An exception is a recent study over almost 500 family members in New York, which compared the views of families of people diagnosed with major depression, schizophrenia or bipolar disorder.[40] Interestingly no differences emerged between these three groups, but experience of ignorance and prejudice were the rule rather than the exception. About a half of the family members agreed with the following statements:

- most people in my community would rather not be friends with families of the relative who is mentally ill living with them
- most people look down on families that have a member who is mentally ill living with them
- most people believe that their friends would not visit them as often if a member of the family were hospitalized with serious mental illness
- most people would rather not visit families that have a member who is mentally ill.

The study concluded that both the people with mental illness and their families feel devalued by their predicament. In other words, their reputation was lower because of the presence of mental illness in the family. This theme, namely the low value attached to people with mental illness and to everyone associated with them, will also be discussed in more detail in subsequent chapters.

Other conditions can also have consequences for the family. A study in London asked family members of people with anorexia nervosa or psychotic disorders about their experiences.[41] Rates of depression and anxiety were significantly higher in the carers of people with anorexia nervosa, while the themes of guilt and shame were identified by both groups. In contrast, almost no information is available about the families of people with personality disorders.[42]

Relatives have repeatedly said that the impact of mental illness on the family can be reduced if they are confident that they can find help in an emergency. In Hong Kong, for example, relatives often reported feeling frustration, anxiety, low self-esteem and helplessness, but this was less for families who expected to receive rapid help if it was needed in a crisis.[23]

Are families discriminated against in the same way in different countries? Unfortunately there are no studies which have looked at this in a careful and comparative way. However, there are indications that some of the reactions to family members are surprisingly consistent between different cultures. One survey in urban and rural areas of Ethiopia questioned almost 200 relatives of mentally ill people with diagnoses of schizophrenia, bipolar disorder, or major depression. About 75 per cent said that they were stigmatized due to mental illness in the family[43] (compared with 43 per cent in a New York study[40]), while 37 per cent wanted to conceal the fact that a relative was ill. Urban residents in Ethiopia were more likely to report stigma as a major problem. The condition was attributed to supernatural forces by 27 per cent of the family members, and two-thirds preferred to deal with the problem through prayer.

> It's a long-term process, this illness isn't going to get cured overnight. I think you have to accept that it is going to take a long time. I've always relied on my faith to some extent. I've always prayed and I always have got through.
>
> Gemma, wife of Mark

Another way in which family members find support is from self-help groups, which have developed in many countries over the last 20 years or so. These groups usually arrange meetings for family members to share information about the conditions affecting their relatives, to discuss their own thoughts and feelings about the situation, and to campaign for better mental health care. In some cases they offer voluntary or paid counsellors, such as Rachel.

> It's important to talk, to be able to talk to someone who's trod the same path. If they see a diagnosis, for example, of schizophrenia for a relative, they go totally shell shocked, because schizophrenia is not only a terrible word to say, and to spell, and to come to terms with, but to think that it is a label now attached to somebody in your family is a very overwhelming thing and people are so totally overwhelmed by this that they become kind of frozen with the horror of their situation. So they need time to get to grips with it. There is such a lot the carer needs to learn about. They need to learn about the medication, any possible side-effects, where to go for help. It's like walking through treacle in boots, to sort out the benefits maze. I often hear parents say they feel they've lost their child, but equally I hear parents say, for someone who's been on the latest medication, saying that they've come back from the dead.
>
> Rachel

From family support groups, many relatives gain confidence by getting to know other people in a similar situation.

I met Ann three years ago and we quickly found out that our husbands are in the same boat, and we would talk about just how our husbands are, and things like benefit. She is usually one step ahead of me when it comes to benefits and she's been very helpful.

Sarah, wife of Peter

Housing

Mental illnesses can also have profound effects on housing. For people who are most disabled by mental illnesses, the pattern for much of the last century in many countries has been to provide completely segregated housing in long-stay psychiatric hospitals.[44,45] In Europe, for example, there is a clear divide between the Western countries, which have now largely completed the process of deinstitutionalization, and the situation in most Central and Eastern European states, in which the transition from institutional care to more locally based services only began after 1989[44,46-53] (see Figures 1.1 and 1.2).

Over the last half century, countries which have closed their large psychiatric institutions, or have at least reduced their scale, have commonly provided long-stay residential care in the community to receive patients transferred from asylums.[54-56] For those who were previously treated as long-stay patients in psychiatric hospitals, the evidence is that residential care provided in the community settings is more cost-effective, and is greatly preferred by service users.[57-60]

Before thinking about how stigma and discrimination are evident in relation to housing, it's important to recognise that the types of housing available, and the patterns of family living, show great variations. Just within different counties in Europe, for example, a recent study showed between 7–65 per cent of people with a diagnosis schizophrenia lived alone. The custom in Mediterranean countries is for adult children to be able to live with their parents indefinitely (see Table 1.1).[61]

Housing problems can occur at any stage of life. Some of the more severely disabling types of mental illness often begin in the teenage years or in early adulthood, at just the time when young people tend to leave home and establish their own families. Often one consequence of the illnesses is that parents will continue to provide accommodation for their unwell adult child for many years longer than they had expected.

Bit by bit over the last six years that I have been taking tablets I've been trying to piece my life together, it's been very difficult and it's really as if I'm 10 years younger now - I mean I am 32 but really it is as if I'm 22.

Tania

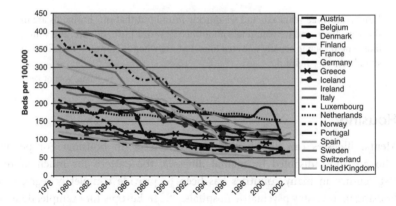

Figure 1.1 Number of psychiatric beds in Western Europe

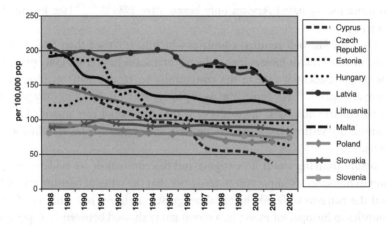

Figure 1.2 Psychiatric beds new EU member countries 1988–2002

Is there their any evidence that people with mental illness face discrimination in terms of housing? The answer is yes. A large survey of almost 2000 service users with severe mental illness across eight of the United States asked about their experiences of discrimination. Almost a quarter (22 per cent) said that they had been homeless, and another 32 per cent said that they had experienced housing discrimination.[62]

As we shall see at many points in the course of this book, there is an important difference here between issues which are highlighted from the point of view of service users/consumers, and those which are identified in research. While housing is frequently mentioned by people who use mental health services, who described their lack of choice, provision of temporary

Table 1.1 Living situation of people with a diagnosis of schizophrenia in five European cities

Living situation	Amsterdam, Holland (n = 61) per cent	Copenhagen, Denmark (n = 52) per cent	London, England (n = 84) per cent	Santander, Spain (n = 100) per cent	Verona, Italy (n = 107) per cent
Alone	49	65	42	7	15
With spouse/partner	8	12	17	17	25
With relatives	20	4	20	72	50
With others	23	19	21	4	10

accommodation, and feelings that they receive low quality provision because of their mental illness, nevertheless there is very little published work about these issues.[63–67]

Perhaps the most visible display of discrimination against people with mental illness in terms of housing is the so-called 'not in my back yard (NIMBY)' phenomenon. This describes the tendency for people to object to proposals to locate a facility for mentally ill people in their own neighbour-hood.[68] For example *The Star*, a local newspaper in Sheffield (England) featured a large picture of placards held aloft by members of a protesting crowd declaring 'Paranoid Schizophrenic Out!' 'Keep Our Children Safe!' and 'Find Another Community!' The article described a march by local people who opposed plans to create a new nursing home for people with a history of mental illness.[69] The secretary of the Highwoods Tenants and Residents Association, in Doncaster in northern England, said:

> We don't have a problem with people needing rehabilitation for psychiatric problems, but this is 50 yards from a play park and 100 yards from Highwoods Junior and Infants School. We are appalled that this can go ahead without any community consultation.

The chief executive of Cambian Healthcare Ltd, proposing to establish the new unit, replied 'Our clients do not pose a risk to anyone.'

There is a real dilemma about what people living near to a proposed new community residential home should be told of these plans. On the one hand it seems reasonable to argue that the medical histories of the new residents are as confidential as, for example, they would be if the new residents suffered from diabetes or epilepsy.[70] In this case it would be unethical of staff to breach such confidential details to any third party, such as potential neighbours, without the consent of the individuals involved. On the other hand, it may be mistaken to underestimate the strength of feeling of neighbours to such local develop-ments, without what they see as a fair process of consultation. One study of such protesting neighbours in Montreal, for example, found that many were against deinstitutionalization in principle,[71] and concluded that it was neces-sary to actively engage neighbours before establishing new facilities in order to increase the likelihood that the new homes would succeed.[72] This view is supported by a study from Scotland which showed that the objections of neighbours may sometimes be more against the lack of consultation than the actual plans for new homes.[73]

In terms of my own experience, I have been directly involved in establishing a day-care centre, a residential home, and three community mental health centres in south London. On each occasion neighbours were initially very worried about these plans.[74] Their background knowledge about mental illnesses was extremely limited. In fact, as we shall see in Chapter 6 on the media, the reaction of neighbours could be seen as fairly reasonable, based upon the information directly available to them, since about three quarters of all news items about mental illness in newspapers focus on violence.[75,76] One study in south London, for example, interviewed the neighbours of a newly opened hostel for people with mental illness and found that less welcoming attitudes were held by people with less knowledge about mental illness,[77] and by the parents of young children.[78]

One of the primary concerns of people in this situation is their personal safety.[79,80] As a consequence, in my view it is usually important, with the agreement of the potential users of the new facility, to actively engage with neighbours from the earliest stages. There is a remarkable paradox here because up to half of all adults will have some mental illness in their own lifetime, and indeed about one in five do so in any given year. Also, about three-quarters of all adults are likely to know someone directly who has had a mental illness.[81] Yet when people feel that their core interests are threatened, they act as if mental illness were an entirely alien concept.

One particular concern, which helps to stimulate organized opposition to new mental health facilities in the community, is the value of property or real estate. One example of this occurred at Worthing on the south coast of England. A couple planned to convert their home into a residential care home for former psychiatric inpatients. All of their immediate neighbours brought a legal action against them on the grounds that such a change would breach restrictive covenants on the proper use of the property. To estimate what they said was the decreased value of their homes (if the residential care home went ahead), they employed a property valuation expert. He noted that there were no direct precedents to make an exact calculation of the potential lost value, so that he would have to draw parallels, for example, with having a malodorous factory or a sewage works next door. Local legal processes could not resolve the dispute, which was then taken to the highest property court in England, the Lands Tribunal. This set a landmark ruling in permitting the couple to go ahead with their plans, on the grounds that the 'public interest' of providing community care outweighed the claims of the neighbours.[82]

Similar issues have been identified in the United States where Congress enacted the Fair Housing Amendments Act of 1988.[83] This law aims to eliminate discrimination in accessing housing for people with physical or mental disability and to support their right to live in the community of their choice. It has been used to test the lawfulness of special restrictions applied only to people with mental disabilities, and other practices that create barriers to proper housing for people with mental illness.[84]

Neighbours

People with mental illness commonly report adverse reactions, especially verbal abuse, from neighbours.[85]

> I've found to my disadvantage that if you stick up for yourself, they throw the fact you have been under psychiatric care in your face. I stuck up for a friend who was being bullied by her neighbour. So I tried to reason with the neighbour, but she said I was mental as well...
>
> ... the people along her road presumed we would be dangerous and violent. I am really upset at being labelled, and people thinking I am violent and highly strung. It's a really lonely feeling and makes me feel a bit isolated. But I will explain it to anyone who wants to listen, as I did to Jane's neighbours.
>
> Eva

> If I am out and neighbours say 'There goes that mad woman!' What right have they to make that judgement, just because I don't conform to their ideas. It's like if people make fun of you and you say something back to them. They always say 'Oh you're mad or paranoid'. Well maybe, but it doesn't mean you are deaf.
>
> Louise

Sometimes such opposition turns to acts which are offensive in the extreme.

> The next type of stigma that hit me was from strangers. A forensic hostel was proposed near me and all of a sudden I'm a target for their anger. I live in a special mental health project flat (apartment), that came under attack. I had dog mess pushed through my letterbox, closely followed by paint stripper thrown over the door causing a lot of damage that took me weeks to sort out.
>
> Maria

While such experiences are sometimes reported by people with mental illness, they do not feature in the scientific literature.[67] Nor do other experiences which often cause severe distress to mentally ill people, such as frustration with the poor quality of public housing available to them. What is clear is that housing problems can make mental illness worse.

> I had problems every month, after that, hot flushes, mood swings, no periods, and my marriage ended due to the way I was. My husband couldn't put up with it. I was crying constantly getting paranoid ... I decided to move from my house and make a new start. I done an exchange with another family, and I was living in this property for two months, and my property started to smell of damp. My bed went green with mould. Electrics blew. Windows were black. I got in touch with my housing and it took ages for them to come out. I contacted Environmental Health and they done something about it. I felt because I can't explain myself properly I was ignored. I had to live in there for a year. My housing [department] knew I wasn't a well lady.
>
> Gina

Such difficulties can easily get out of control and form a cascade of challenges which seem impossible to escape from. From the point of view of professionals, these problems are usually seen as issues to be dealt with by many, separate agencies: health care, social services, housing department, environmental health organizations, social security and welfare benefits agencies, banks and financial services, debt repayment and repossession institutions, the police and criminal justice system. While dealing with any combination of these at the same time can present a challenge to a well person, people experiencing the symptoms of mental illness can find dealing with these agencies difficult or impossible without coordinated support to navigate the system.

> They threw stones at my windows, my nerves were very bad. I phoned my housing and told them 'I can't take this anymore, please help me', and all they could say to me was 'I'm sorry, I know we shouldn't have put you there.' I phoned nearly every day to see if they had found me a new home, but all I could do was keep waiting. My son started getting depressed. He got to the stage where he felt suicidal . . . the psychiatrist said he would write a letter for me to the housing because my son needed an urgent move. My other son started to get ill with his psoriasis it was very inflamed and I just felt like my family was going downhill. I was tortured for a year in this property. I felt like I was losing my mind. I had 25 parking tickets while I was waiting for my mobility stickers. Bailiffs clamped my car, and when they knew it was a disabled car they took it off and made me pay £300. I told them I am not a well person physically and mentally, but they took advantage of me and threatened me with police. I was very scared and gave them this money . . . I feel bullied and I can't express myself very well. People who are ill like myself shouldn't be treated different. I feel I have been because of my illness.
>
> Gina

One important element, often forgotten, are the housing preferences of people with mental illness themselves. For example, there have been several studies about the discharge of long-term psychiatric inpatients to community care. After leaving hospital such surveys, mostly from the UK and the USA, have consistently found that about three-quarters of such people prefer living in the community, and would recommend this to other people who are still long-stay patients in hospital.[5,86–88]

Is the quality of care necessarily better in smaller than in larger homes or institutions? One of the main reasons for beginning the policy of hospital closure was clear evidence that large hospitals produced the so-called syndrome of 'institutionalism'.[89] This describes the state of social withdrawal, apathy, hopelessness and inactivity that characterizes many people who spent most of their adult life in large psychiatric hospitals. There is now good evidence from several countries that smaller nursing and care homes generally do offer a better quality of life than the large hospitals.[54,90–98]

On the other hand, we need to be cautious as neglect occurs in institutions of any size. Nevertheless, in general larger facilities are more often dehumanizing. In most western European countries, and in Australia and New Zealand, 'mental health nursing home' usually means a building providing care for up to 20 or 30 people, while a residential or group home would usually accommodate up to 10 or 15 people. In contrast, most former Soviet countries in Eastern Europe continue to provide 'social care homes' (sometimes called 'internats') which house up to 500 people and which are in most respects identical to large psychiatric hospitals, except that the staff do not have nursing or medical qualifications.

Similarly, so-called nursing homes or social care homes in some parts of the United States are in fact re-designated 'single room occupancy' hotels, containing up to 1000 people each. The *New York Times*, for example, has published a series of scandals over 30 years highlighting financial fraud, under-staffing, neglect, and higher-than-expected rates of death from heat-stroke, suicide and untreated medical conditions. The nature and extent of this form of systematic neglect, often applied to people who have recently been homeless as well as having symptoms of mental illness,[99–101] again gives us an indirect but accurate estimate of the value that our societies place upon people in this predicament.[102]

Not only are people with disabling mental illnesses often brought together in such housing units, in some countries it is common for these buildings to be crowded together in the poorer parts of town, creating what has been described as 'mental health ghettoes'. Despite the provisions of the Fair Housing Amendment Act, which is largely applied to individuals or organisations, we can see in some urban areas of United States that a combination of housing market forces, town planning regulations and unspoken assumptions (about which types of neighbourhood are suitable for which categories of resident)[103] can produce such 'landscapes of despair'.[104] As we shall see in more detail in Chapter 9, this is yet another example of 'structural discrimination' against people with mental illness.[105]

References

1. Caruso DR, Hodapp RM. Perceptions of mental retardation and mental illness. *Am J Ment Retard* 1988; 93(2):118–124.
2. Corrigan PW. Mental health stigma as social attribution: implications for research methods and attitude change. *Clinical Psychology: Science and Practice* 2000; 7(1):48–67.
3. Crocker J, Cornwell B, Major B. The stigma of overweight: affective consequences of attributional ambiguity. *J Pers Soc Psychol* 1993; 64(1):60–70.
4. Greenberg JS, Kim HW, Greenley JR. Factors associated with subjective burden in siblings of adults with severe mental illness. *Am J Orthopsychiatry* 1997; 67(2):231–41.

5. Leff J. *Care in the Community. Illusion or reality?* London: Wiley; 1997.

6. Howard L, Leese M, Thornicroft G. Social networks and functional status in patients with psychosis. *Acta Psychiatr Scand* 2000; 102(5):376–385.

7. Leggatt M. Carers and carer organisations. In: Thornicroft G, Szmukler G, eds., *Textbook of Community Psychiatry*, pp. 475–486. Oxford: Oxford University Press; 2001.

8. Shepherd G, Murray A, Muijen M. Perspectives on schizophrenia: A survey of user, family carer and professional views regarding effective care. *Journal of Mental Health (UK)* 1995; 4(4):403–422.

9. Kuipers L, Bebbington P. Relatives as a resource in the management of functional illness. *Br J Psychiatry* 1985; 147:465–470.

10. Jackson D, Block J, Block J, Patterson V. Psychiatrists' conceptions of the schizophrenogenic parent. *AMA Arch Neurol Psychiatry* 1958; 79(4):448–459.

11. Hartwell CE. The schizophrenogenic mother concept in American psychiatry. *Psychiatry* 1996; 59(3):274–297.

12. Parker G. Re-searching the schizophrenogenic mother. *J Nerv Ment Dis* 1982; 170(8):452–462.

13. Mitchell KM. Social class and the schizophrenogenic mother concept. *Psychol Rep* 1969; 24(2):463–469.

14. Meyer RG, Karon BP. The schizophrenogenic mother concept and the TAT. *Psychiatry* 1967; 30(2):173–179.

15. Brown G, Bone M, Birley J, Wing J. *Schizophrenia and Social Care.* Oxford: Oxford University Press; 1966.

16. Rutter M, Brown G. The reliability and validity of measures of family life and relationships in families containing a psychiatric patient. In: Kiev A, ed,. *Social Psychiatry Volume 1* pp. 148–182. New York: Science House; 1969.

17. Mari JJ, Streiner DL. An overview of family interventions and relapse on schizophrenia: meta-analysis of research findings. *Psychol Med* 1994; 24(3):565–578.

18. Barrowclough C, Hooley JM. Attributions and expressed emotion: a review. *Clin Psychol Rev* 2003; 23(6):849–880.

19. Kuipers L. Expressed emotion: a review. *Br J Soc Clin Psychol* 1979; 18(2):237–243.

20. Leff J. Working with the families of schizophrenic patients. *Br J Psychiatry* Suppl 1994;(23):71–76.

21. Siegler M, Osmond H. *Models of Madness. Models of medicine.* New York: Harper Colophone; 1976.

22. Wasow M. Parental perspectives on chronic schizophrenia. *J Chronic Dis* 1983; 36(4):337–343.

23. Tsang HW, Tam PK, Chan F, Cheung WM, Chang WM. Sources of burdens on families of individuals with mental illness. *Int J Rehabil Res* 2003; 26(2):123–130.

24. Phelan JC, Bromet EJ, Link BG. Psychiatric illness and family stigma. *Schizophr Bull* 1998; 24(1):115–126.

25. Struening EL, Perlick DA, Link BG, Hellman F, Herman D, Sirey JA. Stigma as a barrier to recovery: The extent to which caregivers believe most people devalue consumers and their families. *Psychiatr Serv* 2001; 52(12):1633–1638.

26. Warner R. Schizophrenia and the environment: speculative interventions. *Epidemiol Psichiatr Soc* 1999; 8(1):19–34.

27. Angell B, Cooke A, Kovac K. First-person accounts of stigma. In: Corrigan PW, ed., *On the Stigma of Mental Illness* pp. 69–98. Washington, DC: American Psychological Association; 2005.

28. Wahl OF, Harman CR. Family views of stigma. *Schizophr Bull* 1989; 15(1):131–139.

29. Ostman M, Kjellin L. Stigma by association: psychological factors in relatives of people with mental illness. *Br J Psychiatry* 2002; 181:494–8.

30. Angermeyer MC, Schulze B, Dietrich S. Courtesy stigma – a focus group study of relatives of schizophrenia patients. *Soc Psychiatry Psychiatr Epidemiol* 2003; 38(10):593–602.

31. Lefley HP. Family burden and family stigma in major mental illness. *Am Psychol* 1989; 44(3):556–560.

32. Perlick DA, Rosenheck RA, Clarkin JF, Maciejewski PK, Sirey J, Struening E *et al*. Impact of family burden and affective response on clinical outcome among patients with bipolar disorder. *Psychiatr Serv* 2004; 55(9):1029–1035.

33. Perlick D, Clarkin JF, Sirey J, Raue P, Greenfield S, Struening E *et al*. Burden experienced by care-givers of persons with bipolar affective disorder. *Br J Psychiatry* 1999; 175:56–62.

34. Berry D, Szmukler G, Thornicroft G. *Living with Schizophrenia: the carers story*. Brighton: Pavillion Press; 1997.

35. Joyce J, Leese M, Kuipers E, Szmukler G, Harris T, Staples E. Evaluating a model of caregiving for people with psychosis. *Soc Psychiatry Psychiatr Epidemiol* 2003; 38(4): 189–195.

36. Szmukler GI, Burgess P, Herrman H, Benson A, Colusa S, Bloch S. Caring for relatives with serious mental illness: the development of the Experience of Caregiving Inventory. *Soc Psychiatry Psychiatr Epidemiol* 1996; 31(3–4):137–148.

37. Szmukler GI, Wykes T, Parkman S. Care-giving and the impact on carers of a community mental health service. PRiSM Psychosis Study 6. *Br J Psychiatry* 1998; 173:399–403.

38. Martens L, Addington J. The psychological well-being of family members of individuals with schizophrenia. *Soc Psychiatry Psychiatr Epidemiol* 2001; 36(3):128–133.

39. Phelan JC, Bromet EJ, Link BG. Psychiatric illness and family stigma. *Schizophr Bull* 1998; 24(1):115–26.

40. Struening EL, Perlick DA, Link BG, Hellman F, Herman D, Sirey JA. Stigma as a barrier to recovery: The extent to which caregivers believe most people devalue consumers and their families. *Psychiatr Serv* 2001; 52(12):1633–8.

41. Treasure J, Murphy T, Szmukler G, Todd G, Gavan K, Joyce J. The experience of caregiving for severe mental illness: a comparison between anorexia nervosa and psychosis. *Soc Psychiatry Psychiatr Epidemiol* 2001; 36(7):343–347.

42. Lewis G, Appleby L. Personality disorder: the patients psychiatrists dislike. *Br J Psychiatry* 1988; 153:44–49.

43. Shibre T, Negash A, Kullgren G, Kebede D, Alem A, Fekadu A *et al*. Perception of stigma among family members of individuals with schizophrenia and major affective disorders in rural Ethiopia. *Soc Psychiatry Psychiatr Epidemiol* 2001; 36(6):299–303.

44. Grob G. *From Asylum to Community. Mental health policy in modern America*. Princeton, New Jersey: Princeton University Press; 1991.

45. Shorter E. *A History of Psychiatry: From the era of the asylum to the age of Prozac*. New York: John Wiley & Sons; 1997.

46. Tomov T. Central and Eastern European countries. In: Thornicroft G, Tansella M, eds., *The Mental Health Matrix. A Manual to Improve Services* pp. 216–227. Cambridge: Cambridge University Press; 2001.

47. World Health Organisation. *Mental Health in Europe. Country Reports from the WHO European Network on Mental Health*. Copenhagen: World Health Organisation; 2001.

48. Thornicroft G, Tansella M. Components of a modern mental health service: a pragmatic balance of community and hospital care: overview of systematic evidence. *Br J Psychiatry* 2004; 185:283–290.

49. Thornicroft G, Bebbington P. Deinstitutionalisation – from hospital closure to service development. *Br J Psychiatry* 1989; 155:739–753.

50. Goffman I. *Asylums.* Harmondsworth: Pelican Books; 1968.

51. Rothman D. *The Discovery of the Asylum.* Boston: Little, Brown & Company; 1971.

52. Morrissey JP, Goldman HH. The enduring asylum: in search of an international perspective. *Int J Law Psychiatry* 1981; 4(1–2):13–34.

53. Stallard J. Pauper lunatics and their treatment. *Transactions of the National Association for the Promotion of Social Science* 1870;465.

54. Shepherd G, Muijen M, Dean R, Cooney M. Residential care in hospital and in the community – quality of care and quality of life. *Br J Psychiatry* 1996; 168(4):448–456.

55. Shepherd G, Murray A. Residential care. In: Thornicroft G, Szmukler G, eds, *Textbook of Community Psychiatry* pp. 309–320. Oxford: Oxford University Press; 2001.

56. Trieman N, Smith HE, Kendal R, Leff J. The TAPS Project 41: homes for life? Residential stability five years after hospital discharge. Team for the Assessment of Psychiatric Services. *Community Ment Health J* 1998; 34(4):407–417.

57. Chilvers R, Macdonald G, Hayes A. *Supported housing for people with severe mental disorders* (Cochrane Review). Oxford: Update Software; 2003.

58. Nordentoft M, Knudsen HC, Schulsinger F. Housing conditions and residential needs of psychiatric patients in Copenhagen. *Acta Psychiatr Scand* 1992; 85(5):385–389.

59. Hafner H. Do we still need beds for psychiatric patients? An analysis of changing patterns of mental health care. *Acta Psychiatr Scand* 1987; 75(2):113–126.

60. Thornicroft G. *Measuring Mental Health Needs,* 2nd edn. London: Royal College of Psychiatrists, Gaskell; 2001.

61. Thornicroft G, Tansella M, Becker T, Knapp M, Leese M, Schene A *et al.* The personal impact of schizophrenia in Europe. *Schizophr Res* 2004; 69(2–3):125–132.

62. Corrigan P, Thompson V, Lambert D, Sangster Y, Noel JG, Campbell J. Perceptions of discrimination among persons with serious mental illness. *Psychiatr Serv* 2003; 54(8):1105–1110.

63. Dunn S. *Creating Accepting Communities: Report of the MIND Inquiry into Social Exclusion and Mental Health Problems.* London: MIND; 1999.

64. Prior C. Housing component of mental health services. In: Thornicroft G, Strathdee G, eds, *Commissioning Mental Health Services,* pp. 177–192. London: HMSO; 1996.

65. Greater London Authority. *Getting a Move On. Addressing the Housing and Support Issues Facing Londoners with Mental Health Needs.* London: Greater London Authority; 2003.

66. Ryan CS, Robinson DR, Hausmann LR. Stereotyping among providers and consumers of public mental health services. The role of perceived group variability. *Behav Modif* 2001; 25(3):406–42.

67. Read J, Baker S. *Not Just Sticks and Stones. A Survey of the Stigma, Taboos, and Discrimination Experienced by People with Mental Health Problems.* London: MIND; 1996.

68. Herrmann J. NIMBY (not-in-my-back-yard) – the lingering stigma of mental illness. *Rev Fed Am Health Syst* 1990; 23(4):10–11.

69. Kessen D. Fury over home for mentally ill. *The Star* 2004; 11 November.

70. Zippay A. Trends in siting strategies. *Community Ment Health J* 1997; 33(4):301–310.

71. Piat M. The NIMBY phenomenon: community residents' concerns about housing for deinstitutionalized people. *Health Soc Work* 2000; 25(2):127–138.

72. Piat M. [Group homes and the 'not in my back yard' phenomenon (NIMBY) – it happened close to home: a pilot study]. *Sante Ment Que* 2004; 29(1):151–172.

73. Cowan S. NIMBY syndrome and public consultation policy: the implications of a discourse analysis of local responses to the establishment of a community mental health facility. *Health Soc Care Community* 2003; 11(5):379–386.

74. Reynolds A, Thornicroft G. *Managing Mental Health Services.* Buckingham: Open University Press; 1999.

75. Philo G. The media and public belief. In: Philo G, ed., *Media and Mental Distress* pp. 82–103. London: Longman; 1996.

76. Wahl O. *Media Madness.* New Brunswick, New Jersey: Rutgers University Press; 1995.

77. Wolff G, Pathare S, Craig T, Leff J. Community knowledge of mental illness and reaction to mentally ill people. *Br J Psychiatry* 1996; 168(2):191–198.

78. Wolff G, Pathare S, Craig T, Leff J. Community attitudes to mental illness. *Br J Psychiatry* 1996; 168(2):183–190.

79. Huxley P, Evans S, Leese M, Gately C, Rogers A, Thomas R *et al.* Urban regeneration and mental health. *Soc Psychiatry Psychiatr Epidemiol* 2004; 39(4):280–285.

80. Thomas R, Evans S, Huxley P, Gately C, Rogers A. Housing improvement and self-reported mental distress among council estate residents. *Soc Sci Med* 2005; 60(12):2773–2783.

81. Crisp A, Gelder MG, Goddard E, Meltzer H. Stigmatization of people with mental illnesses: a follow-up study within the Changing Minds campaign of the Royal College of Psychiatrists. *World Psychiatry* 2005; 4:106–113.

82. Thornicroft G, Halpern A. Legal landmark for community care of former psychiatric patients. *BMJ* 1993; 307(6898):248–250.

83. Petrila J, Ayers K. Enforcing the Fair Housing Amendments Act to benefit people with mental disability. *Hosp Community Psychiatry* 1994; 45(2):156–160.

84. Blackwood DP. The Fair Housing Act: Sword or Shield? Contemporary Longterm Care 1997; 20(12): 65–66.

85. Dinos S, Stevens S, Serfaty M, Weich S, King M. Stigma: the feelings and experiences of 46 people with mental illness. Qualitative study. *Br J Psychiatry* 2004; 184:176–181.

86. Thornicroft G, Gooch C, O'Driscoll C, Reda S. The TAPS Project. 9: The reliability of the Patient Attitude Questionnaire. *Br J Psychiatry Suppl* 1993;(19):25–29.

87. Hanrahan P, Luchins DJ, Savage C, Goldman HH. Housing satisfaction and service use by mentally ill persons in community integrated living arrangements. *Psychiatr Serv* 2001; 52(9):1206–1209.

88. Thornicroft G, Bebbington P, Leff J. Outcomes for long-term patients one year after discharge from a psychiatric hospital. *Psychiatr Serv* 2005; 56(11):1416–1422.

89. Wing JK, Brown G. *Institutionalism and Schizophrenia.* Cambridge: Cambridge University Press; 1970.

90. Hobbs C, Tennant C, Rosen A, Newton L, Lapsley HM, Tribe K *et al.* Deinstitutionalisation for long-term mental illness: a 2-year clinical evaluation. *Aust N Z J Psychiatry* 2000; 34(3):476–483.

91. D'Avanzo B, Barbato A, Barbui C, Battino RN, Civenti G, Frattura L. Discharges of patients from public psychiatric hospitals in Italy between 1994 and 2000. *Int J Soc Psychiatry* 2003; 49(1):27–34.

92. Kaiser W, Hoffmann K, Isermann M, Priebe S. [Long-term patients in supported housing after deinstitutionalisation – part V of the Berlin Deinstitutionalisation Study]. *Psychiatr Prax* 2001; 28(5):235–243.

93. Trauer T, Farhall J, Newton R, Cheung P. From long-stay psychiatric hospital to Community Care Unit: evaluation at 1 year. *Soc Psychiatry Psychiatr Epidemiol* 2001; 36(8):416–419.

94. Tansella M. Community psychiatry without mental hospitals – the Italian experience: a review. *J R Soc Med* 1986; 79(11):664–669.

95. Goldman HH, Adams NH, Taube CA. Deinstitutionalization: the data demythologized. *Hosp Community Psychiatry* 1983; 34(2):129–134.

96. Aeschleman SR, White AJ. Maintaining deinstitutionalisation: a profile of a community support team. *N Z Med J* 1987; 100(827):418–420.

97. Priebe S, Hoffmann K, Isermann M, Kaiser W. Do long-term hospitalised patients benefit from discharge into the community? *Soc Psychiatry Psychiatr Epidemiol* 2002; 37(8):387–392.

98. Lesage AD, Morissette R, Fortier L, Reinharz D, Contandriopoulos AP. Downsizing psychiatric hospitals: needs for care and services of current and discharged long-stay inpatients. *Can J Psychiatry* 2000; 45(6):526–532.

99. Abdul HW, Wykes T, Stansfeld S. The homeless mentally ill: myths and realities. *Int J Soc Psychiatry* 1993; 39(4):237–254.

100. Herman DB, Susser ES, Jandorf L, Lavelle J, Bromet EJ. Homelessness among individuals with psychotic disorders hospitalized for the first time: findings from the Suffolk County Mental Health Project. *Am J Psychiatry* 1998; 155(1):109–113.

101. Shern DL, Felton CJ, Hough RL, Lehman AF, Goldfinger S, Valencia E *et al.* Housing outcomes for homeless adults with mental illness: results from the second-round McKinney program. *Psychiatr Serv* 1997; 48(2):239–241.

102. Link BG, Schwartz S, Moore R, Phelan J, Struening E, Stueve A *et al.* Public knowledge, attitudes, and beliefs about homeless people: evidence for compassion fatigue. *Am J Community Psychol* 1995; 23(4):533–555.

103. Harvey D. *Justice, Nature and the Geography of Difference.* Oxford: Blackwell; 1996.

104. Dear M, Wolch J. *Landscapes of Despair.* Princeton, New Jersey: Princeton University Press; 1992.

105. Corrigan PW, Markowitz FE, Watson AC. Structural levels of mental illness stigma and discrimination. *Schizophr Bull* 2004; 30(3):481–491.

Blackboard menu in a café. New York City, 2004.

Chapter 2 Getting personal
Friendships, intimate relationships and childcare

I have lost all my friends since the onset of my mental illness. My ex-colleagues at work have also ceased all contact with me. I lost my career, my own flat, my car. Mental illness has destroyed my life.

Fiona

Narayan is a 28-year-old man who was born in Nepal, studied at university in India, and then moved to London. Four years ago he developed what he calls 'paranoid delusions', and since then he's been admitted to hospital three times. He now attends a mental health outpatient clinic, and many of the symptoms have improved.

My thought process and memory has been damaged, I'm not able to think as fast as before I was ill. My memory is definitely better than when I was in hospital, but it is taking its toll, all the time.

His social recovery has been slower and more limited than his recovery from these symptoms, for example he hasn't worked since becoming unwell, and he expects that his diagnosis would be a clear liability when applying for a job. As he puts it:

An employer would see my diagnosis of schizophrenia as a disadvantage, and so I would be reluctant even to apply for a job. I would expect myself to be in a more disadvantaged position than a normal person. People have a general idea, a stereotype of schizophrenia, from what is reported on the news. A very dangerous condition, you know, where people often become violent and aggressive, even to the extent of murdering people. Personally, as a schizo-phrenic myself, it's not what I would say. I feel frustrated about the stereotype because I know myself, and I know other people with the same condition, doesn't fall into the stereotype. So I'm reluctant to tell other people that I have schizophrenia. I wouldn't actually hide the fact. I wouldn't let people know if I don't have to do.

He has also had some positive experiences as a consequence of having a diagnosis of schizophrenia. At one of his lowest points he became homeless. He found that the diagnosis helped him to be re-housed much more quickly than if he had not been mentally ill.

It's been a strong advantage in terms of housing. As soon as I'd left hospital they helped me find new housing. I was prioritized in terms of housing provision. I got housing faster than if I didn't have mental illness.

His period of illness has had very damaging effects on his friendships.

When I was really ill, I completely cut myself off from socializing with my friends. About girlfriends, well I'm not very confident anymore. It's a lot more difficult to meet people now. They might see my illness as a burden. Now, I don't stop myself socializing altogether, but it's much less. Also because I don't have the money. Some friends have shunned me a bit, and some have stopped seeing me completely. I'm not sure of the reason, but I think the mental illness must be a part of it.

Perhaps his greatest regret since becoming mentally ill is the effect this has had on his most intimate relationships.

My last girlfriend, she left me because I got ill. Because I'd been ill, and because she couldn't cope with my illness ... I was behaving irrationally. There was no particular event or instance, it was just ongoing ... I wasn't violent or anything or aggressive. So it built up over time, and then she left. She was very understanding initially, but over time it got too much for her. We were very close. When I got better and I could think about it, I couldn't understand why she left me.

These themes (fearful misunderstandings of the illness by others, separating from intimate partners and loss of confidence in trying to develop new relationships) recur time and again in the stories of people talking about their experience of severe mental illness. For many, the endpoint is reaching the conclusion 'why try'. In other words, expecting failure, humiliation and emotional pain, they decide not to even try to form close relationships again. This theme will be discussed in more detail in Chapter 8, in relation to self-stigmatisation, avoidance and social withdrawal.

Friends

Friendship has been described by some as more highly valued than 'family and children, or freedom and independence, or justice, or loyalty, or work, or the sense of duty, or love, or honour, or success and climbing the social ladder, or money, or sacrifice and devotion, or marriage, or sex, or patriotism, or religion'.[1] How can mental illnesses affect friendships? How far are these changes in some ways realistic, because of actual changes in behaviour, or how far do they indicate more intimate forms of discrimination? To start at the beginning, like family members many friends will initially react to changing behaviour by treating it as amusing.

> When I got sick for the first time I was seventeen and I was at high school. My behaviour was awkward and my friends and classmates were making fun of me. I was feeling really bad about this. Then I was hospitalised. When they found out about this, they all abandoned me. I lost my friends.
>
> Dimitris

Although issues of friendship may be important for users of mental health services,[2] this is another area which has excited very little interest among researchers.[3,4] It is clear that people with mental illnesses can be profoundly affected in relation to meeting or keeping friends. People who develop depression, for example, report that their 'mate value' is lowered, in other words they feel they have reduced choice for people with whom they could realistically make friends.[5] *'I don't have any friends and I don't want to. I have my family. In the neighbourhood they don't talk to me'* (Stauros).

To summarize the research that has been done in this field, people with more severe forms of mental illness have smaller social networks than others, have relatively more family members than friends in their social circle, and have relationships that are more dependent rather than interdependent.[6,7] *'I have friends only from the day centre and I don't know why'* (Fanis).

It also seems to be true that people with larger and more supportive social networks are also less likely to be admitted to hospital for mental health reasons.[8] There is a tendency, especially among people who have had long periods of hospital treatment, for social contacts to consist mostly of relationships to other users of mental health services, and with staff, even after discharge from long-term admission.[9–14]

> Society at large stigmatises and misunderstands mental health problems and issues like self-harm are often seen as taboo and to be feared. I still find it hard to admit to being someone who self-harms outside a close circle of friends and health professionals and negative attitudes have cost me dearly in terms of lost opportunities and friendships.
>
> Sandra

While mental illness can have a negative effect on the size and quality of social networks, it is also possible that social networks can influence the cause of some mental illnesses. In the British National Household Survey, for example, socially isolated men, with fewer than four close social contacts, were more likely to have a period of mental illness in the 18 months following the survey.[15]

At the same time it is clear that simply being with someone during a period of severe mental illness can be difficult. Some find that they cannot tolerate to see a person suffering in such a way, especially if they feel powerless to do anything to help.

The only discrimination would be with family and friends. That certain hesitancy, coldness where there was warmth, but this is understandable, being with a depressed person is no fun. Depression robs you of life and interest and people do not like to be with unresponsive company.

David

Such feelings can apply equally to people with a mental illness in their reactions to other people in a similar situation.

I've run into a number of fallacies in my own probing, one of which is that depression could be contagious. When I suffered from depression I never wanted to go out because I found it difficult to enjoy myself and could make an atmosphere less fun for others, but I didn't believe for a second that if I kept going out that my friends might 'catch' my depression. I have a friend who is always depressed and frankly I don't encourage him that I want to spend time with him. He does bring me down and frustrate me, but his problems can't affect me because they are to do with things very personal to him for example men's rights and the fact that he's very bored. It will upset me to be with him.

Robert

Intriguingly, people with a diagnosis of mental illness report that, in general, friends and family often react either in a strongly supportive or a strongly avoidant way, but that they could not have predicted who would fall into which category. Some of those who had been warm and kind before the start of their mental health problems cooled noticeably or disappeared from their life, while others who had only been acquaintances or distant relatives showed unexpected empathy and practical support after the mental illness began. There is no scientific literature on who is likely to stand by you or to desert you when life gets tough in this way. *I do not have friends. I had a friend from my childhood who was close in the beginning of my illness. Now we don't see each other*' (Zafeiris).

Lack of friends does not necessarily lead to loneliness.[16,17] Nevertheless, a large scale general population survey of young adults in Australia[18] found that men tended to be lonelier than women throughout adulthood. This was especially true for men living alone, and for single fathers with young children. The social and emotional isolation of these men was associated with unsocial neighbourhoods and poor physical and mental health. In terms of mutual support the report concluded: 'in short, men need women more than women need men'. This survey also recommended ways to avoid loneliness: 'engagement in paid work, caring for others (including involuntary or charitable work), and participation in clubs and sporting groups'. While social isolation can cause loneliness, this may be a two-way process. A study of Canadian students, for example, found that lonely people were less likely to be seen as desirable friends or acquaintances.[19–21]

But being alone is not the same as loneliness. In an unusual study which asked service users directly about their social life, an intricate balance emerged between the needs for friendship and to be alone.[3] Conversely, living closely next to others, such as in a large psychiatric hospital, should not be confused with a satisfying social life. Interviews with long-term inpatients in Wisconsin, for example, showed that many patients experienced the hospital as an 'island' and even planned escape attempts.[22]

Not only are people with mental illness often avoided by others, but their families may also lose some degree of social support. A careful study of family supports in Italy compared the reactions in families in which an individual developed a heart, brain, diabetes, kidney, lung or mental illness.[23] Social support and help in emergencies was dramatically lower in families with a person diagnosed as having schizophrenia, and this was linked to adverse effects on the mental health of other family members.

> I don't think a person like me can have friends. I tried, I tried hard to keep some, but in vain. The psychosis makes people afraid of me. I don't know. Perhaps they are right.
>
> Ioannis

As we shall see later in Chapters 8 and 10, a common reaction under these circumstances is for service users to heavily censor what they say about their condition to friends, in the hope that not disclosing information will prevent others from learning about the diagnosis. This social survival tactic, requiring constant vigilance, may be more successful in larger than in smaller communities.

> At university people would say things behind my back. Nobody would be open to me, but they would whisper behind my back. People would make comments about me. In my village nobody knew, but because it is a small community people would start saying things. Even though they do, I don't pay them any attention. In my neighbourhood in Athens nobody knows, and I avoid speaking to anyone. Only with the lady at the grocery, but I somehow told her that I am on medication and since then she started to be more distant towards me.
>
> Mihalis

Intimate relationships

If friendships can be difficult for people with mental illnesses, what do we know about intimate relationships? Again, there is little research on this question and we need to pay attention to what people with mental illnesses say about their most personal experiences.

> Well the person I was friendly with, she ended it after I was in treatment here. We were friends for like seven years. First, she kept her distance. We didn't have

an argument. After that I stopped dating. I think about the fear when they find out eventually. I don't want to sit through that again. Once you get close to someone, you start talking. You might talk about what pills you take. For example, if they come to my house or I go to their house … they might see the pills and ask what it's for. I think that they would worry and stop the relationship.

Leroy

These are challenges which particularly affect people in young adulthood, at the same time when some types of mental illness begin.[24] A survey of almost 200 young people with mental illnesses in Finland, for example, found that their problems

could be identified in all central spheres of life as difficulties in relation to the self, school, parents, peers, dating and the future … focus should be made on the inner world of the young person, as well as on their behaviour within the different spheres of life.[25]

Specific conditions may affect close relationships in different ways. Some people with bipolar disorder, for example, say that their links with friends and family are harmed more by manic than by depressive episodes.

I once made a list of everything I could think of that I'd done that was notably embarrassing or problematic when I was high, and there were about 35 items, every one affecting a person I knew and the relationship I have with them. I found that after depression people are generally just happy to 'have you back', whereas after mania everything seems to have changed, been damaged somehow. I think that I scared a number of people to death with the sort of things that I talked about and the sort of mind games that I tried to get people to play. Then, when the dust settles, you have to hold your head up and return back to normal. There's an intense embarrassment about everything, and worse than that, the feeling that you are now 'branded' mentally ill for life, and that you are facing stigma from all directions.

Robert

Parents may also have strong views about who would be a suitable partner for their son or daughter, and people with a diagnosis of mental illness are often seen as clearly unsuitable.

I had once a friend and we've been to his place a few times. His parents afterwards told him not to bring me again to his place, because probably they noticed that I had some sort of problem.

Sotiris

In Japan, for example, before a possible marriage the parents of one of the partners may choose to hire a private investigator to scrutinize the whole family, and family tree, of a potential son or daughter-in-law to establish if there is any 'bad blood' in the ancestry. It is understood that finding a history of mental illness in the family is enough to forbid the marriage,[26] and such attitudes are not confined to Japan.

> During that time I got married to a State Registered Nurse, a single parent with a two year-old son, and we were doomed to argue and row about this and that. Seldom did we pull in the same direction at the same time. I desperately wanted us to have a baby, but she always refused citing the risk that one of my 'bad genes' could give our child schizophrenia (that was my self-diagnosis of what I had suffered from).
>
> Paul

Similarly, neighbours may have strong and negative views, which can limit the dating opportunities of people with mental illness. *'When I tried to flirt with a young woman, other men assaulted me. If I had no mental illness they could not do it'* (Ali).

Sexual relationships

In many ways patterns of sexual behaviour can be changed by mental illness, but it is usually very difficult to know how far this reflects direct or indirect discrimination. There is evidence that among young people with a diagnosis of mental illness risky sexual behaviours are more common than in the general population. A survey of almost 1000 young people in New Zealand, for example, found that young people diagnosed with drug dependence, schizophrenia-related, or antisocial disorders were more likely to engage in risky sexual intercourse, contract sexually transmitted diseases, and have sexual intercourse before 16 years old. Surprisingly, so were young people with depressive disorders. Young people with mania were even more likely to report risky sexual intercourse and have sexually transmitted diseases.[27]

Relatively little is known about whether the use of contraception by people with mental illnesses is similar to that of the general population or not.[28] A study of men with a diagnosis of a psychotic disorder in Texas found that most had fathered children, and that 60 per cent of these children under 16 years old were not being parented by their biological father. Nearly half (41 per cent) of the people included in this study had had sexual intercourse during the preceding year, had not wanted children, and reported that they or their sexual partner had not used contraception at the time of their last inter-course.[29] A parallel assessment of women with long-term psychiatric disabilities showed that, compared with women without mental illness, they had more induced abortions and were also more likely to have given up their own children for fostering or adoption. These women were more likely to have had more than one male sexual partner, and to report having been pressurized into unwanted sexual intercourse.[30]

There is fairly strong evidence that women with diagnoses of severe mental illnesses are less well informed about contraception than women in general. In a North American study of pregnant women with a diagnosis of a psychotic disorder, there was no record of whether birth control had been discussed.[31] In the Texan study just mentioned, only 10 per cent of women concerned said that family planning had been discussed with them.[32] Further, a large-scale assessment of women attending primary care in the UK showed that women with psychotic disorders were more likely to be prescribed injectable contraception, the post-coital pill, the coil, or to have had a termination of pregnancy.[33]

The finding of a relatively higher number of sexual partners for women with a diagnosis of a psychotic disorder was also made in Maryland. Compared with women included in a national survey, women with mental illness had fewer pregnancies and live births, were more likely to have had a pregnancy that did not result in a live birth, and had more lifetime sexual partners.[34]

When mental health staff try to help people with mental illness deal with questions of contraception, they find this an ethical and legal minefield. The history of psychiatry has tragic examples of psychiatric patients being subjected to involuntary sterilization or worse, enforced on eugenic grounds,[35–37] and this leads many staff to be very reluctant to do any more than offer factual advice to people with mental illness. Perhaps more often, clinical staff simply do not discuss contraception with service users at all.[38]

Even so, there are times when it may be in the best interest of someone with a mental illness to have effective contraception, for example when that person does not have the capacity to make such a decision. In many countries laws or regulations are either not directly relevant (for example referring largely to people with learning disabilities/mental retardation) or are ineffective.[39] Some countries in Eastern Europe have a system of registering people with mental illness as legally 'incapable'. One consequence of this is that women can be given a method of contraception, such as depot injections, without their consent, and there is considerable concern about whether these practices are compatible with the relevant international conventions on human rights.[40]

One serious consequence of risky sexual behaviour is human immunodeficiency virus (HIV) infection, and it is clear that some groups of people with mental illness have a relatively high risk of being HIV-positive. Among male psychiatric patients in a New York City shelter for homeless men, for example, almost a fifth (19.4 per cent) were HIV-positive.[41] For mentally ill men and women living in such homeless shelters the use of protective measures is not common. Among mentally ill homeless men who were sexually active in New York, most had sex without a condom and with non-monogamous partners.[42] Among such men AIDS was the leading cause of death.[43]

Where pregnancies do go ahead, women with severe mental illness start antenatal care later than most women, and are more likely to have obstetric complications, including foetal and neonatal deaths.[44–50] Yet there is no clear evidence that this indicates any form of direct discrimination by services. Nevertheless nothing is published directly reporting the view of such women on this subject.

Another serious risk faced particularly by women with more severely disabling mental illnesses is of sexual coercion or abuse. Awareness of this problem has emerged particularly during the last decade. One survey compared the sexual experience of psychiatric outpatients in New Zealand, compared with a similar group of people who had never been treated for psychiatric illness.[51] Abuse in adulthood was reported by almost a third of the people with a diagnosis of mental illness. Compared with the control group, patients were more likely to report a history of sexual abuse during adulthood, and female patients were also more likely to have been sexually abused than male patients. For some, these may have been retraumatizing events, because those who were sexually abused as adults were also more likely to report a history of sexual abuse during childhood.

These findings suggest that some women with forms of severe mental illness may be trying to survive both the mental illness and their experiences of prolonged or repeated trauma.[52] Although the question of post-traumatic stress disorder among people with psychotic disorders is now widely discussed in some centres in North America,[53] there is evidence that they may be common elsewhere. A series of studies in India, for example, showed that about a third of women admitted to a hospital in Bangalore reported coercive sexual experiences. In half these cases the perpetrator was the husband, and in 10 per cent of cases it was a person in a position of authority in the local community.[54] Most of these women said that before the study they had not disclosed their experience to anyone else, and that they had not sought help.[55]

Sexual relations in psychiatric institutions raise particular challenges, both for inpatients and for staff. Historically, there have been swings in staff attitudes on whether psychiatric wards should be mixed- or single-sex.[56] After several decades of a policy supporting mixed-sex wards in England, for example (in the name of normalization) there has been a trend back towards same-sex wards. This follows reports by female inpatients of their feelings of vulnerability, especially in acute wards.[57] Despite this, sexual contact within psychiatric hospitals may well be common. One study among acute inpatients in London showed that 10 per cent had sexual intercourse with other patients while admitted to hospital, and 2 per cent had used condoms.[58] There is a balance here between an individual's right to sexual expression and the need to protect vulnerable patients. Psychiatric staff are usually aware of this conflict and a survey of long-stay mental health facilities in the USA found that 60 per cent had a policy on sexual relations, and that 83 per cent had sex education programmes for residents.[59] Often staff are faced with considerable ambiguity, and there are no clear national or state regulations about who has capacity to give valid consent to consensual sexual relations, not least because the condition of many inpatients changes rapidly. Under these circumstances it is common for acute inpatient units, in particular, to prohibit all sexual contact between patients, as is the case at Bellevue Hospital in New York.[60] Such a policy could be seen either as a discriminatory infringement of basic human rights, or as a sensible protection against exploitation and abuse.

In terms of the direct effects of treatment, many of the drugs used to treat mental illnesses have important effects to limit sexual feelings or relations. In particular medications used to treat psychotic disorders, depression or anxiety often produce reduced sexual desire, or problems of arousal, erection, ejaculation and orgasm. These are common reasons for people to chose not to take these drugs,[61] although this is rarely discussed with doctors.[38] Indeed mental health staff frequently shy away from the taboo area of sexual relations, even if this may cause the person with mental illness not to take medication and to suffer worse symptoms as a consequence.[62–64]

Although, as we saw in the previous chapter, people with more severely disabling mental illnesses tend to socialize with people with similar problems, this can also bring complexities.

> As a single person, it's very difficult to broach the subject of mental illness if you have just met someone you like. I've met people who have their own illness problems, and whilst they understand my difficulties better, now we find there's two sets of problems lurking, and a feeling that things could be very difficult if we both became ill. I find it hard to tolerate illness in a girl I've just met, so I know that people will find it hard to tolerate in me.
>
> Robert

Such difficulties in forming and keeping close relationships do not only result from discrimination by others. Even before making contact with mental health services, and being offered a diagnosis, young people in the 'prodromal' period (when symptoms are developing) may also have greater difficulties in intimacy. A study in Finland, for example, spoke with over 200 young people who had recently been diagnosed as having schizophrenia. In general the men had been more unsocial, withdrawn and less confident in close personal relationships, compared with women, before contacting mental health services. After receiving treatment the men also coped less well in their social and intimate relationships.[65] So such partnerships are complex, involve subtle aspects of behaviour and expectations, and may only partly reflect discrimination.

Marriage

I inhibit myself on topics of close relationships with women, and marriage.

Ali

While marriage, or a long-term partnership, is central to the aspirations of most people, with or without mental illness, we need to tread carefully here. Patterns of marriage vary to an astonishing extent between different countries, and have changed rapidly in recent decades. A study of people with a diagnosis of schizophrenia in five different European countries, for example, found that two-thirds were effectively single, and only 17 per cent were married, but with large international variations. The proportions of people with mental illness who were married (compared with the general population in each country) were: Amsterdam in Holland 10 per cent (compared with 28 per cent), Copenhagen in Denmark 11 per cent (compared with 21 per cent), London in England 16 per cent (compared with 22 per cent), Santander in Spain 16 per cent (compared with 47 per cent) and Verona in Italy 24 per cent (compared with 55 per cent). So it is clear that having a diagnosis of mental illness can reduce a person's chances of marrying or staying married, especially in the Mediterranean countries of Southern Europe.[66] By comparison a study in Chennai in Southern India found that 70 per cent of young adults with a diagnosis of schizophrenia went on to marry in the following ten years.[67] *'Once I had a partner and when I told her that I have schizophrenia, she started shaking. I never saw her again. After that I hide it'* (Emanouil).

Within marriage, the effects of mental illness can add pressures which are hard to withstand. In a large nationwide study in the United States, for example, married men and women who had a diagnosis of severe depression said that they had fewer positive and more negative interactions with their spouse or partner, compared both with people with other types of mental illness, and with people with no mental illness. The researchers concluded that poor quality intimate relationships are characteristic of people with severe depression.[68] But it is wrong to over-generalize.

I was still very ill. I could tell via the fiction and self-portraits I was doing at the time. But out of all this morbidity and inky blackness, my door was unlocked by a woman that I only knew for six months yet changed my life. Rebecca, a former art student and model, was the first person to see and recognise that I had artistic talent and that I should go to Art College. She helped me prepare a portfolio to take to the interview. More than this she wasn't phased by my revelation that I had had a breakdown. In fact, she told me many artists, poets, and writers have breakdowns.

Paul

Once again we come to an issue which is seen to be of crucial importance in the eyes of many people with mental illness, but is a topic on which most books and scientific journals are silent.[69–71]

> I have not read anything regarding persons who marry while living with serious, persistent mental illness. I married in the 1960s when persistent mental illness was considered a 'nervous breakdown' and not an ongoing disease. With this article, I want to educate and explore thought in other persons who might share the same problems I experienced. I want to give a voice to the isolation I felt while married, coping with my illness. I felt so different from other married women with my closeted illness. I have two beautiful daughters who suffered a tragedy in their young lives when I became ill, yet our love seems to have survived and our relationship each day grows. With this article I want to give a voice to one marriage and mental illness. I want someone who reads this to say, 'Yes, I feel like that; I know I'm not alone.'[72]

As we will find at several points throughout this book, contradictory things often happen at the same time. For example, while mental illness for a spouse can bring extra strain to a marriage, being married can also be a clear advantage for a person with mental illness. The Finnish study of young adults with a diagnosis of schizophrenia, referred to earlier, also found that positive changes in symptoms and social activities were most common among people with mental illness who were living with a spouse. Strikingly the worst outcome was for men living alone, who more often lose their social contacts than do women with mental illness.[73]

> I open my heart to people, but a friend has hurt me deeply. 'You are on medication' he said, 'You are not ok, go and take your pills. Just leave'.
>
> Vasilis

Divorce

Mental illness can both precede and follow divorce and separation.[74] First, divorce can increase the risk of mental illness starting. A survey of over 2000 adults in the National Survey of Health and Development in Britain found that divorce and separation were associated with increased subsequent levels of anxiety, depression and alcohol use. This was true even though half of those separated or divorced were re-married or reunited with their spouses by the time they were assessed. Such pain can persist. There was no reduction over time in the symptoms of mental illness among divorced and separated people.[75]

Divorce can also slow down recovery for people who had a mental illness before separating. Among about 5000 people in the British Household Panel Survey, divorce decreased the rate of recovery from anxiety and depression. As we saw earlier, low social support also decreased the chances of recovery, and again this applied more often to men.[76] For women, by comparison, being a single parent after divorce was more likely to lead to depression.[77] On the other hand, rates of depression are not increased for those who escape marriages which have serious long-term problems, such as domestic violence, and which allow people to make a fresh start.[78]

Such reactions to divorce can go far beyond the usual levels of adjustment that most people experience following separation. In Denmark, for example, a recent divorce was found to increase the risk of being admitted to hospital for depression or hypomania,[79] no matter at what age the divorce took place.[80–82]

Can having a mental illness itself increase the chance of separation or divorce? The evidence suggests that the answer is yes. Another large-scale survey, this time of almost 6000 people in the United States, showed that a prior mental illness in one partner substantially increased the risk of divorce. It has been estimated that among the US population there are approximately 23 million lost years of marriage among men, and 48 million lost years of marriage among women, as a consequence of mental illness.[83] *'My husband plans to divorce and despises me because of my illness'* (Faiza).

Patterns of separation can also show striking cultural patterns. Interviews with women with a diagnosis of schizophrenia in Southern India found that despite no longer living in the marital home, many of them had not separated legally, nor were they receiving any maintenance from their husbands. The stigma attached to separation was as poignant as that of being mentally ill, if not more so. Even several years after the separation, these women still harboured hope that they would eventually reunite with their husbands.[84] In most cases the women returned to live with their parents, who felt intense distress and were especially concerned about the long-term social and financial security of their daughters.[85]

Children

Most published work on mentally ill parents refers to mothers:[86–90] fathers are almost invisible. Although childbirth can trigger particular types of mental illness, particularly postnatal depression or puerperal psychosis, our focus here is on how pre-existing mental illness is related to fertility, childbirth and parenting.

In some respects mental illnesses can have an important influence on childbearing. For women with a diagnosis of mood-related psychosis (bipolar disorder and psychotic depression), for example, their fertility rate is lower than for similar women without mental illness, and this does not seem to be because of prescribed medication.[91] Women with a diagnosis of a psychotic illness have higher rates of complications during pregnancy, and there may be a greater risk of stillbirth or neonatal death.[92,93] They also faced an increased risk of relapse of a psychotic condition, and twice the risk of becoming depressed in the year after birth.[94] The situation may well be even worse for mothers whose mental illness starts during pregnancy.[95]

In terms of parenting we find a mixed picture. A review of this literature concluded that a significant proportion of mothers with psychotic disorders have parenting difficulties or lose custody of their infant.[96] On the other hand, the physical health of babies who live with mothers with psychotic disorders is not significantly different from that of other babies.[97] A diagnosis of schizophrenia for a mother is associated with receiving social services supervision. Some interventions are effective. One British study found that preventative measures targeting social and financial problems, the early treatment of symptoms, and assessing the father's health needs, can lead to better parenting.[98]

In sum, there is little clear evidence to suggest that women diagnosed with a mental illness cannot parent. One study of admissions to psychiatric mother and baby units in the UK found that two-thirds did not need social services support on discharge.[99] However, there is considerable evidence to show that women with severe mental illness lose custody of their children far more often than most parents. Among a group of Danish parents with mental illness, a quarter had children placed in institutions or foster care, while 40 per cent had never received professional help related to their children, and a third said that their requests for parenting support had not been responded to.[100] Similarly, in Australia a study found that most of the children of parents diagnosed as having a psychotic illness no longer lived with their parents. Over 10 per cent of these parents described childcare interventions which had taken place against their will, and nearly a third said that they were reluctant to seek help with childcare because they were frightened that their children would be taken away.[101] According to one Canadian report, parents with mental illness lose custody for reasons that would rarely be used for other parents.[102] In general it seems to be fair to say that these findings suggest that there may be some degree of discrimination against mentally ill parents in relation to childcare, but that this has not yet been established.

Despite this, mental health services seem to pay scant attention to childcare problems among the people they treat,[103] and usually they leave such needs unmet.[104] A North American study found that up to a third of the children of mothers with a diagnosis of severe mental illness received formal help during childhood, either from school or mental health agencies.[105] It may take too long for services to recognise when to offer support: among mothers in their first admission to psychiatric hospital one study found that 'there was virtually no evidence that any form of educational or family-oriented treatment was offered'.[106]

What do we know about the perspective of such parents themselves?[107] Fifty mothers who were admitted to psychiatric hospital in Denmark were asked about childcare. Most were already preoccupied with their children's situation and were relieved to discuss these issues. Half of these people had emotional difficulties with their children, among whom half suffered from physical or mental health problems. Most of the children had parents who had been mentally ill all their life, and family discord was common.[100] The effects on the children seem to be greater if both parents have mental illness.[108]

In such families the views of the children themselves are rarely discussed.[109] One intriguing study in Michigan asked 22 children to describe their experiences living in a family where a parent has a diagnosis of mental illness. They spoke of their parents' 'bad days' and 'good days' (when they got more attention). They had little detailed information about their parents' conditions, and tellingly their main recommendation to their parents was 'Get help earlier'.[110]

Services can help. A specific support programme in New Hampshire offering adult and children's mental health care, home-based parent training and practical community supports showed good results.[111] But this is the exception. Although most women with mental illness in South London are mothers (63 per cent), this role is not one that is usually recognised or supported,[112] at least until things go wrong.

Losing custody of a child is more common for parents with mental illness.[113] Losing a child under these circumstances can cause profound distress. A study in Pennsylvania concluded that many such women did not know how to gain custody or how to maintain contact with their children, nor how to navigate legal and social services.[114] Having a child taken away while unwell with mental illness, can be a traumatic event in its own right. Not surprisingly, losing custody seems to occur more often for women who are compulsorily admitted to hospital, or who enter a forensic treatment programme.[112]

Another consequence of mental illness is that other family members may see the person as incompetent to share normal family childcare responsibilities, both on an informal day-to-day basis, and also in longer-term formal ways.

> One situation that cropped up was when my sister delegated to my younger sibling the custody as the carer/guardian if anything were to happen in the future. I queried why I had not been appointed. Yes, the depression thing came up. I often feel alienated when some of my family will talk to me as if I'm stupid and say. 'Snap out of things'.
>
> Tania

So we have seen that mental illness can have important effects on making and keeping friends, on dating and forming intimate relationships, on marriage, separation, divorce, pregnancy and childcare. How far are these different experiences discriminatory, and how far do they reflect the reality of how the symptoms of mental illness affect people? Here we need to pause to appreciate the recent historical context. Forced sterilization laws for people with mental disabilities were only repealed in Sweden and several American states during the last 30 years.[115] More recently, a British survey of mental health service users found that a half of women and a quarter of men felt that they had had their parenting abilities unfairly questioned.[116] Indeed, fear of losing custody or access to their children dominated the accounts of a group of mentally ill mothers in London, and influenced all their meetings with mental health and social services, so that they were reluctant to disclose any parenting difficulties they did have. They reported a widespread assumption that mentally ill women are poor parents, regardless of the facts of an individual case. They saw services as offering little continuing support for parenting, and intervening only in crises.[117]

As we see many times in the course of this book, people with mental illness repeatedly encounter the assumptions of others about what they should and should not do, where often these assumptions go well beyond the actual consequences of the mental illness. It is therefore worth keeping in mind some core issues. Among women who have a severe form of mental illness most are mothers, and the majority describe motherhood as rewarding and central to their lives.[117] Despite all of these challenges many people with mental illness, often after long discussion, do choose to have children and do succeed as parents. This is the experience of one couple in London.

> We were discussing whether to have children, and for a long time we decided not to. The problems seemed to be too great, there was no money. He felt he couldn't cope with having children, and we talked about it and argued and discussed and eventually I said 'Okay that's it', and I thought I'd accepted it, but I hadn't really! There was a bit of me underneath that hadn't accepted it one little bit, and I got myself very depressed at that point. Our then parish priest was a great help to me. Somehow he managed to see what was going wrong. He said 'Don't give up on the idea of having children,' He said 'You need to have children, you want to have children.'
>
> Sarah, wife of Peter

> In a way I didn't want to have children because I was so worried about how we were going to cope, but obviously Sarah was so unhappy about not having children. After a while I agreed, and I'm glad I did.
>
> Peter, husband of Sarah

References

1. Zeldin T. *An Intimate History of Humanity.* London: Vintage; 1998.

2. Dunn S. *Creating Accepting Communities: Report of the MIND Inquiry into Social Exclusion and Mental Health Problems.* London: MIND; 1999.

3. Boydell KM, Gladstone BM, Crawford ES. The dialectic of friendship for people with psychiatric disabilities. *Psychiatr Rehabil J* 2002; 26(2):123–131.

4. Thornicroft G, Rose D, Huxley P, Dale G, Wykes T. What are the research priorities of mental health service users? *Journal of Mental Health* 2002; 11:1–5.

5. Kirsner BR, Figueredo AJ, Jacobs WJ. Self, friends, and lovers: structural relations among Beck Depression Inventory scores and perceived mate values. *J Affect Disord* 2003; 75(2):131–148.

6. Beels CC, Gutwirth L, Berkeley J, Struening E. Measurements of social support in schizophrenia. *Schizophr Bull* 1984; 10(3):399–411.

7. Buchanan J. Social support and schizophrenia: a review of the literature. *Arch Psychiatr Nurs* 1995; 9(2):68–76.

8. Becker T, Albert M, Angermeyer MC, Thornicroft G. Social networks and service utilisation in patients with severe mental illness. *Epidemiol Psychiatr Soc* 1997; 6(1 Suppl):113–125.

9. Dunn M, O'Driscoll C, Dayson D, Wills W, Leff J. The TAPS Project. 4: An observational study of the social life of long-stay patients. *Br J Psychiatry* 1990; 157:842–8, 852.

10. Dayson D. The TAPS project 15: The social networks of two group settings: a pilot study. *Journal of Mental Health* 1992; 1:99–106.

11. Borge L, Martinsen EW, Ruud T, Watne O, Friis S. Quality of life, loneliness, and social contact among long-term psychiatric patients. *Psychiatr Serv* 1999; 50 (1):81–84.

12. Evert H, Harvey C, Trauer T, Herrman H. The relationship between social networks and occupational and self-care functioning in people with psychosis. *Soc Psychiatry Psychiatr Epidemiol* 2003; 38(4):180–188.

13. Howard L, Leese M, Thornicroft G. Social networks and functional status in patients with psychosis. *Acta Psychiatr Scand* 2000; 102(5):376–385.

14. Thesen J. Being a psychiatric patient in the community – reclassified as the stigmatized 'other'. *Scand J Public Health* 2001; 29(4):248–255.

15. Brugha TS, Weich S, Singleton N, Lewis G, Bebbington PE, Jenkins R *et al.* Primary group size, social support, gender and future mental health status in a prospective study of people living in private households throughout Great Britain. *Psychol Med* 2005; 35(5):705–714.

16. Olds J, Schwartz RS. What is the psychiatric significance of loneliness? *Harv Ment Health Lett* 2000; 16(10):8.

17. Joiner TE, Jr, Lewinsohn PM, Seeley JR. The core of loneliness: lack of pleasurable engagement – more so than painful disconnection – predicts social impairment, depression onset, and recovery from depressive disorders among adolescents. *J Pers Assess* 2002; 79(3):472–491.

18. Flood M. *Mapping Loneliness in Australia.* Canberra: The Australia Institute; 2005.

19. Rotenberg KJ, MacKie J. Stigmatization of social and intimacy loneliness. *Psychol Rep* 1999; 84(1):147–148.

20. Wing JK, Brown G. *Institutionalism and Schizophrenia.* Cambridge: Cambridge University Press; 1970.

21. Curson DA, Pantelis C, Ward J, Barnes TR. Institutionalism and schizophrenia 30 years on. Clinical poverty and the social environment in three British mental hospitals in 1960 compared with a fourth in 1990. *Br J Psychiatry* 1992; 160:230–241.

22. Lee H, Coenen A, Heim K. Island living: the experience of loneliness in a psychiatric hospital. *Appl Nurs Res* 1994; 7(1):7–13.

23. Magliano L, Fiorillo A, De RC, Malangone C, Maj M. Family burden in long-term diseases: a comparative study in schizophrenia vs. physical disorders. *Soc Sci Med* 2005; 61(2):313–322.

24. Burke KC, Burke JD, Jr., Regier DA, Rae DS. Age at onset of selected mental disorders in five community populations. *Arch Gen Psychiatry* 1990; 47(6):511–518.

25. Alestalo A, Munnukka T, Pukuri T. Problems of young people in community psychiatric care. *J Psychiatr Ment Health Nurs* 2002; 9(1):33–40.

26. Desapriya EB, Nobutada I. Stigma of mental illness in Japan. *Lancet* 2002; 359(9320):1866.

27. Ramrakha S, Caspi A, Dickson N, Moffitt TE, Paul C. Psychiatric disorders and risky sexual behaviour in young adulthood: cross-sectional study in birth cohort. *BMJ* 2000; 321(7256):263–266.

28. Jones KP, Wild RA. Contraception for patients with psychiatric or medical disorders. *Am J Obstet Gynecol* 1994; 170(5 Pt 2):1575–1580.

29. Coverdale JH, Schotte D, Ruiz P, Pharies S, Bayer T. Family planning needs of male chronic mental patients in the general hospital psychiatry clinic. *Gen Hosp Psychiatry* 1994; 16(1):38–41.

30. Coverdale JH, Turbott SH, Roberts H. Family planning needs and STD risk behaviours of female psychiatric out-patients. *Br J Psychiatry* 1997; 171:69–72.

31. Rudolph B, Larson GL, Sweeny S, Hough EE, Arorian K. Hospitalized pregnant psychotic women: characteristics and treatment issues. *Hosp Community Psychiatry* 1990; 41(2):159–163.

32. Coverdale J, Falloon I. Home or hospital-based emergency care for chronic psychiatric patients? *New Zealand Medical Journal* 1993; 106(957):218–219.

33. Howard L. PhD Thesis: The fertility, and medical and psychosocial outcomes of pregnancy, for women with psychosis. University of London; 2004.

34. Dickerson FB, Brown CH, Kreyenbuhl J, Goldberg RW, Fang LJ, Dixon LB. Sexual and reproductive behaviors among persons with mental illness. *Psychiatr Serv* 2004; 55(11):1299–1301.

35. Gottesman II, Bertelsen A. Legacy of German psychiatric genetics: hindsight is always 20/20. *Am J Med Genet* 1996; 67(4):317–322.

36. Roelcke V. [Mentalities and sterilization laws in Europe during the 1930s. Eugenics, genetics, and politics in a historic context]. *Nervenarzt* 2002; 73(11):1019–1030.

37. Burleigh M. *Death and Deliverance. 'Euthanasia' in Germany 1900–1945*. Cambridge: Cambridge University Press; 1994.

38. McLennan JD, Ganguli R. Family planning and parenthood needs of women with severe mental illness: clinicians' perspective. *Community Ment Health J* 1999; 35(4):369–380.

39. Coverdale JH, Bayer TL, McCullough LB, Chervenak FA. Respecting the autonomy of chronic mentally ill women in decisions about contraception. *Hosp Community Psychiatry* 1993; 44(7):671–674.

40. Mental Disability Advocacy Center. *Russia's Guardianship System Challenged at the European Court of Human Rights*. Budapest: Mental Disability Advocacy Center; 2005.

41. Susser E, Valencia E, Conover S. Prevalence of HIV infection among psychiatric patients in a New York City men's shelter. *Am J Public Health* 1993; 83(4):568–570.

42. Susser E, Valencia E, Miller M, Tsai WY, Meyer-Bahlburg H, Conover S. Sexual behavior of homeless mentally ill men at risk for HIV. *Am J Psychiatry* 1995; 152(4):583–587.

43. Susser E, Colson P, Jandorf L, Berkman A, Lavelle J, Fennig S *et al.* HIV infection among young adults with psychotic disorders. *Am J Psychiatry* 1997; 154(6):864–866.

44. Bennedsen BE, Mortensen PB, Olesen AV, Henriksen TB. Congenital malformations, still-births, and infant deaths among children of women with schizophrenia. *Arch Gen Psychiatry* 2001; 58(7):674–679.

45. Bennedsen BE, Mortensen PB, Olesen AV, Henriksen TB, Frydenberg M. Obstetric compli-cations in women with schizophrenia. *Schizophr Res* 2001; 47(2–3): 167–175.

46. Bennedsen BE, Mortensen PB, Olesen AV, Henriksen TB. Preterm birth and intra-uterine growth retardation among children of women with schizophrenia. *Br J Psychiatry* 1999; 175:239–245.

47. Bennedsen BE. Adverse pregnancy outcome in schizophrenic women: occurrence and risk factors. *Schizophr Res* 1998; 33(1–2):1–26.

48. Sacker A, Done DJ, Crow TJ. Obstetric complications in children born to parents with schizophrenia: a meta-analysis of case-control studies. *Psychol Med* 1996; 26(2):279–287.

49. Rieder RO, Rosenthal D, Wender P, Blumenthal H. The offspring of schizophrenics. Fetal and neonatal deaths. *Arch Gen Psychiatry* 1975; 32(2):200–211.

50. Howard L, Shah N, Salmon M, Appleby L. Predictors of social services supervision of babies of mothers with mental illness after admission to a psychiatric mother and baby unit. *Soc Psychiatry Psychiatr Epidemiol* 2003; 38(8):450–455.

51. Coverdale JH, Turbott SH. Sexual and physical abuse of chronically ill psychiatric outpatients compared with a matched sample of medical outpatients. *J Nerv Ment Dis* 2000; 188(7):440–445.

52. Harris M. Modifications in service delivery and clinical treatment for women diagnosed with severe mental illness who are also the survivors of sexual abuse trauma. *J Ment Health Adm* 1994; 21(4):397–406.

53. Mueser KT, Salyers MP, Rosenberg SD, Goodman LA, Essock SM, Osher FC *et al.* Interper-sonal trauma and posttraumatic stress disorder in patients with severe mental illness: demographic, clinical, and health correlates. *Schizophr Bull* 2004; 30(1):45–57.

54. Chandra PS, Deepthivarma S, Carey MP, Carey KB, Shalinianant MP. A cry from the darkness: women with severe mental illness in India reveal their experiences with sexual coercion. *Psychiatry* 2003; 66(4):323–334.

55. Chandra PS, Carey MP, Carey KB, Shalinianant A, Thomas T. Sexual coercion and abuse among women with a severe mental illness in India: an exploratory investigation. *Compr Psychiatry* 2003; 44(3):205–212.

56. Grob G. *From Asylum to Community. Mental health policy in modern America.* Princeton, New Jersey: Princeton University Press; 1991.

57. Shepherd G, Beadsmoore A, Moore C, Hardy P, Muijen M. Relation between bed use, social deprivation, and overall bed availability in acute adult psychiatric units, and alternative residential options: a cross sectional survey, one day census data, and staff interviews. *BMJ* 1997; 314(7076):262–266.

58. Warner J, Pitts N, Crawford MJ, Serfaty M, Prabhakaran P, Amin R. Sexual activity among patients in psychiatric hospital wards. *J R Soc Med* 2004; 97(10):477–479.

59. Dobal MT, Torkelson DJ. Making decisions about sexual rights in psychiatric facilities. *Arch Psychiatr Nurs* 2004; 18(2):68–74.

60. Ford E, Rosenberg M, Holsten M, Boudreaux T. Managing sexual behavior on adult acute care inpatient psychiatric units. [Review] [24 refs]. *Psychiatric Services* 2003; 54(3):346–350.

61. Segraves RT. Psychiatric illness and sexual function. *Int J Impot Res* 1998; 10 Suppl 2:S131–S133.

62. Clayton DO, Shen WW. Psychotropic drug-induced sexual function disorders: diagnosis, incidence and management. *Drug Saf* 1998; 19(4):299–312.

63. Demyttenaere K, De FJ, Sienaert P. Psychotropics and sexuality. *Int Clin Psychopharmacol* 1998; 13 Suppl 6:S35–S41.

64. Strauss B, Gross J. [Psychotropic drug-induced changes in sexuality–frequency and relevance in psychiatric practice]. *Psychiatr Prax* 1984; 11(2):49–55.

65. Salokangas RK, Stengard E. Gender and short-term outcome in schizophrenia. *Schizophr Res* 1990; 3(5–6):333–345.

66. Thornicroft G, Tansella M, Becker T, Knapp M, Leese M, Schene A *et al.* The personal impact of schizophrenia in Europe. *Schizophr Res* 2004; 69(2–3):125–132.

67. Thara R, Srinivasan TN. Outcome of marriage in schizophrenia. *Soc Psychiatry Psychiatr Epidemiol* 1997; 32(7):416–420.

68. Zlotnick C, Kohn R, Keitner G, la Grotta SA. The relationship between quality of interpersonal relationships and major depressive disorder: findings from the National Comorbidity Survey. *J Affect Disord* 2000; 59(3):205–215.

69. Forthofer MS, Kessler RC, Story AL, Gotlib IH. The effects of psychiatric disorders on the probability and timing of first marriage. *J Health Soc Behav* 1996; 37(2):121–132.

70. Birtchnell J. Psychiatric disorders in marriage. *Br J Hosp Med* 1986; 35(6):409–412.

71. Dominian J. Marriage and psychiatric illness. *BMJ* 1979; 2(6194):854–855.

72. Fox V. Marriage and mental illness. *Psychiatr Rehabil J* 2001; 25(2):196–198.

73. Salokangas RK. Living situation, social network and outcome in schizophrenia: a five-year prospective follow-up study. *Acta Psychiatr Scand* 1997; 96(6):459–468.

74. Wade TJ, Pevalin DJ. Marital transitions and mental health. *J Health Soc Behav* 2004; 45(2):155–170.

75. Richards M, Hardy R, Wadsworth M. The effects of divorce and separation on mental health in a national UK birth cohort. *Psychol Med* 1997; 27(5):1121–1128.

76. Pevalin DJ, Goldberg DP. Social precursors to onset and recovery from episodes of common mental illness. *Psychol Med* 2003; 33(2):299–306.

77. Wade TJ, Cairney J. Major depressive disorder and marital transition among mothers: results from a national panel study. *J Nerv Ment Dis* 2000; 188 (11):741–750.

78. Aseltine RH, Jr, Kessler RC. Marital disruption and depression in a community sample. *J Health Soc Behav* 1993; 34(3):237–251.

79. Kessing LV, Agerbo E, Mortensen PB. Does the impact of major stressful life events on the risk of developing depression change throughout life? *Psychol Med* 2003; 33(7):1177–1184.

80. Kessing LV, Agerbo E, Mortensen PB. Major stressful life events and other risk factors for first admission with mania. *Bipolar Disord* 2004; 6(2):122–129.

81. Svedin CG, Wadsby M. The presence of psychiatric consultations in relation to divorce. *Acta Psychiatr Scand* 1998; 98(5):414–422.

82. Kessing LV, Agerbo E, Mortensen PB. Major stressful life events and other risk factors for first admission with mania. *Bipolar Disord* 2004; 6(2):122–129.

83. Kessler RC, Walters EE, Forthofer MS. The social consequences of psychiatric disorders, III: probability of marital stability. *Am J Psychiatry* 1998; 155(8):1092–1096.

84. Thara R, Kamath S, Kumar S. Women with schizophrenia and broken marriages – doubly disadvantaged? Part I: patient perspective. *Int J Soc Psychiatry* 2003; 49(3):225–232.

85. Thara R, Kamath S, Kumar S. Women with schizophrenia and broken marriages – doubly disadvantaged? Part II: family perspective. *Int J Soc Psychiatry* 2003; 49(3):233–240.

86. Mowbray CT, Oyserman D, Zemencuk JK, Ross SR. Motherhood for women with serious mental illness: pregnancy, childbirth, and the postpartum period. *Am J Orthopsychiatry* 1995; 65(1):21–38.

87. Bosanac P, Buist A, Burrows G. Motherhood and schizophrenic illnesses: a review of the literature. *Aust N Z J Psychiatry* 2003; 37(1):24–30.

88. Park RJ, Senior R, Stein A. The offspring of mothers with eating disorders. *Eur Child Adolesc Psychiatry* 2003; 12 Suppl 1:I110–I119.

89. Miller LJ, Finnerty M. Sexuality, pregnancy, and childrearing among women with schizophrenia-spectrum disorders. *Psychiatr Serv* 1996; 47(5):502–506.

90. Ramsay R, Howard L, Kumar C. Schizophrenia and safety of parenting of infants: a report from a U.K. mother and baby service. *Int J Soc Psychiatry* 1998; 44(2):127–134.

91. Howard LM, Kumar C, Leese M, Thornicroft G. The general fertility rate in women with psychotic disorders. *Am J Psychiatry* 2002; 159(6):991–997.

92. Howard LM. Fertility and pregnancy in women with psychotic disorders. *Eur J Obstet Gynecol Reprod Biol* 2005; 119(1):3–10.

93. Howard LM, Goss C, Leese M, Thornicroft G. Medical outcome of pregnancy in women with psychotic disorders and their infants in the first year after birth. *Br J Psychiatry* 2003; 182(1):63–67.

94. Howard LM, Goss C, Leese M, Appleby L, Thornicroft G. The psychosocial outcome of pregnancy in women with psychotic disorders. *Schizophr Res* 2004; 71(1):49–60.

95. Mowbray CT, Bybee D, Oyserman D, Macfarlane P. Timing of mental illness onset and motherhood. *J Nerv Ment Dis* 2005; 193(6):369–378.

96. Howard LM. Fertility and pregnancy in women with psychotic disorders. *Eur J Obstet Gynecol Reprod Biol* 2005; 119(1):3–10.

97. Howard LM, Goss C, Leese M, Thornicroft G. Medical outcome of pregnancy in women with psychotic disorders and their infants in the first year after birth. *Br J Psychiatry* 2003; 182(1):63–67.

98. Howard LM, Goss C, Leese M, Appleby L, Thornicroft G. The psychosocial outcome of pregnancy in women with psychotic disorders. *Schizophr Res* 2004; 71(1):49–60.

99. Howard LM, Thornicroft G, Salmon M, Appleby L. Predictors of parenting outcome in women with psychotic disorders discharged from mother and baby units. *Acta Psychiatr Scand* 2004; 110(5):347–355.

100. Wang AR, Goldschmidt VV. Interviews of psychiatric inpatients about their family situation and young children. *Acta Psychiatr Scand* 1994; 90(6):459–465.

101. Hearle.C, McGrath J. Motherhood and Schizophrenia. In: Castle D, McGrath J, Jayashri K, eds., pp. *Women and Schizophrenia.* Cambridge: Cambridge University Press; 2000; 79–94.

102. British Columbia Minister of Health Advisory Council on Mental Health. *Discrimination Against People with Mental Illnesses and Their Families: Changing attitudes, opening minds.* Vancouver: British Columbia Minister of Health Advisory Council on Mental Health; 2002.

103. Mowbray CT, Oyserman D, Bybee D, Macfarlane P, Rueda-Riedle A. Life circumstances of mothers with serious mental illnesses. *Psychiatr Rehabil J* 2001; 25(2):114–123.

104. Chernomas WM, Clarke DE, Chisholm FA. Perspectives of women living with schizophrenia. *Psychiatr Serv* 2000; 51(12):1517–1521.

105. Mowbray CT, Lewandowski L, Bybee D, Oyserman D. Children of mothers diagnosed with serious mental illness: patterns and predictors of service use. *Ment Health Serv Res* 2004; 6(3):167–183.

106. Craig T, Bromet EJ. Parents with psychosis. *Ann Clin Psychiatry* 2004; 16(1):35–39.

107. Thomas L, Kalucy R. Parents with mental illness: lacking motivation to parent. *Int J Ment Health Nurs* 2003; 12(2):153–157.

108. Burke L. The impact of maternal depression on familial relationships. *Int Rev Psychiatry* 2003; 15(3):243–255.

109. Mordoch E, Hall WA. Children living with a parent who has a mental illness: a critical analysis of the literature and research implications. *Arch Psychiatr Nurs* 2002; 16(5):208–216.

110. Riebschleger J. Good days and bad days: the experiences of children of a parent with a psychiatric disability. *Psychiatr Rehabil J* 2004; 28(1):25–31.

111. Brunette MF, Dean W. Community mental health care for women with severe mental illness who are parents. *Community Ment Health J* 2002; 38(2):153–165.

112. Howard LM, Kumar R, Thornicroft G. Psychosocial characteristics and needs of mothers with psychotic disorders. *Br J Psychiatry* 2001; 178:427–432.

113. Coverdale JH, Turbott SH. Family planning outcomes of male chronically ill psychiatric outpatients. *Psychiatr Serv* 1997; 48(9):1199–1200.

114. Sands RG, Koppelman N, Solomon P. Maternal custody status and living arrangements of children of women with severe mental illness. *Health Soc Work* 2004; 29(4):317–325.

115. Stefan S. Whose egg is it anyway? Reproductive rights of incarcerated, institutionalized and incompetent women. *Nova Law Review* 1989; 12:406–456.

116. Read J, Baker S. *Not Just Sticks and Stones. A Survey of the Stigma, Taboos, and Discrimination Experienced by People with Mental Health Problems.* London: MIND; 1996.

117. az-Caneja A, Johnson S. The views and experiences of severely mentally ill mothers – a qualitative study. *Soc Psychiatry Psychiatr Epidemiol* 2004; 39(6):472–482.

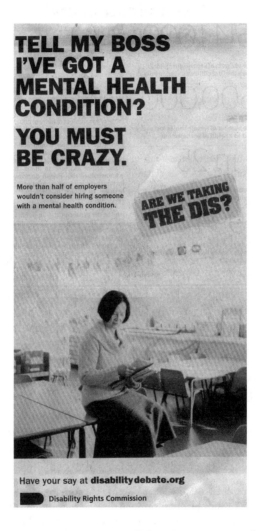

Newspaper advertisement placed by the UK Disability Rights Commission, 2006.

Chapter 3 It's not working

Discrimination and employment

There is widespread evidence that many people with mental illness suffer unjustified restrictions in getting and keeping work.[1-10] This is our focus in Chapter 3.

> Unfortunately I have never suffered from such cruelty because when applying for jobs I never admitted to my own depression. If I had, I would never have stood a chance. People are frightened about anything to do with mental illness, they just do not understand the malady.
>
> David

People always said that Rachel was very clever. For some this made it more difficult to understand her when she began to develop mental health problems. 'When I was ill at university they really didn't know what to do about it.' Her parents also struggled to know what her changing behaviour really meant. 'My mother, she gets over-anxious which is very debilitating. She just worries, worries, worries which just exacerbates the whole thing. And my dad used to say 'You ought to pull yourself together.' Initially her doctors did not tell her the diagnosis. 'That was in 1983 and it was not until 1986 that I got my diagnosis. That was what they used to do in those days, not give your diagnosis in your first episode.'

Not knowing what her condition was, she was reluctant to continue to take medication. 'So I went to my GP, and he said it's very dangerous to come off the drugs. So I came off the drugs and got psychotic again and that's when I lost another two jobs.' Eventually one of her doctors did disclose her diagnosis.

> I went to see a psychiatrist and he said 'You've got paranoid schizophrenia. Do you think you're causing plane crashes and that the television is talking to you?' I said yes, yes, yes, yes, yes, and he said 'Well you're schizophrenic'. It was so enormously helpful to think: (a) this was something diagnosable, and (b) there are self-help groups. I don't think I've lost the job since then, partly because I was medicated. At least it was something that you thought people understood.

Rachel's mental illness has affected many aspects of her life. Finding boyfriends has been hard.

> There was one bloke I took home and at one point I said 'I'm schizophrenic' and he said 'You know how to flatter a guy!' I manage my illness. It's something

I deal with. Its very much a part of me. It's not something I go on about. Nice men are afraid of upsetting you and are a bit wary which is extremely frustrating. I would rather they thought, 'Well you're managing this and it's your choice'.

She has suffered financially from her condition, for example by having to pay higher premiums for insurance. *'My endowment policy from my mortgage is a higher rate. I pay more because I'm ill. I think it's 15–20 per cent more. I disclosed my condition because otherwise you end up not being covered at all.'* Travel insurance is also a continuing problem. *'I had to ring a special line and she said 'Well in that case you are not covered for schizophrenia'. If I broke a leg I would be covered, but not for a previously existing condition.'*

Rachel is sure that discrimination against her at work has been worse than any other consequence of her mental illness. Her dilemmas started in knowing whether to disclose her medical history when applying for jobs.

There is a whole issue about whether you tell people or not. If you tell people, they turn you down at interview unless it's public sector, when they have a quota. Sometimes they say 'We won't touch that'. In the librarian's job, if I had said about my mental illness I might not have got the job. I would say disclose and discuss it, but knowing that you might not get the job because of it. It's horrible. That's the worst thing for everybody.

Despite this she has successfully found many jobs, but she feels she was not always treated fairly when she was unwell. On one occasion she was working abroad for a multinational corporation.

I got deported from (country). I lost my job because I was ill, and then my visa ran out. I was put in a deportation jail for two weeks, and the embassy sorted me out a flight. I was psychotic and nobody treated me there.

On the other hand, looking back she thinks that her employers sometimes had good reasons to sack her when she was unwell, but she regrets how they dismissed her.

I had 20 jobs in five years, and I was being sacked because I really wasn't very well. For the librarian's job, they should have had a proper chat with me rather than just sack me. But at that point I went off my medication and from their point of view I just wasn't doing the job properly. So I didn't complain, but I think it could have been handled differently. I've been sacked from two or three jobs, some without any real explanation.

She now works where her personal experience of mental illness is positively valued. *'In my current job it was explicitly stated in the advertisements that knowledge of mental health was an advantage.'* Still, she feels that her promotion prospects are damaged by declaring that she has a mental illness.

If you put that you are in a wheelchair it's fine, but for mental illness there are subtle ways that you are treated differently. You can't put your finger on it really. I applied for a job on a government advisory committee, and I didn't get it. You can't help feeling that they would rather have someone in a wheelchair, or blind people or deaf people. They don't know quite where to pigeonhole you.

With experience Rachel has developed ways to cope with her problems.

I have learned mechanisms of coping with other people in the office, and I don't go around telling other people usually, and people don't notice so it must be all right. You learn to accommodate things. I'm articulate, and you get a sort of alley-cat attitude, and instinct about situations and about sensing things. I've made a huge effort with friends and I have loads of friends. Because interpersonal relationships are difficult when you are ill I have really concentrated on it, and now it's one of my major skills, I think! You overcompensate in a way.

Before becoming unwell she expected that 'educated' people would be better informed about mental illness than the general population, but she has learned to her cost that this was wrong.

Even the 'concerned' middle classes, even you, would think 'Maybe she's not up to it.' It does show you just how little the 'informed' middle classes know about mental illness. Everybody knows very little about it. Because most of the publicity is negative, about violence and so on. There's no information for people, is there? Also they don't like talking about it, and half of them are worried they got a little bit of something themselves.

The significance of work

Work can promote good mental health by: opportunities for control and using skills, externally generated goals, variety, environmental clarity, money, physical security, interpersonal contact, and a valued social position.[11] As one person has put it, 'This is my workplace. This is where I earn my definition, the place that tells me what I am'.[12] Yet the simple fact is that a diagnosis of mental illness is one of the most potent ways to remove a person from the workforce.[13] A review in England, for example, using the standard National Labour Force Survey, found that in recent years the proportion of the whole adult population who were employed was about 75 per cent, for people with physical health problems the figure was about 65 per cent while for people with more severe mental health problems only about 20 per cent were employed.[1] Even for people with more common types of mental illness, such as depression, only about half are competitively employed.[14]

Although these are average figures they hide great variations. In a study of people with a diagnosis of schizophrenia in five European countries, the lowest employment rate was in England (5 per cent), compared with 20 per cent and

23 per cent in the Spanish and Italian sites.[15] So it is clear that although the primary disability can affect a person's ability to find and keep work, the flexibility of the employment environment also plays a large part in shaping how far people with diagnoses of mental illness are included within or excluded from the workforce. The figures are formidable: in England one third of people with mental health problems say that they have been dismissed or forced to resign from their jobs,[16] 40 per cent say that they were denied a job because of their history of psychiatric treatment,[16] and about 60 per cent say that they have been put off applying for a job as they expect to be dealt with unfairly. Indeed for some people with mental illness discrimination in the work place is far greater than in any other domain.

> I am now 59 years living in a flat, which I own, and I am very happy and contented. I have not experienced a stigma or discrimination since leaving work.
>
> Stephen

Even so, such discrimination does not necessarily signal resignation. One survey in Britain found that people with mental disorders had the highest 'want to work' rate: while overall 52 per cent of the disabled people interviewed wanted to find a job, among people with 'mental illness, phobias and panics' this figure rose to 86 per cent.[17] Another UK report found as many as 90 per cent of service users wanted to return to the workplace.[18] Similar findings have emerged from a study in Indianapolis in which two-thirds of people with severe mental illness said that they wanted to work in competitive employment.[19] At the same time many people with mental illness come to think that their symptoms are not compatible with holding down a steady job.

> I haven't worked for a long time. Unfortunately when the emetophobia (that's a fear of vomiting) sets in I panic and get really bad panic attacks. I can't be in buildings with loads of people, in case anyone has a stomach bug. In which case I would get up and leave there and then. I do understand that no-one can employ me like this. As all businesses need employees they can rely on. So I'm on benefits, which I hate. People look down on you like you're lazy. Which is so far from the truth, but I don't want to explain why I'm on benefits. I'm intelligent, and bubbly and I'd love to work and meet people, but I can't see anyway around it at the moment.
>
> Eva

Repeated service user surveys support the view these very low rates of employment represent one of worst barriers that stem from discrimination.[16,20] A large study in Germany, for example, found that the most powerful ways in which stigma was actually experienced was in relation to interpersonal interactions, structural discrimination, public images of mental illness and access to meaningful social roles, especially at work.[21] So it is plain that for many people with mental health problems there is a vast mismatch between their wish to work and their actual experiences in the job market. This gap may be getting worse: employment rates for people with a diagnosis of schizophrenia, for example, seem to have fallen during the last 50 years in many economically developed countries.[22] Indeed, the need for a meaningful link to society through work may be even more for some people with mental illness if they experience isolation or exclusion in other areas of their lives.[5]

Finding Work

> Somebody like me can never expect to work again.
>
> Leroy

The challenge of finding work is one that many people with mental illness come to believe is beyond them. Some have heard the fatal words from their doctor 'You'll never be capable of holding a job',[23] and conclude that they should adjust to permanent unemployment. Others reach the same conclusion after unsuccessful attempts to find a job.[24]

Why is finding and keeping a job so difficult for so many people with a diagnosis of mental illness? One explanation is that employers discriminate against applicants who declare a history of psychiatric treatment. In a study of 200 Human Resource Officers in UK companies, vignettes of job applicants were submitted which were identical except for the presence or absence of a diagnosis of depression. The mention of a mental illness significantly reduced the chances of employment, compared with a history of diabetes. This differential treatment was based upon perceptions of potential poor work performance, rather than expectations of future absenteeism.[25]

Similar results came from another study of employers throughout Britain. Fewer than 40 per cent said that they would consider employing a person with a history of mental health problems, compared with 60 per cent for people with a physical disability, and about 80 per cent for long-term unemployed people and lone parents.[1,26,27] Possible checks to such direct discrimination are the policies of Occupation Health departments, but fewer than half of employers in the UK, for example, have such staff.[28]

It may come as a shock to see just how reluctant many employers are to take on people who have a diagnosis of mental illness. Two studies in California asked employers about who they would offer a retail sales job to. People with mental illness were seen to be just as undesirable as ex-convicts, or as 'marginally adjusted individuals'. The only group whom the employers were even more reluctant to hire were people with active tuberculosis.[29]

Many employers remain reluctant to hire disabled people even when they are required to do so by law.[30] A survey in the Southern United States of 117 businesses found that only 15 per cent had specific policies for implementing the Americans with Disabilities Act (ADA), and just a third had actually employed disabled people. Although larger companies were more likely to know the provisions of the ADA (which will be discussed in more detail in Chapter 11), nevertheless most companies did not see it as their responsibility to take a lead in employing disabled people.[31,32]

What does seem to work in helping companies both to abide by disability laws and to act as fair employers for disabled people? Revealingly, compliance with the ADA was greater for those companies which had received formal information about the details of the law, which had previously employed people with 'mental disabilities', or which had received a threat of legal sanction.[33] Perhaps most importantly, one study found that stigmatising attitudes did not predict compliance. In other words it may not be necessary to change stigma-related attitudes (prejudice) in order to reduce unfair behaviour (discrimination) towards people with mental illness.[31,32] Indeed, the central argument of this book is that it is behaviour change (reduced discrimination) that is the most important challenge.

A second barrier to work stems from the attitudes of mental health staff who may discourage job applications by service users.[34] This may be well-intentioned in the belief that a job rejection might be sufficient stress to trigger a relapse: it is also related to how far staff are optimistic or pessimistic about the outlook for the people they treat.[35] But perhaps more important is that in most countries work preparation and support is simply not seen as a core task for mental health services.[36]

Further powerful deterrents against entering the workforce in many countries are the effects of the welfare benefits payments. Where there are welfare entitlements for people who have severe or long-lasting disabilities, often this is the sole source of income for most people with such disabilities.[37] Very often the application process is so complex and time-consuming that service users are realistically reluctant to give up this type of financial security in case a new job does not last. In addition, the rules on additional earning may be restrictive and difficult to understand.[13] These factors combined act as powerful incentives not to look for work.

A real dilemma faced by people with a history of psychiatric treatment is whether to disclose this when applying for a job. From what we have just seen, there are strong reasons to believe that mentioning this will reduce the likelihood of success. On the other hand, failure to disclose will mean that the person is not able to ask for modifications to the job to make it more manageable (often called 'reasonable adjustments' or 'reasonable accommodations').[38,5] So there is no easy solution to this dilemma. One approach is to make a balance sheet of the advantages and disadvantages of disclosing a history of mental illness, and to use this in making a decision,[2] and this is discussed in more detail in Chapter 10.

> I was working in a solicitor's as a trainee receptionist. I couldn't tell my boss I had to see a psychiatrist every week, so I told him I was on a training scheme one day a week. When I had to tell him I was being taken into hospital his reaction said it all. He sat back in his seat wanting to keep as far away from me as possible. As soon as mental illness is mentioned people literally back off from you.
>
> Jo[4]

Such decisions are far from trivial and can affect a person's most intimate sense of him or herself. One study in New York State asked groups of service users about this and they said that a critical issue was how far they saw their core identity as a disabled person. Where the mental illness was not so central to people in defining who they fundamentally were, then they were much less likely to disclose their treatment history.[39]

> An employer would see my diagnosis of schizophrenia as a disadvantage, and so I would be reluctant even to apply for a job. I would expect myself to be in a more disadvantaged position than a normal person.
>
> Raj

Keeping Work

> I've been a victim of stigma for most of my life, from a variety of sources from employers to total strangers and even to some degree from my own family. Mental illness is seen in such a negative way that it should be a four letter word with all the connotations they conjure up. I lost a job because of my mental illness and the time I had to take off work because of it. I'm a capable person - even my reference said so - but my mental illness and the stigma attached to it got in the way.
>
> Maria

While finding work may be difficult, this is only half the battle. It can be just as hard to keep a job when you have a mental illness. In a large survey of over 500 working people with mental illnesses, they were asked to describe their main problems. The difficulties they described were: loss of confidence, feeling isolated (and this leading to poor work performance), lack of understanding from colleagues, fear of disclosing the diagnosis, being bullied or given demeaning jobs with poor prospects of promotion, struggling to cope with the social aspects of the workplace and frequent stress and anxiety.[40]

I was transferred to another section in 1980, and worked for a male Senior Executive Officer who was a friend of the woman supervisor bully. He pressurized me by picking on me, giving me horrible jobs. I was placed in a basement cellar without windows to work on my own packing parcels and store work. The pressure was so much that I was unhappy and took another overdose of psychiatric drugs.

Stephen

For those who have not disclosed their diagnosis, there can be a continuing fear that someone will find out, and a fear of the consequences. Commonly people describe how colleagues discover the diagnosis of mental illness and react (as we saw with friends in Chapter 2) in polarized ways that they could not have anticipated, either showing unexpected sympathy and support, or avoidance and rejection.

I had a cleaning job for three years, but when I mentioned an appointment with a psychiatrist I received a letter the next week to say my services were no longer required.[16]

Other hurdles can be put in front of people known to have a history of mental illness, which can affect their promotion prospects, for example, or how they are dealt with during periods of reorganization at work.

I have suffered from depression for 14 years and my employer has been aware of this since the onset. I had not had any problems as a result of my depression until my division reorganized and I found myself without a post. Initially I coped with the support of friends and colleagues but my managers ignored my obviously deteriorating state of health. I was often tearful during work, unable to concentrate and constantly seeking reassurance regarding the work I had to undertake. My manager's response to this was to tell me not to be so stupid as I was an experienced officer and should be capable of coping.

Thomas

There are also some accounts by employees whose psychiatric disabilities are known, where they are employed with some reluctance, at lower pay rates, or on worse terms and conditions.[14,41,42]

My first experience of stigma was when my Supervisor dictated a letter to the Union and I heard him say that they were forced to employ people direct from mental hospitals because the pay was so low.

Stephen

Vietnam veterans, for example, who suffered from post-traumatic stress disorder (PTSD) on returning home, were 8 per cent less likely to work than Vets who did not have a mental illness. Among those who were employed, people with PTSD earned about $3 less per hour, and roughly the same disadvantage was found for those with anxiety or depression. But the effect was even greater for people with severe depression, as their wages were about $7 less per hour than veterans who were well.[43]

> I passed the Clerical Assistant's exam at the first attempt, and was made 'permanent unestablished' because of my ill health in spite in the first 11 years only taking less than 20 days sick leave (I can verify this). I was excluded from pension rights and possible promotion. I was never invited to apply for high positions. My desk was put behind a pillar and I remained there for about seven years until I moved sections.
>
> Stephen

Another dimension of the relationship between work and mental health concerns people who take time off work because of stress or anxiety or depression. In the UK, for example, 176 million working days were lost in 2003 because of sickness-related absence, and every week 1 million people report sick. Long-term sickness accounts for more than a third of total days lost and about 75 per cent of absence costs.[44] Mental illness is now one of the most common causes of sick leave, and levels of absence because of stress have doubled in the UK in the last decade.[45,46] Most of the days lost to work relate to what are called 'common mental disorders' (mainly anxiety and depression) rather than to what are often seen as the more disabling psychotic conditions.[47]

Returning to work after a period of absence because of mental illness is often described by service users as a particularly difficult transition. Common reactions from colleagues include brief superficial questions, lack of comfort talking about the cause for absence, not discussing the difficulties directly, or ignoring the issues altogether. There is often a sense that the person has now become unpredictable.[48] '*We're not accepted when we go back to work, no matter that you can do the job. They don't treat you as an equal, they're always a bit wary.*'[49]

Service users also describe other more sinister reactions, such as being demoted to a lower level of responsibility, or being put into a temporary or supernumerary post. This may be intended to ease the person back into a work routine or to be a temporary measure during a period of organisational change. Nevertheless some people with mental illness feel that they are deliberately put into positions which are either well below or beyond their capabilities, so that they will fail and be fired.

> (I was) forced by occupational health to forfeit (my) appointment as Finance Director because of manic depression.[50]
> I was then told that I had to take a post on a supernumerary basis until something more permanent was found for me. I duly reported and was given work that had previously been undertaken by staff two grades lower than myself.

Although I was anxious about my position I tried to focus on the posting being temporary until a permanent post was found. Unfortunately this did not happen and I ended up having a blazing row with my manager when he tried to force me into the temporary post on a permanent basis. Following this I was extremely distressed to the extent that my girlfriend left her office to collect me and take me home. She then contacted my GP and arranged for an emergency prescription of tranquillizers to be phoned through to the chemist. The following day she took me as an emergency patient to see my GP who increased my anti-depressant medication. I was off work for almost four months.

Thomas

Where managers are uncomfortable to see people return to work after having a period of mental illness, this often remains unsaid. In fact many co-workers will be unsure about what to say, if anything, about the period of absence, perhaps from embarrassment, but also from a concern not to say anything to upset their colleague who has returned to work. On the other hand, prejudiced attitudes are sometimes expressed quite directly.

This supervisor told the Section in my presence that she had a cousin who was put into a mental hospital, and she had been asked to visit her but she said that she would not go near the place and said that that was where they all belong. At another time she told the Section in a loud voice, again in my hearing, that he (meaning me) has no mind, he is very stupid and completely un-trainable.

Stephen

At its most extreme, such prejudice on the part of managers or supervisors can mean that they will not even consider re-employing a person who has been unwell with mental illness.

I feel that I have been a victim of unfair discrimination from other people because of mental illness. It started seven years ago when I went through a trauma. I always had my boss following my every move and he made sure I was at my desk from 8 a.m.–5 p.m. If I wasn't he would find me. This was before I had help from the local mental health centre. The next thing I know I'm in a room with the boss and my mother only to hear I can't do my job and got sacked on the spot. My boss verbally abused me. In a way it was a relief I got sacked because it meant I didn't have to see him. I've been to job interviews and they ask what I've been doing since then, and when I say I've been in hospital twice I don't get anywhere. The interviewers always are patronizing.

Barbara

A cycle can be established in which a person returns to work, becomes unwell again, is seen as unreliable and not able to bear stress. Employers may offer, for genuine and sometimes legally imposed reasons, a less stressful post, and unless this is carefully negotiated the offer may be seen by the service user as humiliating and a further cause of stress and worry. This can then slow down recovery or even precipitating a further episode of being unwell. Such cycles can seem impossible to escape from, and lead some service users to take retirement on medical grounds rather than face what seems to be an endless prospect of work-related discrimination.

> Once I had recovered from that acute period of depression I informed my managers that I was fit to return to work, but I was not permitted to do so. I have since remained away from work for two years, despite applying for 20 different posts. I also asked to do work of a lower grade until a suitable post arose and applied to undertake generic training. Both of these requests were refused. The reason I have been given for being rejected for all of the posts applied for is that I could not cope with the pressure of the post. However none of the managers asked me whether I felt able to cope with the pressures likely to come with the posts or what I thought had triggered my last severe period of depression. They have simply refused to take me because I suffer from chronic depression. No assessment has be carried out as to what reasonable adjustment could be made within the terms of the Disability Discrimination Act to allow me to return to work in any post. I could see no point in carrying on existing, and attempted to take an overdose of various tablets because I was convinced that it would solve everyone's problems if I were dead. Following a period of hospitalisation I was declared fit to work and I am back to square one.
>
> Thomas

A key role can be played by Occupational Health departments, which are now an integral part of many large organisations.[51–54] Nevertheless service users sometimes find that Occupational Health staff are more orientated to physical than to mental disorders,[55] and interventions to offer psychological treatments in the work place are still rare. One example is a Dutch project in which about four sessions of psychological treatment were given at work for people with anxiety and depression who had been away from work for at least two weeks. The treatment reduced time off work and also fewer people had the same problems again in the following year.[56] Even so, in practice many service users say that they find Occupational Health staff unsympathetic towards people with mental illnesses, and they are confused by the fact that such staff are contractually required to act both for the interests of the employees and of the employer.

> I was an Approved Social Worker working for the local authority when I developed a mental illness. As I took a considerable amount of time off work, I was requested to have an assessment by the Occupational Doctor. Unfortunately, I was too unwell to attend an appointment and requested the doctor assess me at home. This request was refused and I was medically retired, based on one psychiatric report on my mental illness.
>
> Fiona

One particular group may have a special reason for feeling discriminated against, namely health professionals who are mentally ill. Paradoxically, there is evidence that mental health staff may be especially unforgiving when their own members suffer from mental illness.[57,58] One leading psychologist in England puts it like this:

> I've encountered all those hushed conversations along the lines of 'Is she really all right? Is she really able to work? ... particularly from other clinical psychologists, who have difficulties with a high-profile member of their own profession being open about having mental health problems.[4]

Punitive reactions have been described by one General Practitioner (Family Physician) in England who was treated in hospital for bipolar disorder.

> The problem starts once you go through the gates of a psychiatric hospital. Once you're labelled the notes start building up. Psychiatrists won't retract anything, change the diagnosis, amend the notes. If you disagree with them, they say you lack insight. I was Sectioned (compulsorily admitted to hospital), and then I was sacked because it was written into my General Practice agreement that if a colleague is Sectioned under the Mental Health Act they can be removed from the practice.[4]

Even during treatment, some service users report that they receive worse care *because* they are mental health professionals.

> I have also been discriminated against because of my position as a social worker, by people looking after my care. When I became very unwell, I was referred to a psychiatric unit in the community. Following an assessment, I was informed that I should be admitted providing I did not tell the other patients that I was a social worker. This put a great strain on me as other patients did ask my occupation and I had to lie. I was assessed for a day centre. I was accepted for the service. However a couple of days later the day care provision stated that they discussed my case and decided that as I was a social worker, it would not be 'appropriate' for me to attend day care as my position may affect the other clients.
>
> Fiona

> It has taken several years to return to work after appalling experiences in medical school, where I was employed as a medical researcher. I became ill with depression, was bullied, intimidated, harassed until I resigned ... a technician pinned up offensive articles about mentally ill people in my lab and one person refused to speak to me.[59]

Conclusion

There is widespread agreement that work can provide a core stability and meaning to the lives of many people, and that its absence can increase the chance of becoming or staying mentally ill.[11,13,18] Yet there is little systematic research on whether and how workplace discrimination (direct or indirect) takes place against people with mental illnesses. It is also clear that some types of mental illness can severely compromise core skills needed at work, for example, attention, memory and interpersonal relations. One survey in the USA found that people who were depressed showed impairment of task focus and productivity that was the equivalent to 2.3 days lost to work each month.[60] At the same time little is known about the extent to which work contributes to recovery. Indeed the situation in some countries seems to be deteriorating, for example, the employment rate in schizophrenia has declined over the last 50 years in the UK'.[22]

On many occasions in this book we shall need to adopt binocular vision: to see the world both through the eyes of researchers (describing the evidence base) and through the eyes of service users (describing the experience base). In relation to discrimination at work the experience base at present is stronger than the evidence base. In one survey of mental health service users in the UK a staggering 95 per cent said that their mental health problems had considerable negative effects on their employment prospects.[61] A further study in Britain found that 37 per cent of service users reported experiences of discrimination in seeking work, while 47 per cent described experiences of discrimination at work.[61,62] A survey carried out by UK MIND produced similar results: 34 per cent reported being dismissed or forced to resign from their jobs for reasons related to mental illness.[16] Unsurprisingly this leads most people with mental illness (75 per cent in one New York study)[63] to be very reluctant to disclose a psychiatric history when applying for a job. As we shall see in Chapter 11, in the UK for example, employees or job applicants are not obliged to disclose a mental health problem, and employers can only enquire about such difficulties if their questions are constructive and specifically relate to their ability to do the job or the need to make 'reasonable adjustments'. At the same time, under the UK Disability Discrimination Act, an employer has no duty to an employee until disclosure is made about a disability.[64]

It was a concern with such issues that led another UK charity, the Mental Health Foundation, to conduct a large-scale survey specifically about work-related experiences among people with a diagnosis of mental illness. In total 411 people took part in this survey and these were the main findings:

- over half believed that they had definitely or possibly been turned down for a job in the past because of their mental health problems
- only one-third felt confident in disclosing their experience of mental health problems on job application forms.
- people with anxiety or depression were more likely to be employed, but still fewer than 60 per cent were employed full-time or part-time

- fewer than half of the people who responded with psychosis, schizophrenia, bipolar disorder or phobias were in full-time or part-time employment
- one in five of people with mental health problems do voluntary work, and the groups who are least likely to be paid for their work (particularly people with bipolar disorder or schizophrenia) are those most likely to be working in a voluntary capacity
- nine out of ten people in employment had informed somebody in the workplace about their experience of mental health problems
- of those who had been open about their mental health problems in the workplace, over half usually had support when they needed it, and two-thirds reported that people at work were always or often very accepting
- about a quarter reported that sometimes too much account was taken of their mental health problems, and that they felt more patronized or monitored than other colleagues
- over 15 per cent believed that they had been passed over for promotion because of their mental health problem
- 10 per cent believed that colleagues made sarcastic remarks or that colleagues avoided them because of their mental health problem.
- a third believed that bullying at work had caused or added to their mental health problems.[59]

These findings cannot be ignored. They indicate at least that such experiences need further careful exploration, and at worst that systematic discrimination is taking place against the whole category of people who have a history of mental illnesses or psychiatric treatment. We shall see in Chapters 10 and 11 what we know about how such discrimination can be minimized or reversed.

References

1. Social Exclusion Unit. *Mental Health and Social Exclusion*. London: Office of the Deputy Prime Minister; 2004.
2. Corrigan P, Lundin R. *Don't Call Me Nuts*. Tinley Par, Illinois: Recovery Press; 2001.
3. Becker DR, Drake RE. *A Working Life for People with Severe Mental Illness*. Oxford: Oxford University Press; 2003.
4. Dunn S. *Creating Accepting Communities: Report of the MIND Inquiry into Social Exclusion and Mental Health Problems*. London: MIND; 1999.
5. Repper J, Perkins R. *Social Inclusion and Recovery*. Edinburgh: Balliere Tindall; 2003.
6. Pozner A, Ng M, Hammond J, Shepherd G. *Working it Out*. Brighton: Pavilion; 1996.
7. Crowther RE, Marshall M, Bond GR, Huxley P. Helping people with severe mental illness to obtain work: systematic review. *BMJ* 2001; 322(7280):204–208.
8. Perkins R, Selbie D. Decreasing employment discrimination against people who have experienced mental health problems in a mental health trust. In: Crisp A, edr., pp. 350–355. *Every Family in the Land*. London: Royal Society of Medicine; 2004.

9. Boardman J, Grove B, Perkins R, Shepherd G. Work and employment for people with psychiatric disabilities. *Br J Psychiatry* 2003; 182:467–468.

10. Glozier N. Changing minds: the Workplace Project. In: Crisp A, edr., *Every Family in the Land*, pp. 392–393. London: Royal Society of Medicine; 2004.

11. Warr P. *Work, Unemployment and Mental Health.* Oxford: Oxford University Press; 1987.

12. Galloway J. *The Trick is to Keep Breathing.* London: Minerva; 1991.

13. Warner R. *Recovery from Schizophrenia: Psychiatry and political economy.* Hove: Brunner-Routledge; 2004.

14. Meltzer H, Gill B, Petticrew M, Hinds K. *OPCS Surveys of Psychiatric Morbidity in Great Britain. Report 3: Economic activity and social functioning of adults with psychiatric disorders.* London: HMSO; 1995.

15. Thornicroft G, Tansella M, Becker T, Knapp M, Leese M, Schene A *et al.* The personal impact of schizophrenia in Europe. *Schizophr Res* 2004; 69(2–3):125–132.

16. Read J, Baker S. *Not Just Sticks and Stones. A Survey of the Stigma, Taboos, and Discrimination Experienced by People with Mental Health Problems.* London: MIND; 1996.

17. Stanley K, Maxwell D. *Fit for Purpose?* London: IPPR; 2004.

18. Grove B. Mental health and employment. Shaping a new agenda. *Journal of Mental Health* 1999; 8:131–140.

19. Bond GR, Becker DR, Drake RE, Rapp CA, Meisler N, Lehman AF *et al.* Implementing supported employment as an evidence-based practice. *Psychiatr Serv* 2001; 52(3):313–322.

20. Becker DR, Drake RE, Farabaugh A, Bond GR. Job preferences of clients with severe psychiatric disorders participating in supported employment programs. *Psychiatr Serv* 1996; 47(11):1223–1226.

21. Schulze B, Angermeyer MC. Subjective experiences of stigma. A focus group study of schizophrenic patients, their relatives and mental health professionals. *Soc Sci Med* 2003; 56(2):299–312.

22. Marwaha S, Johnson S. Schizophrenia and employment – a review. *Soc Psychiatry Psychiatr Epidemiol* 2004; 39(5):337–349.

23. Rogers J. Work is key to recovery. *Psychosocial Rehabilitation Journal* 1995; 18:5–10.

24. Perkins R, Evenson E, Davidson B. *The Pathfinder User Employment Programme.* London: South West London and St George's Mental Health NHS Trust; 2000.

25. Glozier N. Workplace effects of the stigmatization of depression. *J Occup Environ Med* 1998; 40(9):793–800.

26. Department for Work and Pensions. *Recruiting Benefits Claimants: Quantitative Research with Employers in ONE Pilot Areas.* Research Series Paper No. 150. London: Department for Work and Pensions; 2001.

27. Manning C, White P. Attitudes of employers to the mentally ill. *Psychiatr Bull* 1995; 19:541–543.

28. CBI (Confederation for British Industry). *Their Health in Your Hands. Focus on Occupational Health Partnerships.* London: Confederation for British Industry, CBI Publications; 2002.

29. Brand RC, Jr, Clairborn WL. Two studies of comparative stigma: employer attitudes and practices toward rehabilitated convicts, mental and tuberculosis patients. *Community Ment Health J* 1976; 12(2):168–175.

30. Britt TW. The stigma of psychological problems in a work environment: Evidence from the screening of service members returning from Bosnia. *Journal of Applied Social Psychology* 2000; 30(8):1599–1618.

31. Scheid TL. Employment of individuals with mental disabilities: business response to the ADA's challenge. *Behav Sci Law* 1999; 17(1):73–91.

32. Scheid TL. The Americans with Disabilities Act, mental disability, and employment practices. *J Behav Health Serv Res* 1998; 25(3):312–324.

33. Mechanic D. Cultural and organisational aspects of the ADA to persons with psychiatric disabilities. *Millbank Quarterly* 1998; 76:5–23.

34. Rinaldi M. *Insufficient Concern*. London: Merton MIND; 2000.

35. Landeen J, Kirkpatrick H, Woodside H, Byrne C, Bernardo A, Pawlick J. Factors influencing staff hopefulness in working with people with schizophrenia. *Issues Ment Health Nurs* 1996; 17(5):457–467.

36. Evans J, Repper J. Employment, social inclusion and mental health. *J Psychiatr Ment Health Nurs* 2000; 7(1):15–24.

37. Slade M, McCrone P, Thornicroft G. Uptake of welfare benefits by psychiatric patients. *Psychiatr Bull* 1995; 19:411–413.

38. Corrigan PW. *On the Stigma of Mental Illness: Practical strategies for research and social change*. Washington, DC: American Psychological Association; 2004.

39. Dalgin RS, Gilbride D. Perspectives of people with psychiatric disabilities on employment disclosure. *Psychiatr Rehabil J* 2003; 26(3):306–310.

40. Bird L. Poverty, social exclusion and mental health: a survey of people's personal experiences. *A Life in the Day* 2001; 5:3.

41. Huxley P, Thornicroft G. Social inclusion, social quality and mental illness. *Br J Psychiatry* 2003; 182:289–290.

42. Office for National Statistics. *Labour Force Survey*. London: Stationery Office; 2002.

43. Savoca E, Rosenheck R. The civilian labour market experiences of Vietnam-era veterans: the influence of psychiatric disorders. *Journal of Mental Health Policy and Economics* 2001; 4:199–207.

44. Henderson M, Glozier N, Holland EK. Long term sickness absence. *BMJ* 2005; 330(7495):802–803.

45. Jones J, Huxtable C, Hodgson J, Price M. *Self-reported work-related illness in 2001/2002*. London: Health and Safety Executive; 2003.

46. Health and Safety Executive. *Tackling Work-related Stress. A manager's guide to improving and maintaining employee health and well-being*. London: Health and Safety Executive; 2001.

47. Henderson M, Glozier N, Holland EK. Long term sickness absence. *BMJ* 2005; 330(7495):802–803.

48. Glozier N. The Disability Discrimination Act 1995 and psychiatry: lessons from the first seven years. *Psychiatr Bull* 2004; 28:126–129.

49. Knight M, Wykes T, Hayward P. 'People don't understand': an investigation of stigma in schizophrenia using Interpretative Phenomenological Analysis (IPA). *Journal of Mental Health* 2003; 12(3):209–222.

50. Warner L. *Out of Work: a Survey of Experiences of People with Mental Health Problems with the Workplace*. London: Mental Health Foundation; 2002.

51. Fingret A. Occupational mental health: a brief history. *Occup Med (Lond)* 2000; 50(5):289–293.

52. Felton JS, Swinger H. Mental health outreach of an occupational health service in a government setting. *Am J Public Health* 1973; 63(12):1058–1063.

53. Felton JS. Role of the occupational physician in mental health services. *Occup Med* 1988; 3(4):707–717.

54. Felton JS. Occupational health in the USA in the 21st century. *Occup Med* (*Lond*) 2000; 50(7):523–531.
55. Putnam K, McKibbin L. Managing workplace depression: an untapped opportunity for occupational health professionals. *AAOHN J* 2004; 52(3):122–129.
56. Van der Klink J, Blonk R, Schene A, van Dijk F. Reducing long term sickness absence by an activating intervention in adjustment disorders: a cluster randomised controlled design. *Occupational and Environmental Medicine* 2003; 60:437.
57. Reid Y, Johnson S, Morant N, Kuipers E, Szmukler G, Thornicroft G *et al*. Explanations for stress and satisfaction in mental health professionals: a qualitative study. *Soc Psychiatry Psychiatr Epidemiol* 1999; 34(6):301–308.
58. Prosser D, Johnson S, Kuipers E, Dunn G, Szmukler G, Reid Y *et al*. Mental health, 'burnout' and job satisfaction in a longitudinal study of mental health staff. *Soc Psychiatry Psychiatr Epidemiol* 1999; 34(6):295–300.
59. Mental Health Foundation. *Out at Work. A Survey of the Experiences of People with Mental Health Problems within the Workplace*. London: Mental Health Foundation; 2002.
60. Wang PS, Beck AL, Berglund P, McKenas DK, Pronk NP, Simon GE *et al*. Effects of major depression on moment-in-time work performance. *Am J Psychiatry* 2004; 161(10):1885–1891.
61. Mental Health Foundation. *An Uphill Struggle: Poverty and Mental Health*. London: Mental Health Foundation; 2001.
62. DePonte P. *Pull Yourself Together! A Survey of the Stigma and Discrimination Faced by People who Experience Mental Distress*. London: Mental Health Foundation; 2000.
63. Link BG, Struening EL, Rahav M, Phelan JC, Nuttbrock L. On stigma and its consequences: evidence from a longitudinal study of men with dual diagnoses of mental illness and substance abuse. *J Health Soc Behav* 1997; 38(2):177–190.
64. MindOut for Mental Health. *Working Minds Toolkit. A Practical Resource to Promote Good Workplace Practice on Mental Health*. London: Department of Health; 2003.

Do any of the following apply to you? *(Answer Yes or No)*

A. Do you have a communicable disease; physical or mental disorder; or are you a drug abuser or addict? ☐ Yes ☐ No

B. Have you ever been arrested or convicted for an offense or crime involving moral turpitude or a violation related to a controlled substance; or been arrested or convicted for two or more offenses for which the aggregate sentence to confinement was five years or more; or been a controlled substance trafficker; or are you seeking entry to engage in criminal or immoral activities? ☐ Yes ☐ No

C. Have you ever been or are you now involved in espionage or sabotage; or in terrorist activities; or genocide; or between 1933 and 1945 were you involved, in any way, in persecutions associated with Nazi Germany or its allies? ☐ Yes ☐ No

D. Are you seeking to work in the U.S.; or have you ever been excluded and deported; or been previously removed from the United States; or procured or attempted to procure a visa or entry into the U.S. by fraud or misrepresentation? ☐ Yes ☐ No

E. Have you ever detained, retained or withheld custody of a child from a U.S. citizen granted custody of the child? ☐ Yes ☐ No

F. Have you ever been denied a U.S. visa or entry into the U.S. or had a U.S. visa canceled? If yes, when?_____where?_____ ☐ Yes ☐ No

G. Have you ever asserted immunity from prosecution? ☐ Yes ☐ No

IMPORTANT: If you answered "Yes" to any of the above, please contact the American Embassy **BEFORE** you travel to the U.S. since you may be refused admission into the United States.

_____   _____
Family Name *(Please Print)*   First Name

_____   _____
Country of Citizenship   Date of Birth

WAIVER OF RIGHTS: I hereby waive any rights to review or appeal of an immigration officer's determination as to my admissibility, or to contest, other than on the basis of an application for asylum, any action in deportation.

CERTIFICATION: I certify that I have read and understand all the questions and statements on this form. The answers I have furnished are true and correct to the best of my knowledge and belief.

Application form for an Immigration Visa Waiver Form for entry into the USA, requiring disclosure of mental illness history, 2005

Chapter 4 By a process of exclusion

Discrimination in civil and social life

Veronica qualified as a librarian. After finishing her first degree she went on to complete her PhD. But after the start of her mental health problems she began to learn from her own experience about how her 'record' would limit where and how she could travel.

> My problem is actually about insurance and driving. I used to live in my car, I used to drive everywhere. And then I lost my driving licence, and there was a long set of questions and one of the questions said 'Have you ever suffered from mental illness?' and like an idiot I said yes. Most of the people I know lie. So I lost my driving licence. One of the executives of the local mental health group was a barrister and she agreed to appeal it for me. We had to go to court for the appeal and they renewed my licence for a year.

Her experience of trying to regain her licence proved relentlessly frustrating.

> This went on for some time, and I just got fed up of applying, and I wasn't able to drive any more, and actually about 18 months ago I decided I was going to apply again. The same thing happened again, I had to complete a medical form. Then I heard nothing, and I heard nothing, and I assumed they were just not going to renew it and then one day this letter came saying that they had renewed my licence for three years. I was stunned, and I was very pleased. And then about two months later another letter came, saying that they had sought further medical advice and that they were only going to renew it for one year after all, which was very disappointing. So basically I was denied my main means of transport, and it's now 20 years since I drove last. I was just very, very angry. I thought, you know, I've never had an endorsement. I had one accident when I was a very new driver. There are all these people driving around who've got endorsements. They drive when they're drunk. Younger men who are totally reckless, and I'm a very safe driver, and they won't give me a licence, but they do give these other people licences. So it just feels very unfair. So I gave up trying to get my licence back.

Veronica's freedom to travel has also been severely compromised by limits on her ability to buy travel insurance.

> I had planned to go to Australia for four months, so had to get a visa. In order to get the visa I had to get travel insurance and health insurance. They had a blanket ban on people with mental health problems, and they said 'Psychiatric disorders are exempt from this policy'. They use blanket exclusion clauses, not

for high-risk individuals, but for the category of mental illness. I don't see why having a mental illness should make you any more of a risk than having cancer or diabetes or heart disease. Now, for visas to travel to other countries I lie, and nothing happens, and they don't find out. I don't know what would happen if I ticked the 'Yes' box.

Not being able to buy insurance has also stopped Veronica exercising other important civil rights, such as owning property.

> After that, I had given up trying to get insurance, because the whole thing was just so difficult, and I also found it very humiliating. Always rubbing my face in the fact that I had this psychiatric disorder, which meant that I was an inferior sort of being. So my partner and I did buy a flat, and we were told that if we wanted a joint mortgage that we needed joint health insurance, and I thought 'well, I'm just not doing this, I'm just not going to put myself through it all again', but that did mean that I was not an owner of the flat. It was sole-owned by my partner. Because we weren't married, I don't know what would have happened if, say, he had died, or what rights I would have had.

Veronica has even found her credibility as a victim of crime questioned because of her mental illness.

> I was once in a psychiatric hospital for quite a period of time, and I was living in a maisonette. The people downstairs were well-known criminals, and they broke into my flat, and stole everything and sold it on including some very valuable pieces of jewellery. I went home for the weekend, my first visit home from hospital, and my place was devastated. It was dreadful. To make an insurance claim for a burglary you need a police report number. So eventually, when I got discharged from hospital, a Detective Sergeant came around, and he said 'Why has it taken you so long to get in touch with us?', and I said 'I've been in hospital', and he said 'Oh dear what's the matter?', so I told him, and he said 'Well if you've got a mental record ...', and I said, 'It's not a criminal record!', and then he said 'Oh, but I believe everything you say', so obviously he thought that people with mental records were not to be believed. But he also said, 'You won't make a credible witness. No Crown Prosecution Service is going to put you on the stand with the record that you have got.' It wasn't until this Detective Sergeant agreed that I was 'to be believed', despite my record, that I could make an insurance claim.

So far we have seen that discrimination seeps into the most intimate and important aspects of the lives of people with a diagnosis of mental illness: family, home and work. How far is the same true for participation in the wider social world? Is there evidence that full membership of what is sometimes called 'civic society' is jeopardized? In practice are there open or even subtle restrictions which stand in the way? Is it true that normal social venues such as clubs and leisure facilities are fully open to those with mental health problems? Are travel, financial services or legal entitlements at all compromised? Is there good evidence that the basic human rights guaranteed to all citizens are actually honoured in practice for people with mental illness? These are the questions we shall consider in this chapter.

> For the last three years I have had episodes of hypomania about every six months or so, these episodes seem to come on through stress and lack of sleep. I even had an episode in the States when on a business trip. I was put in jail, and when I was released the next day, my hotel had kicked me out, and I had to return to the UK.
>
> Emile

Leisure and Recreation

To make a leisurely start, we can consider access to mainstream sport and social facilities by people with mental illnesses. This is another aspect of life that has been by-passed by researchers. Although possible limitations in accessing leisure activities have been described for over two decades,[1] no detailed information is available on how common these problems are, nor about how far people with mental illnesses are limited by such barriers. One survey in North Carolina interviewed people with a range of physical and psychiatric disabilities and concluded that three responses were common when faced with limited access to community recreational facilities: yielding to helplessness, embracing their situation, or resisting the stigma.[2]

Occasionally more clear-cut evidence emerges that mental illness is used systematically to exclude people from general leisure and sports facilities, even though it is becoming recognised that physical exercise may be an effective intervention for some types of mental illness.[3,4] The Japanese family organisation, Zenkaren, for example, has shown that in Yokohama about 10 per cent of fitness clubs and swimming pools implemented discriminatory regulations to prevent mentally disabled people from using their facilities, and that many other facilities nationwide, including those run by large companies, have similar regulations. One such club, for example, did not allow mentally ill people to join, along with people with tattoos or those with infectious diseases. When Zenkaren and the Yokohama Municipal Government asked the club to reform its discriminatory rules, the firm said, 'We didn't intend to be discriminatory at all, but had simply made our regulations based on those by other firms in the industry.' This was not the first such case of discrimination. The Japanese Ministry of Land, Infrastructure and Transport had found that three major airlines were refusing to allow mentally ill people on flights unless they were accompanied by psychiatrists or met other conditions.[5]

We need to distinguish between any degree of exclusion which may be reasonable (for example to exclude a person who has frequent episodes of seizures and unconsciousness from swimming unaccompanied) from situations in which the exclusion is either entirely unwarranted or grossly disproportionate to any risk involved. There is no convincing evidence that any diagnosis of mental disorder, in itself, justifies being banned from social or leisure centres which are open to other members of the general public.

> The other night I went to the cinema with a friend. Great I thought, it's half empty but suddenly it filled up, people talking, laughing, I started to sweat and shake then I got a violent headache. I had to leave the cinema after 20 minutes.
>
> Louise

Travel and Transport

In many ways it can be more difficult for people with mental illness to travel than for others. As we saw in the last chapter, rates of unemployment among people with some types of mental illness are extraordinarily high, and so most people with the more severe forms of illness depend upon their families or upon welfare benefits for basic needs and to meet everyday costs. Discretionary travel, for example, to take a holiday is simply not affordable for most people with psychotic disorders. For the same reason, rates of car ownership are very low among people with severe mental disorders compared with the general population. Indeed owning a car is often taken as a measure of poverty in epidemiological studies.[6,7]

Beyond this, people with mental illness can have problems keeping a driving licence. Many countries have regulations which place limits on when a mentally ill person can drive. By law, in Britain people need to inform the Driver and Vehicle Licensing Agency (DVLA) if they have 'any mental ill-health condition (including depression)', or 'any psychiatric illness requiring hospital admission'. Failure to notify the DVLA means that the person is not able to drive legally and that car insurance will probably be invalid. Under these circumstances failure to disclose a mental illness could have very serious consequences. In the UK, for example, people with anxiety or depression can continue to drive, while those with 'more severe anxiety states or depressive illnesses (with significant memory or concentration problems, agitation, behavioural disturbance or suicidal thoughts)' must stop driving until medically assessed. People with acute psychotic episodes (including hypomania) must usually stop driving until all of the following conditions are satisfied: '(a) has remained well and stable for at least 3 months, (b) is compliant with treatment, (c) has regained insight, (d) is free from adverse effects of medication which would impair driving, and is (e) subject to a favourable specialist report.'[8] Such conditions are not in themselves unreasonable, if applied with care on a case-by-case basis, but where they are simply used to bar a whole class of people from driving, they may be discriminatory in practice.

While we can imagine that any one of these conditions might not be fully met in the eyes of a doctor, whose recommendations are usually followed by the licensing authority, one study found that many psychiatrists are reluctant to enter this arena because it might infringe upon patients' ability to drive, obtain insurance, or earn a livelihood.[9] A study in Switzerland, for example, compared psychiatrists' and lay opinions about restrictions on mentally ill people and showed that fewer than 7 per cent of the doctors felt that withdrawal of a driving licence was routinely necessary for people with mental illness, whereas 54 per cent of the general public agreed with such restrictions.[10]

Another reason for the reluctance of many doctors to be involved in these decisions may simply be ignorance. A survey of psychiatrists in England found that only 40 per cent could correctly advise people with a diagnosis of bipolar disorder about driving, and none could correctly advise a person with a diagnosis of schizophrenia.[11] How accurate are such predictions of driving safety? Little is known about this, but another study in Switzerland did examine this question by following up 100 drivers who had been psychiatric inpatients. Twelve were judged by their doctors to be unfit to drive, and subsequently the police withdrew licences for seven other people. Among the 100 people followed up there were three road traffic accidents, with no injuries.[12]

Another barrier to travel that can be discriminatory is the need to declare a mental illness to obtain a visa. Entrants to the United States are asked: 'do you have a communicable disease; physical or mental disorder; or are you a drug abuser or addict?' Other screening questions refer to 'moral turpitude', being a 'controlled substance trafficker', or being 'involved with espionage, or sabotage; or in terrorist activities; or in genocide'. These demeaning bedfellows, used alongside mental illness, categorize undesirable entrants.

There is a further important limit to travel, namely insurance.[13,14] One survey in Britain found that a quarter of the people with mental illness said that they had been refused insurance or other financial services.[15] This may well be unlawful. In the UK the Disability Discrimination Act 1995 makes it illegal to provide goods, facilities and services to a disabled person (including people with mental health problems) on terms which are unjustifiably different from those given to other people. Since 1996, this Act has made it illegal to refuse insurance, or charge higher premiums, unless the company can demonstrate statistically higher risks as a direct result of a specific mental health condition for that *particular individual*. However, people are reluctant to take out legal steps against big institutions and only a small handful of such cases brought under the Disability Discrimination Act have been successful.

Because of widespread concerns that discriminatory practices were making access to different types of insurance more difficult for disabled people, the Association of British Insurers (ABI) has produced a Code of Practice for its members on how to interpret the 1995 Disability Discrimination Act. In general, an insurance company must be fair and reasonable in its dealings with disabled people (including people with mental health problems) and must account for any difference in treatment between disabled and non-disabled people. Insurers' decisions must be based on information relevant to the assessment of the risk to be insured and from a reliable source. These may include: actuarial or statistical data, medical research information, a medical report, or an opinion on an individual from a reliable source. Insurers must make sure that the information is accurate and that their use of it is reasonable. It must be shown that the disabled individual has a higher risk; if not, there should be no differentiation in their treatment. But in fact many insurance application forms ask for details of any pre-existing conditions, and may refuse cover if such conditions are present.[16] As many mental illnesses are either long-lasting or have cycles of relapse and remission, this disqualifies many people with mental illness from buying insurance cover.[17]

Money

One of the central characteristics of people with the more severe types of mental illness is their material poverty.[18,19] One study of people, mainly with diagnoses of psychotic disorders, living in Los Angeles concluded that the most powerful factor that shaped their identities and their everyday opportunities was their subsistence income.[20] Among the many consequences of a low income is not being able to afford what most people in that population would consider basic necessities, such as new clothes or holidays.[21] *'Due to medication I have put on a lot of weight and I have outgrown my clothes. Due to my income I cannot afford to buy new ones.'*[21]

A second implication of living on a low income is that it may be impossible to afford usual social activities, for example to go out to a bar or café, and this can have a progressively demoralizing effect.[22,23]

> All in all I find the experience of being on a low income degrading. I feel I am being punished for being ill and as if it is my fault, which in turn makes me more depressed. You see others buying such lovely things and I can have none of it. It really hurts.[21]

Even though, as we saw in Chapter 3, employment rates are especially low among people with mental illness, in countries where welfare benefits are available, many people do not receive their full entitlement. A survey in South London found that two-thirds of people treated at a community mental health centre were receiving less money from welfare benefits than they were entitled to.[24] Specialist welfare benefits advisors then offered detailed support to claim benefits and after a year had increased their income on average by £3079.[25] Similar results were found from a project in Florida, which offered detailed advice and help to mentally ill people who were eligible for a particular welfare benefit. The people who received this assistance were twice as likely as others to secure this extra income.[26]

For these reasons debtor bankruptcy can be a serious practical problems for people with mental illness, and a factor that can prevent recovery, or even lead to suicide attempts.[27,28] A national survey in Britain found that those with mental illness were three times more likely to be in debt, and twice as often had problems managing their money compared to the general population.[29] Depression is associated with not having a bank account and people who borrow money from places other than a bank have poorer mental health than those with access to better rates of credit.[30] *My illness, depression and stress, has been exacerbated by my debt problem. As a result I cannot get well enough to go back to work to earn money to pay the debts.*[31]

In every country where this has been studied, most people with the more severe forms of mental illness are relatively impoverished. Under these circumstances money is sometimes used as a powerful incentive to change the behaviour of service users. In five of the United States, for example, a range of methods are commonly used to achieve higher rates of adherence to community mental health care plans. Four particular methods (money, housing, criminal justice arrangements and community treatment orders/outpatient commitment) are used most often, and 44–59 per cent of service users in these five states had at least one of these applied to them. Money was used as a form of leverage for between 7–19 per cent of service users interviewed, and was applied especially for younger people with more long-standing conditions.[32]

The rights of citizenship

An important series of the political and personal rights available to citizens may be withdrawn from people with a mental illness or with a history of psychiatric treatment. Voting is an important example of such political rights, and is available in democratic nations to all adults with a limited number of exceptions.[33] Restrictions to such rights both diminish a person's democratic participation, and reduce social status.[34] An important study was carried out in 1989 and in 1999 in 50 of the United States. This initial survey described the loss of civil and legal rights for mentally ill and mentally incompetent persons, and for people convicted of a felony. Most states applied restrictions to all three categories in terms of these five issues: serving on a jury, voting, holding official positions and in limiting parental or marriage rights. The survey was repeated 10 years later to assess any changes. Interestingly many states made no distinction between a diagnosis of mental illness and a judicial determination of incompetence. In 1989 every state restricted at least one of these rights for people with mental illness, while only three states (Alabama, Mississippi and Nevada) restricted all five rights. A decade later two more states (Georgia and Iowa) also limited all of these rights. No state had removed a restriction on these rights. The overall trend was towards increasingly curtailed rights. In 1999, 19 of these states limited voting rights for mentally ill people and 12 restricted voting for those assessed to be incompetent.[35, 36] In other words mentally ill people in the USA are more often deemed to be unsuitable to exercise their basic political right to vote than people who are assessed as incompetent, although there is evidence of the opposite trend in Canada.[37]

In the UK complex regulations allow inpatients to vote as long as they have a non-hospital address and they have 'capacity' to vote[38] (established at the voting station by the electoral returning officer, if necessary, who asks the question 'Are you the person whose name appears on the register of electors').[39] In practice many compulsorily detained patients are disenfranchised.[18] Once again, the general public may not fully support such civil participation: in a survey of psychiatrists and the lay public, 1 per cent of the former felt that psychiatric patients should lose their right to vote, compared with 17 per cent of the general population.[10]

Even where patients are entitled to vote, their participation in elections may be marginal.[40] One study in Germany found that fewer than 10 per cent of inpatients voted in a regional election. A campaign to inform this group of their electoral rights led to a doubling of the number who voted in the next election.[41] More generally, though, the loss of this vital democratic right can be seen as an important expression of social exclusion.[42] As one commentator has put it, 'I vote, I count.'[43]

Often civil rights are lost as a package. In Lithuania, for example, many people with long-term mental illnesses are placed in residential care homes called 'Internats'. About a quarter of such residents have been classified by psychiatrists as being incompetent, and these people lose their right to vote, to stand for elected office, to own property or to sign legal contracts. There are well-substantiated accounts that the designation of 'incompetence' is applied inconsistently, may sometimes be used on behalf of families seeking to take possession of a resident's property, and that once the 'incompetent' label is applied, it is rarely removed. Similarly in Russia being 'legally incapacitated' means losing rights to manage property, choose where to live, sign contracts, rent an apartment, be employed, vote in elections, marry, or seek any remedy through the courts.[44] The systematic withdrawal of such fundamental rights can be considered a type of 'civil death'.[45]

Another right accorded to most citizens, but often withdrawn from people with mental illness, is jury service. In the USA in 1999, 42 states restricted this form of social participation, five states more than a decade earlier.[36] In England, under the Juries Act of 1974 there is a blanket exclusion so that 'mentally disordered persons' are ineligible to serve on a jury, where this means

> anyone who suffers or has suffered from mental illness, psychopathic disorder, mental disorder, mental handicap, or severe mental handicap and because of that condition; (a) is resident in hospital or other similar institution, regularly attends for treatment by a medical practitioner, or is under guardianship, or has been determined by a judge to be incapable, by reasons of mental disorder, of managing and administering his/her property and affairs.[39]

Since the lifetime prevalence of mental disorders is now understood to be about half of the adult population, such restrictions, consistently applied, might seriously deplete the pool of available jurors![46] By comparison, for people with a physical disabilities, jury service eligibility is considered on a case-by-case basis by the judge concerned. Nevertheless, some people with mental illness see this exception as a clear advantage.

> For jury service, I use mental illness as an excuse, I write on the form 'I'm currently being treated mental disorder', and they just to write back saying 'fine! '
>
> Veronica

Personal safety

> The whole street - they set dogs on me. I'd go in the shops and the children would come and spit on me and stuff like that.[47]

While general concerns about personal security and safety may have increased in recent years, it is clear that people with a diagnosis of mental illness are more likely to be the victims of violence that the general population. This may take the form of physical assault,[47] or other abuse, such as having eggs thrown.[15] The European Convention on Human Rights, for example, paradoxically both makes a 'prohibition on discrimination', and in Article 5.1 qualifies this by stating that although, 'everyone has the right and security of person', those of 'unsound mind' form an exception to this provision under Article 5.1.e.

There is now a great deal of evidence that people with a diagnosis of mental illness may be victimized in public places, and are even far from safe within mental health services. In detailed interviews in with people treated at community and day care mental health services in North London, about a half described experiences of verbal or physical abuse, where the latter occurred much more often for people with psychotic than non-psychotic disorders.[47] Although it may be true that people with mental illnesses are more often the victims than the perpetrators of crimes,[48] and that they are liable to be seen as 'unreliable witnesses' in court,[49] the academic literature contains many thousands of publications on violence by mentally ill people (see Chapter 7), but has almost no interest at all in such people as the victims of violence. In a sense this bias reflects both the interests of researchers and those of the agencies which fund research.

One exception is a careful study of over 300 people in North Carolina who were involuntarily admitted to psychiatric hospital and then placed on 'outpatient commitment' orders after discharge, so that they had to comply with certain treatment requirements while at home.[50] About a quarter were the victims of non-violent crime in a four month period, which was no different to the general population. In contrast, the people with mental illness had a much higher chance of being the victims of violent crime – two-and-a-half times greater than in the general population (8.2 per cent compared with 3.1 per cent). These rates of assault were especially high for people with problems of substance use or transient living conditions (and as we saw in Chapter 1, homelessness itself is relatively more common for people with mental illnesses). There was an unexpectedly high level of resilience (or perhaps resignation) to these threats: only 16 per cent of the people interviewed expressed concerns about their personal safety, although those with a higher level of education more often expressed greater feelings of vulnerability. *'Various gangs in the neighbourhood call me 'nutter' and spit at me. The gangs on the estate know I was a psychiatric patient and so I'm teased and harassed.'*[15]

Psychiatric hospital wards can also be experienced as dangerous places to be.[51,52] A survey of people admitted to psychiatric hospitals in New York found that people going to hospital for a mental health assessment most often said that they accepted admission to get away from problems to do with safety, money, or employment.[53] On the other hand, a study of over 1000 people treated in psychiatric wards in South Australia found high rates of assaults within hospital, mostly by patients upon patients. The perpetrators were more often either long-term inpatients or people with two or more different diagnoses (see Chapter 7 concerning comorbidity).[54]

There seems to be agreement between those offering and receiving care that psychiatric wards in Britain are far too often untherapeutic. A national survey in the UK found that about a quarter of ward managers (senior nurses) felt that their ward environment did not promote positive mental health care.[55] A quarter of inpatients said that they rarely felt safe in hospital.[56] Similar results came from another British survey, this time of over 1000 service users, in which a third of inpatients had experienced violent or threatening behaviour while in hospital, and indeed 18 per cent of hospital visitors had also been threatened.[57]

> The next type of stigma that hit me was from strangers. A forensic hostel was proposed near to me and all of a sudden I'm a target for their anger. I live in a special mental health project flat, that came under attack.
>
> Maria

Human rights

Internationally agreed covenants and declarations have the potential to protect vulnerable groups, including those who are involuntarily detained. Nevertheless, such broad statements of principle are often far from clinical reality. So just how practically useful are lofty statements of principle? First they set out 'in unambiguous terms'[58] agreed prohibitions against the abuses of basic human rights. They also establish a framework to support those who oppose breaches of human rights or who seek to resist pressure to assist in ill treatment. Third, they set boundaries upon actual or potential conflicts of interest, for example, between the autonomy of service users against the protection of the public. In addition, they can act as an integrating statement of the purpose for mental health services, and so assist in the interpretation of local guidelines or laws. Finally such statements can ensure that the ethical aspects of clinical practice are given sufficient emphasis to practitioners, and so reduce the likelihood of abuses of human rights. Given all this, does the evidence presented in this book add up to show a broad respect or disrespect of these human rights for people with mental illness?[39]

> I've been abused in the street. I've had my house broken into twelve times and had a knife put through the door. All in an effort to try and drive me out. And I'm the one who's supposed to be nasty and violent.[18]

The key binding international points of reference for mental health are the Universal Declaration of Human Rights, the International Covenant on Civil and Political Rights, and the International Covenant on Economic, Social and

Cultural Rights. Those countries which have ratified these covenants are consequently obliged under international law to guarantee to every person in its territory, without discrimination, all the rights enshrined within them. Nevertheless it is important to appreciate that international conventions, including international human rights conventions, once ratified by states are legally binding, but only upon states. They are not binding on individuals, such as mental health practitioners. In addition, the impact of such measures depends in large part upon how well their implementation is monitored.

More specifically in relation to mental health, the UN Principles for the Protection of Persons with Mental Illness and for the Improvement of Mental Health Care were adopted in 1991 (more often called 'the Mental Illness Principles'). The first principle sets the foundation for all others:

> All persons with a mental illness, or who are being treated as such persons, shall be treated with humanity and respect for the inherent dignity of the human person ... shall have the right to exercise all civil, political, economic, social and cultural rights as recognised in the United National Universal Declaration of Human Rights, and the International Covenant on Economic, Social and Cultural Rights, International Covenant on Civil and Political Rights, and in other relevant instruments ... all persons have the right to the best available mental health care.[58–60]

The application of such principles can have important implications. Amnesty International (Irish Section), for example, expressed its concern in 2001 that some mentally vulnerable people were placed in isolation cells in prison, often for significant lengths of time, which may have constituted a violation of international standards for humane detention and solitary confinement. In reply the Minister for Justice, Equality and Law Reform gave a commitment that padded cells would be replaced by safety observation cells that would 'fully meet the needs and respect the dignity' of those detained.[59]

Despite such measures, there are many credible reports detailed where even the most basic of human rights are not respected for people with mental illness. In Romania, for example, it has been alleged that in recent years the winter death rate in psychiatric institutions is considerably more than what could be reasonably expected, possibly related to insufficient heating and nutrition on the wards.[61] Just to the northwest of Romania, the use of cage beds have recently been described in the Czech Republic, Slovakia, Hungary and Slovenia, although the last three have now discontinued their use.

The Mental Disability Advocacy Centre has documented a series of abuses of human rights in European and Central Asian countries, for example, the use of forced labour (in which inpatients are compelled to do unpaid work as a form of 'labour therapy'), and the physical and sexual abuse of female patients by male psychiatric patients in the Kyrgyz Republic.[62] At Radnevo, the largest psychiatric hospital in Bulgaria, it has been reported that inpatients are denied the right to vote, in violation both of the Bulgarian Constitution and international law.[63]

If anything there now seem to be too many ethical and legal requirements. Too few of them are well known, and none of them entirely honoured. Psychiatrists, for example, have tried to put their own house in order with the World Psychiatric Association Declaration of Madrid. With this essentially humanitarian set of principles it encourages its members by saying that 'psychiatrists should at all times ... be guided primarily by the respect for patients and concern for their welfare and integrity'.[64]

Despite these libertarian promptings, sometimes such conventions betray a deeper misunderstanding or hostility towards mentally ill people. In England, the Human Rights Act of 1998 incorporated into national law the provisions of the European Convention on Human Rights (ECHR). The ECHR was originally signed in 1950, and in places it reveals older and deeper prejudices against people with mental illness. Article 5, for example, states that groups of persons of 'unsound mind', along with 'vagrants' and 'drug addicts' are exempted from the protections afforded to others. In contrast, Article 14 of the ECHR, its non-discrimination provision, states:

> The enjoyment of the rights and freedoms set forth in this Convention shall be secured without discrimination on any ground such as sex, race, colour, language, religion, political or other opinion, national or social origin, association with a national minority, property, birth or other status.

Breach of this is a violation of the Convention. So while mental illness-related disabilities are not given as a specified ground, they are included in 'any ground', or 'other Status', as was demonstrated in the legal case of Botta *v.* Italy.[65] Paradoxically, in Britain the Human Rights Act has provoked criticism that it 'perpetuates rather than challenges the lesser regard for the autonomy of patients with mental illness than of other medical patients'.[66–68]

> As I understand it the European Convention on Human Rights exempts people who are insane anyway, these are people who don't have basic human rights because they are insane, so that's not a very helpful piece of legislation!
>
> Veronica

In addition, the World Health Organisation has issued a statement of the core civil rights which should be accorded to every person with a diagnosis of mental illness: right to vote, right to marry, right to have children and maintain parental rights, right to own property, right to work and employment, right to education, right to freedom of movement and choice of residence, right to health, right to a fair trial and due process of law, right to sign cheques and engage in financial transactions, right to religious freedom and practice.[69]

So we can see two very different worlds. In the air-conditioned calm of international professional, ethical, legal and diplomatic organisations there now exists a series of binding treaties and laws, or discretionary covenants, conventions and principles, all solemnly issued. Meanwhile in wards, hostels, social care homes and nursing homes in many countries worldwide we know that standards of care fall well below both what is required by law, and below what can reasonably be seen as humane.

Care standards are to a large extent independent of the level of resources available locally. We saw in Chapter 1 how far homeless mentally ill people in New York are neglected. Across the world in India, 25 psychiatric patients were burned to death at Erwadi in 2001 when a fire swept the hospital. Most of the 46 inpatients had been chained to their beds. Erwadi was considered a centre for religious observation and pilgrimage, and in the course of their 'treatment' patients were 'frequently caned, whipped and beaten ... driving away the evil ... during the day they were tied to trees with thick ropes ... at night they were tied to their beds with iron chains'.[70]

> My life was already shamed with my disability which I hold no one to fault ... he did not consider the psychological harm I went through when I was back in Zimbabwe and to make matters worse he is not considering more psychological impairment he is subjecting me to if I return to Zimbabwe. I feel that my rights as a mentally disabled person are being violated, as I am not allowed to live a life away from torture.
>
> Linda

So to answer the central question posed at the start of this chapter, the weight of evidence presented here, along with that detailed elsewhere in this book, propels us relentlessly towards the conclusion that our societies give less value to the category of people called mentally ill than to any other group.

Letter to The Editor, Irish Times, Dublin, 24 November 2003

Madam,

We would like to bring to the attention of your readers the extent of stigma that individuals with mental ill health continue to experience in Ireland

The Irish Advocacy Network is an Ireland-wide movement that fights for the rights of individuals who have experienced mental health problems. Its membership consists of individuals who have used or are continuing to use mental health services throughout Ireland.

Letter to The Editor, Irish Times, Dublin, 24 November 2003 (*cont.*)

IAN set about organising a three-day conference earlier this year. Employees telephoned several hotels asking if they were able to facilitate the conference. They were astounded at several responses and suspect that hotel staff were reluctant to facilitate a conference whose audience for the first two days would consist of people with mental illness.

One hotel quoted an extraordinary price of £126,000. Another was concerned that medical or professional representatives would not be present during the conference to look after the 'ill'. We were finally accepted by Jackson's Hotel, Ballybofey, Co Donegal. Jackson's turned out to be a warm friendly place with excellent staff and a good quality of service.

We are offended that people continue to believe that individuals with mental health problems are unable to be responsible and capable citizens. We believe that this experience confirms the extent of ignorance and against prejudice of mental health that prevails in our society. This should be extremely worrying to us all as mental ill health is increasingly prevalent in our society.

Our conference was a great success. We would like to thank the staff of Jackson's Hotel for their open-mindedness and for treating us as equal citizens in a respectful and courteous manner.
Yours, etc.,

Paddy McGowan, Irish Advocacy Network Management, Committee, Rooskey, Monaghan.

References

1. West P. Social stigma and community recreational participation by the mentally and physically handicapped. *Therapeutic Recreation Journal* 1984; 18:41–49.
2. Bedini LA. Just sit down so we can talk: perceived stigma and community recreation pursuits of people with disabilities. *Therapeutic Recreation Journal* 2000; 34:55–68.
3. Salmon P. Effects of physical exercise on anxiety, depression, and sensitivity to stress: a unifying theory. *Clin Psychol Rev* 2001; 21(1):33–61.
4. Blumenthal JA, Babyak MA, Moore KA, Craighead WE, Herman S, Khatri P *et al*. Effects of exercise training on older patients with major depression. *Arch Intern Med* 1999; 159(19):2349–2356.
5. Mainichi Shimbun. Fitness clubs, pools shutting out mentally disabled with biased rules. *Mainichi Shimbun* 2 May 2004.

6. Koppel S, McGuffin P. Socio-economic factors that predict psychiatric admissions at a local level. *Psychol Med* 1999; 29(5): 1235–1241.

7. Brugha T, Jenkins R, Bebbington P, Meltzer H, Lewis G, Farrell M. Risk factors and the prevalence of neurosis and psychosis in ethnic groups in Great Britain. *Soc Psychiatry Psychiatr Epidemiol* 2004; 39(12):939–946.

8. Driver and Vehicle Licensing Agency. *Chapter 4 Psychiatric disorders.* Swansea: DVLA; 2005.

9. Brown P. Mental illness and motor insurance. *Psychiatr Bull* 1993; 17:620–621.

10. Zogg H, Lauber C, jdacic-Gross V, Rossler W. [Expert's and lay attitudes towards restrictions on mentally ill people]. *Psychiatr Prax* 2003; 30(7):379–383.

11. Wise MEJ, Watson JP. Postal survey of psychiatrists' knowledge and attitudes towards driving and mental illness. *Psychiatr Bull* 2001; 25:345–349.

12. Frei A, Gerhard U, Rummele W. [Catamnesis of psychiatrically evaluated automobile drivers]. *Schweiz Arch Neurol Psychiatr* 1990; 141(2): 123–138.

13. Appelbaum PS. Discrimination in psychiatric disability coverage and the Americans With Disabilities Act. *Psychiatr Serv* 1998; 49(7):875–6, 881.

14. Berman LE. Mental health parity. *Managed Care Interface* 2000; 13(7):63–66.

15. Read J, Baker S. *Not Just Sticks and Stones. A Survey of the Stigma, Taboos, and Discrimination Experienced by People with Mental Health Problems.* London: MIND; 1996.

16. Rossler W, Salize HJ, Biechele U. [Social legislative and structural deficits of ambulatory management of chronic psychiatric and handicapped patients]. *Nervenarzt* 1995; 66(11):802–810.

17. Association of British Insurers. *An Insurer's Guide to the Disability Discrimination Act 1995.* London: Association of British Insurers; 2003.

18. Dunn S. *Creating Accepting Communities: Report of the MIND Inquiry into Social Exclusion and Mental Health Problems.* London: MIND; 1999.

19. Estroff S. *Making it Crazy: Ethnography of psychiatric clients in an American community.* Berkeley, California: University of California Press; 1981.

20. Dear M, Wolch J. *Landscapes of Despair.* Princeton, New Jersey: Princeton University Press; 1992.

21. Bird L. Poverty, social exclusion and mental health: a survey of people's personal experiences. *A Life in the Day* 2001; 5:3.

22. Blenkiron P, Hammill CA. What determines patients' satisfaction with their mental health care and quality of life? *Postgrad Med J* 2003; 79(932):337–340.

23. Thesen J. Being a psychiatric patient in the community – reclassified as the stigmatized 'other'. *Scand J Public Health* 2001; 29(4):248–255.

24. Slade M, McCrone P, Thornicroft G. Uptake of welfare benefits by psychiatric patients. *Psychiatr Bull* 1995; 19:411–413.

25. Frost-Gaskin M, O'Kelly R, Henderson C, Paccitti R. A welfare benefits outreach project to users of community mental health services. *International Journal of Social Psychiatry* 2003; 49:251–263.

26. Dow MG, Boaz TL. Assisting clients of community mental health centers to secure SSI benefits: a controlled evaluation. *Community Ment Health J* 1994; 30(5):429–440.

27. Prahm H. [Increased debts and mental health]. *Gesundheitswesen* 1999; 61(1):27–30.

28. Hatcher S. Debt and deliberate self-poisoning. *Br J Psychiatry* 1994; 164(1):111–114.

29. Meltzer H, Singleton N, Lee A, Bebbington P, Brugha T, Jenkins R. *The Social and Economic Consequences of Adults with Mental Disorders.* London: The Stationery Office; 2002.

30. Payne S. *Poverty, Social Exclusion and Mental Health. Findings from the 1999 PSE Survey.* Working Paper No. 15. Bristol: Townsend Centre for International Poverty Research; 2000.

31. Edwards S. *In Too Deep. CAB clients' experiences of debt.* London: Citizens Advice Bureau; 2003.

32. Monahan J, Redlich AD, Swanson J, Robbins PC, Appelbaum PS, Petrila J *et al.* Use of leverage to improve adherence to psychiatric treatment in the community. *Psychiatr Serv* 2005; 56(1):37–44.

33. Klein MM, Grossman SA. Voting competence and mental illness. *Am J Psychiatry* 1971; 127(11):1562–1565.

34. Thompson B, Hall J. Helping psychiatric inpatients exercise their right to vote. *Hosp Community Psychiatry* 1974; 25(7):441.

35. Burton VS, Jr. The consequences of official labels: a research note on rights lost by the mentally ill, mentally incompetent, and convicted felons. *Community Ment Health J* 1990; 26(3):267–276.

36. Hemmens C, Miller M, Burton VS, Jr, Milner S. The consequences of official labels: an examination of the rights lost by the mentally ill and mentally incompetent ten years later. *Community Ment Health J* 2002; 38(2):129–140.

37. Howard G, Anthony R. The right to vote and voting patterns of hospitalized psychiatric patients. *Psychiatr Q* 1977; 49(2):124–132.

38. Smith H, Humphreys M. Changes in laws are necessary to allow patients detained under Mental Health Act to vote. *BMJ* 1997; 315(7105):431.

39. Peay J, Law and stigma: present, future and futuristic solutions. In: Crisp A, edr., *Every Family in the Land*, pp. 367–372. London: Royal Society of Medicine; 2004.

40. Jaychuk G, Manchanda R. Psychiatric patients and the federal election. *Can J Psychiatry* 1991; 36(2):124–125.

41. Kunze H, Lutze P, Stumme W. [Voting rights of psychiatric patients (author's transl)]. *Psychiatr Prax* 1982; 9(2):42–50.

42. Nash M. Voting as a means of social inclusion for people with a mental illness. *J Psychiatr Ment Health Nurs* 2002; 9(6):697–703.

43. Appelbaum PS. 'I vote. I count': mental disability and the right to vote. *Psychiatr Serv* 2000; 51(7):849–50,63.

44. Mental Disability Advocacy Center. *Russia's guardianship system challenged at the European Court of Human Rights.* Budapest: Mental Disability Advocacy Center; 2005.

45. Burton VS. The consequences of official labels: A research note on rights lost by the mentally ill, mentally incompetent, and convicted felons. *Community Mental Health Journal* 1990; 26:267–276.

46. Kessler RC, Demler O, Frank RG, Olfson M, Pincus HA, Walters EE *et al.* Prevalence and treatment of mental disorders, 1990 to 2003. *N Engl J Med* 2005; 352(24):2515–2523.

47. Dinos S, Stevens S, Serfaty M, Weich S, King M. Stigma: the feelings and experiences of 46 people with mental illness. Qualitative study. *Br J Psychiatry* 2004; 184:176–181.

48. Murphy E. *After the Asylums.* London: Faber and Faber; 1991.

49. Pedler M. *MIND's Response to 'Speaking up for Justice' Report of the Interdepartmental Working Group on the Treatment of Vulnerable or Intimidated Witnesses in the Criminal Justice System.* London: MIND Policy Unit; 1998.

50. Hiday VA, Swartz MS, Swanson JW, Borum R, Wagner HR. Criminal victimization of persons with severe mental illness. *Psychiatr Serv* 1999; 50(1):62–68.

51. Sainsbury Centre for Mental Health. *Acute Problems: a survey of the quality of care in acute psychiatric units.* London: Sainsbury Centre for Mental Health; 1998.

52. Sainsbury Centre for Mental Health. *An Executive Briefing on Adult Acute Inpatient Care for People with Mental Health Problems.* London: Sainsbury Centre for Mental Health; 2002.

53. Perese EF. Unmet needs of persons with chronic mental illnesses: relationship to their adaptation to community living. *Issues Ment Health Nurs* 1997; 18(1):19–34.

54. Miller RJ, Zadolinnyj K, Hafner RJ. Profiles and predictors of assaultativeness for different psychiatric ward populations. *Am J Psychiatry* 1993; 150(9):1368–1373.

55. Sainsbury Centre for Mental Health. *Acute Care 2004: a National Survey of Adult Psychiatric Wards in England.* London: Sainsbury Centre for Mental Health; 2005.

56. Mind. *WardWatch: MIND's Campaign to Improve Hospital Conditions for Mental Health Patients.* London: MIND; 2005.

57. Royal College of Psychiatrists Research Unit. *The National Audit on Violence in Mental Health and Learning Disability Services.* Healthcare Commission, London: 2005.

58. Amnesty International. *Ethical Codes and Declarations Relevant to the Health Professions.* London: Amnesty International; 2000.

59. Amnesty International. *Mental Illness, the Neglected Quarter: Summary Report.* Dublin: Amnesty International; 2003.

60. United Nations. *UN Principles for the Protection of Persons with Mental Illness and for the Improvement of Mental Health Care.* Adopted by UN General Assembly Resolution 46/119 of 18 February 1992. New York: United Nations; 1992.

61. Amnesty International. *Romania: Memorandum to the government concerning inpatient psychiatric treatment.* London: Amnesty International; 2004.

62. Mental Disability Advocacy Center. *Mental Health Law in the Kyrgyz Republic and its Implementation.* Budapest: Mental Disability Advocacy Center; 2004.

63. Mental Disability Advocacy Center. *The Right to Vote at Risk in Bulgaria.* Budapest: Mental Disability Advocacy Center; 2005.

64. World Psychiatric Association. *Declaration of Madrid.* Geneva: World Psychiatric Association; 1996.

65. Fennell P. The third way in mental health policy: negative rights, positive rights, and the Convention. *J Law Soc* 1999; 26(1):103–127.

66. Bindman J, Maingay S, Szmukler G. The Human Rights Act and mental health legislation. *Br J Psychiatry* 2003; 182:91–94.

67. Kingdon D, Jones R, Lonnqvist J. Protecting the human rights of people with mental disorder: new recommendations emerging from the Council of Europe. *Br J Psychiatry* 2004; 185:277–279.

68. Macgregor-Morris R, Ewbank J, Birmingham L. Potential impact of the Human Rights Act on psychiatric practice: the best of British values? *BMJ* 2001; 322(7290):848–850.

69. World Health Organisation. *WHO Resource Book on Mental Health, Human Rights and Legislation.* Geneva: World Health Organisation; 2005.

70. World Health Organisation. *Investing in Mental Health.* Geneva: World Health Organisation; 2003.

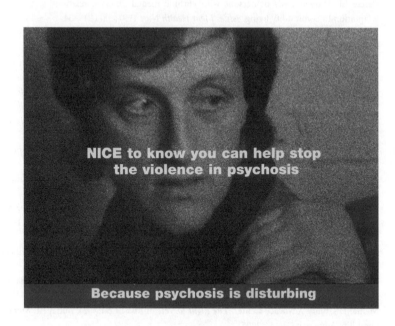

Advertisement by a pharmaceutical company for anti-psychotic medication, Hospital Doctor newspaper, 2005.

Chapter 5 Harmful helpers
Discrimination in health and social care

Diana came to England from Ghana 30 years ago as a young woman, and between raising her children took courses in Chartered Accounting. Suddenly, at the age of 51, she developed the features of a psychotic illness. She began to give credit to odd beliefs, for example she felt that when she crossed the road that cars swerved to try to run her over. She was admitted to a psychiatric ward in a general hospital, but her behaviour was seen as loud, unpredictable and aggressive, so she was transferred to an intensive care unit at a psychiatric hospital. On one occasion she was forcibly injected with medication. Now she is almost fully recovered from the symptoms of the mental illness, nevertheless she is adamant that this episode has irreversibly changed her life.

Other people treat her differently now, 'My friends make me feel like a weakling'. She used to be a central figure in her local community, and was heavily involved, for example, in organising her church and the annual carnival. Although she ties hard to minimize the impact of being unwell, she admits that it has damaged her.

> I used to be very influential in the local community, I was chair of the Education Committee, but I discovered that they don't involve me so much any more. I keep myself to myself more than before. I used to be a very outgoing person, now I'm more withdrawn from society. I'm no longer the person I used to be. I used to be someone who had leadership qualities. I've lost confidence. I don't want to be the centre any more. I shy away from getting too involved. I used to socialize in my community, then they would be looking at me in a funny way, and for a couple of them, it's like you don't exist any more.

On the other hand, Diana has mixed feelings about the effect of her illness on her family life. She feels her family were 'tremendously supportive' when she was unwell. Especially as they had previously taken her for granted. 'It was as if I was the big pillar that would never fall.' But she did fall. Against the grain, her children began to clean up at home and take their share of domestic responsibilities. When she came home they advised her to 'take it easy, and avoid too much stress'. At first she was pleased to slow down, but later on she felt over-protected by her husband and children.

A central dilemma for Diana, while she is urged not to 'over-do it', is to know what level of stress would be too much. In fact she feels caught, as the only way to find this out would be to do too much and become unwell again. Her other choice is to push herself too little, and then to feel that she was under-achieving for the rest of her life. She doesn't talk about this with her family, or about whether is it is helpful to discuss her difficulties. 'My family don't want me talk about my mental problems very much. I think it helps to talk about it here in this country, but they don't think so.'

Before going into hospital Diana had been working full time.

> My boss was very supportive and when I got my job back, he suggested that I agree to reduce my working hours from five working days to three working days. After a short while I wished that it would go back to normal, but he said the funding for my project was reduced.

Now she continues to work part-time, but she doesn't know whether the reason given by her manager is genuine, or if it indicates some degree of discrimination.

Diana thinks that the main reason for her rapid recovery was her strong religious belief. While she was in hospital she prayed often, and on her discharge she decided to tell her congregation about her experiences. 'I gave a kind of testimony in my church when I came out of my illness.' In retrospect she now doubts that this was a good idea. 'Sometimes I do get the feeling that they treat me differently, that people who used to come to you and chat; now they look away.' This is connected to ideas that are common among her community of people from Ghana.

> In Africa, in Ghana, I would not talk about it because of the stigma. There's nothing you can say that convinces people that you're a normal person. You are no longer a credible person. Everything you say is seen from the point of view that you were once mentally unbalanced. They see it as a very, very bad thing. They have a lot of superstitions, a lot of negative attitudes. I could say I was ill, but I could never say the nature of the illness. I might say 'extreme depression', but I would not use the word 'mental'. They look at mental illness from a religious point of view. They see mental illness as something that is demonic, something caused by evil spirits, caused by evil people. People attack people with mental illness. If you're a normal person they believe that someone can send an evil spirit to you. Most times they believe that taking a person to hospital - they never recover. They will always remain a psychiatric patient. They will never get fully treated.

Diana's strongest feelings are about how she was treated by health staff. Although she says that the community psychiatric nurses who visited her at home later were 'brilliant people', this was overshadowed by more negative experiences. When she was transferred to the intensive care (locked) ward she was forcibly injected with medication. Although these events happened over a year ago she is still very distressed when remembering this episode.

> There were between six and eight staff members, I'm not sure, I can't remember too much. I didn't have a very clear vision. I saw people surrounding me, holding me by the hand, holding me by the legs. I don't think it was something they had to do. There was no talking. They would have helped better if they had more understanding and more talking … more respect. I felt really bad. While I was in hospital I tried to complain but I don't know if anybody was listening. It was a nightmare.

After leaving hospital she felt physically unwell and consulted her family doctor.

> I was feeling really tired and I thought I should see my local GP, and I said 'Can you please do a physical examination', because I wasn't feeling very well. At the end of the day he said 'Have you had any mental problems before?' I was really angry. I was really, really angry with him. Was he trying to say that the reason I was coming to see him was because I had had a mental problem? I left medical clinic that day feeling really, really, really bad.

Diana's mixed feelings about mental health care are common among people with mental illness, who both feel that they have been helped and been misunderstood by psychiatric services. It is a paradox that many mentally ill people do not speak highly of mental health staff, who are specifically trained to treat people with such conditions. The experience of people with mental illness is that they often feel patronized, punished or humiliated by such contact. Indeed service users often rate mental health staff as one of the groups which most stigmatises mentally ill people.[1] How is this possible when mental health professionals are especially qualified to understand and offer expert assistance to people with mental health problems? These thorny issues are the centre-point of this chapter.

Access to mental health care

Most people in the general population (in all the countries where this has been studied) have a mixture of little and wrong information about mental illnesses, alongside wary and cautious attitudes about mentally ill people. It is therefore understandable that they are often slow to recognise developing mental health problems in themselves, in family members or in friends, and are reluctant to seek help for fear of the consequences.

It is only recently that we have begun to understand the power of these barriers to finding treatment and care.[2] For examples studies from several countries have consistently found that even after a family member has developed clear-cut signs of a psychotic disorder, on average it is over a year until the unwell person first receives assessment and treatment.[3–5] A survey of almost 10,000 adults in the USA has added more detail to this picture. The results showed that the majority of people with mental disorders eventually contact treatment services, but they often wait a long time before doing so: with average delays before seeking help of eight years for mood disorders, and at least nine years for anxiety disorders. People who wait longer than average before receiving care are more likely to be young, old, male, poorly educated, or a member of a racial/ethnic minority.[6]

Where do people go to try to find help? The detailed US survey just mentioned also asked this question and produced some surprising answers. Only about a third (41 per cent) of people who had experienced mental illness in the previous year had received any treatment: 12 per cent from a psychiatrist, 16 per cent from a non-psychiatric mental health specialist, 23 per cent treated by a general medical practitioner, 8 per cent from a social services professional, and 7 per cent from a complementary or alternative medical provider. In terms of treatment adequacy, mental health specialists provided care that was at least reasonable in about half (48 per cent) of the cases they saw, while in primary care only 13 per cent of people treated received care that was adequate. Unmet needs were greater for the poor: older people, minority ethnic groups, those with low incomes or without insurance and residents of rural areas.[7] The study concluded that 'most people with mental disorders in the United States remain either untreated or poorly treated'.[7]

It is wrong to think that health services are usually the first port of call when people want help for mental illness. In the national survey referred to above, a quarter of people who sought help first went to a member of the clergy. This pattern seems to be remarkably stable: and applied to 31 per cent in the 1950s and to 24 per cent in the 1990s. Indeed more people first went to a faith leader for help than went to a psychiatrist (17 per cent), or to a general medical practitioners (17 per cent).[8]

On what basis do people judge where to go for help? A large national survey in Germany described vignettes of people with depression or schizophrenia and asked about how to find help. Revealingly the general public thought that mental health staff are useful for treating people with schizophrenia, but not for depression. The reason for this is that most people felt that schizophrenia was caused by biological or uncontrollable influences, while they understood depression to be a consequence of 'social disintegration' (including unemployment, drug or alcohol misuse, marital discord, family distress or social isolation) so that people with depression were more often recommended to seek help and social support from a friend or confidant.[9]

This may go some way to explain why depression is essentially untreated in some countries. An international study of depression found that 0 per cent of people with depression in St Petersburg received evidence-based treatment in primary care, and only 3 per cent were referred on to specialist mental health care.[10] But the major barrier to care in that Russian site was money: an inability to afford treatment costs was the main barrier to care for 75 per cent of the depressed Russian patients studied.

Even under better resourced conditions, it known that most people with a mental illness in the United States do not seek assistance. An early national survey found that fewer than one-third of all mentally ill people received assessment and treatment, although the rate rose to 60 per cent for people with a diagnosis of schizophrenia.[7,11,12] Over the last decade the occurrence of mental illnesses each year in the United States has not changed (29.4 per cent between 1990 and 1992, and 30.5 per cent between 2001 and 2003). On the other hand, relatively more people with mental illness were treated, rising over this decade from 20.3 per cent to 32.9 per cent.

It is a paradox that even though two thirds of adults with a mental illness went untreated, a half of those who did receive treatment did not have a clear-cut mental illness.[13] Interestingly the idea that conditions which are less stigmatised (for example depression compared with schizophrenia) are those which are seen to be more treatable is not supported by the findings of these surveys.[14] So no single factor is enough to explain complex patterns of help-seeking. Nevertheless the weight of evidence does suggest that even when there are no major financial barriers to care, that many people do not seek help or minimize their contact with services in an attempt to avoid being labelled as mentally ill.[15]

We saw earlier that particular groups may have even lower rates of treatment for mental disorders, and this applies in particular to African-Americans in the USA or to black Caribbean groups in the UK.[16] Several American studies suggest that African-Americans receive mental health care about half as often as white people,[17–19] even though they have higher rates of some mental disorders.[20,21] Several important barriers to care can increase the impact of mental illnesses among black communities in Britain and the USA. These factors have been described as: sociocultural (health beliefs and mistrust of services), systemic (lack of culturally competent practices in mental health services),[22] economic (lack of health insurance), or individual barriers (denial of mental health problems).[23]

The interplay of these factors produces the contradictory situation in which black groups may have higher rates of many mental illnesses, lower rates of general referral and treatment, but higher rates of compulsory treatment and forensic service contact.[24,25] In the USA patterns of contact with mental health services are in some ways different for black and white people. Black people with a mental illness are more likely to seek help if their families are supportive, and if a family member has had a positive personal experience of mental health care. In one study they did not view mental health on a continuum of well-being, but tended to think of themselves as either mentally healthy or mentally ill. Many interviewees said they did not think they were 'crazy', therefore they did not seek mental-health services.[26] Also there was little information about mental-health services in the African-American community. Most people interviewed did not learn about available mental-health services until their conditions had become severe.[21] There is an important general point here that we shall return to repeatedly in this book: that most people of all cultures have relatively little accurate and useful knowledge about mental illness.

Such feelings, at best of ambivalence, and at worst of deliberate avoidance of treatment and care for fear of stigma, have been found throughout the world. For instance, a study of Muslim Arab female university students in Jordan, the United Arab Emirates and Israel, found that for most of these women their first resort was to turn to God through prayer during times of psychological distress, rather than to seek help from health or social care agencies.[27] A strong reluctance to be seen as mentally ill appears to be a universal phenomenon.

Even in battle-hardened soldiers stigma is a powerful factor. Over 3000 military staff from US Army or Marine Corps units were anonymously surveyed three to four months after their return from combat duty in Iraq or Afghanistan. They were assessed for depression, anxiety, or post-traumatic stress disorder (PTSD). Most of the unwell soldiers (60–77 per cent) did not seek mental health care, largely related to concerns about possible stigmatisation.[28]

Why do so many people try so hard to avoid contacting psychiatric services? As we shall see in more detail in Chapter 9, people who are starting to have symptoms of mental illness are also members of the general population and share the same pool of information about psychiatric disorders. The following common beliefs are likely to reduce their likelihood of seeking help: that psychiatric treatments are ineffective;[29] that others would react with avoidance; or that a person should solve their own problems.[30] At the same time strong family encouragement to go for mental health assessment and treatment does often work.[31]

It is not fair to point only to individual factors in trying to understand the puzzle of under-treatment. In the USA the National Depressive and Manic-Depressive Association undertook an investigation to explore why 'there is overwhelming evidence that individuals with depression are being seriously under-treated'. They concluded that

Reasons for the continuing gap include patient, provider, and health care system factors. Patient-based reasons include: failure to recognize the symptoms, underestimating the severity, limited access, reluctance to see a mental health care specialist due to stigma, noncompliance with treatment, and lack of health insurance. Provider factors include poor professional school education about depression, limited training in interpersonal skills, stigma, inadequate time to evaluate and treat depression, failure to consider psychotherapeutic approaches, and prescription of inadequate doses of antidepressant medication for inadequate durations. Mental health care systems create barriers to receiving optimal treatment.[32]

Two months ago I went to my home village. I went for a coffee at a cafe. Most people there, of those who were aware of my problem, call me 'mad'. More specifically they said 'Here is the lunatic'. That incident made me very sad, I quickly finished my coffee and I left.

Panagiotis

Are people in rural areas better or worse served than those in towns and cities? The evidence here is patchy but a clear outline does tend to emerge. If a person with a mental illness wants to keep personal information confidential, this seems to be more difficult in rural communities. A study in Arkansas, for example, compared over 200 urban and rural residents' views about depression and its treatment. The rural residents with a history of depression labelled people who sought professional help more negatively than their urban counterparts. By the same token, those who labelled depression more negatively were less likely to have sought professional help.[33]

Similar findings also emerged from a study in Iowa where people living in the most rural environments were more likely to hold stigmatising attitudes toward mental health care than people in towns, and such views strongly predicted willingness to seek care.[34] Perhaps for these reasons, a survey of rural residents in Virginia found that over a third of the population had a diagnosed mental disorder, but only 6 per cent subsequently sought help, and those who did not go for treatment said that they 'felt there was no need'.[35] Evidence from Tennessee also showed that among people who were mentally unwell, those more likely to seek help were women, younger people and those who had been treated for a mental illness previously.[36]

In my village they don't know that I am living at a group home and that I am on medication. I have told them that I am working at a shop in Athens. My close relatives know it and some of them were more supportive after I got sick than before. In my village I don't want them to know about it because I don't want people to say things about me.

Dionisis

There is some evidence that these factors also prevent rural children with mental illness from having access to mental health care. A study of parents in rural areas of North Carolina concluded that although as many as 20 per cent of children had some type of treatable mental illness, only about one-third of them received help from the mental health system.[37, 38] The researchers found that one of the main barriers to care was stigma toward the use of the mental health care system.

So it seems to be true that stigma about mental illness is no less in many rural areas, and may be even stronger than in towns and cities. In part this may be based upon fears that a rural community will learn details about a period of mental illness, while it is easier in cities to remain anonymous. But relatively little research has been done in rural areas to understand these processes in more detail. This is especially important because there are relatively high rates of suicide among male farmers in many countries.[39–46]

> At university people would say things behind my back. Nobody would be open to me, but they would whisper behind my back. People would make comments about me. In my village nobody knows, because it is a small community and people would start saying things. Even though they do, I don't give any attention. In my neighbourhood in Athens nobody knows and I avoid speaking to anyone. Only with the lady at the grocery, but I somehow told her that I am on medication and since then she started to be more distant towards me, so I became more 'normal'. A friend that I've got from the university comes and sees me when he's got some time. We keep in touch.
>
> Mihalis

Being known as a psychiatric patient

For several decades it has been recognised that having been admitted to a psychiatric hospital can have an adverse effect on a person's reputation.[47–49] How can we understand such a powerful blemish on a person's identity? In part this damage is linked to popular views of psychiatrists: who they are, what they do and what they represent.[50] It is widely believed that psychiatrists use diagnostic labels in a cavalier way.[51] Similarly it is often believed that psychiatrists tend to use medications rather than psychological treatments, and that these drugs have unpleasant or even dangerous side-effects.[52]

At the same time popular opinion often goes well beyond the facts. We can take mental health medications as an example. A study in Germany tried to understand the reasons why people would accept or reject the psychotropic drugs they had been prescribed, compared with their views about taking drugs for cardiac conditions. The researchers found that psychiatric drugs were generally not well accepted because they were believed to cause more severe side-effects than cardiac drugs. Direct experience of contact with people taking psychiatric medications was limited, and so most people drew on other sources of information, mainly reports in the mass media, which gave an overwhelmingly negative account of mental illness and its treatments.[53] We shall return to the question of how mental illness is shown in the print, broadcast and film media in Chapter 6, but it is interesting to see that these representations can have an impact on whether psychiatric treatments are accepted or not.

Perceptions by service users of healthcare staff

Is it possible that staff trained specifically to treat people with mental illnesses can be seen by service users to be stigmatising themselves? Strangely enough, the answer seems to be yes.[54] A survey in South Australia, for example, compared the attitudes of over 250 mental health staff and the general public about the likely outcomes of cases of people with depression and schizophrenia. Professionals were generally more pessimistic about the chances of recovery than the general public, and psychiatrists were even less optimistic than nurses. In an important observation, the study found that most staff base their attitudes upon their personal experience of treating people with mental disorders.[55]

This 'physician bias' is understandable, as doctors will tend to draw upon their own clinical experience when advising patients. In many specialist mental health services the service users who recover quickly are discharged from care, and so, over time, doctors will tend to accumulate most of their clinical experience in trying to treat patients who do not fully recover, or who recover and then relapse again. They simply do not keep in touch with those who recover and stay well.

Perhaps an extreme version of this process applies to forensic psychiatrists whose working life consists of assessing and treating mentally ill offenders, often people who have committed serious crimes. As a consequence such psychiatrists tend to be even more cautious and pessimistic about therapeutic outcomes than general psychiatrists.[56] Interestingly, in recent years a number of studies of schizophrenia have been published which indicate that the long-term outlook for this condition is considerably better than used to be believed.[57–59] A more charitable view of this issue is that mental health staff often feel a strong personal responsibility for doing everything that they can to prevent a relapse of mental illness for the people they treat, and so they are reluctant to encourage service users to take on potentially stressful activities, for example full-time work, in case the person's condition deteriorates.[60]

People with some particular mental disorders are less favoured by psychiatric staff, especially people with a diagnosis of 'personality disorder'. Paradoxically, although service users with such a diagnosis claim to be especially rejected by healthcare staff, there are few investigations of stigma against people with a personality disorder.[61–64] These studies do suggest that people with this diagnosis are felt by staff to be difficult, less deserving of care, manipulative, attention-seeking, annoying and in control of their suicidal urges.[65] The diagnosis is therefore interpreted by some mental health staff as pejorative,[66] and one that does not arouse their empathy.[67]

Other diagnostic groups also appear to be less popular with heath staff. Chronic fatigue syndrome is bitterly contested in terms of its status as a physical, psychiatric or psychosomatic condition, and arouses controversy about its causation and treatment. People who have been given or assumed this diagnosis often describe experiences of rejection by both general and mental health staff.[68–71]

> Some of the worst experiences I have had have been in psychiatric hospitals. I recognise the need to be kept safe but often I have felt that my rights and dignity have been stripped away. Being intimately searched again and again and constantly followed whilst under 'close observation' just leaves me feeling singled out and perceived as little more then a nuisance ('there's to be no trouble on my shift'). I have seen, unofficially, my hospital notes and there is more than one occasion when nurses have actually lied to cover their own backs after I have self-harmed. After I have self-harmed, just when I feel at my most vulnerable, I have encountered a wall of silence as if talking about it will only encourage me to do it again. This is without the stigma attached to self-harm by many of my fellow patients. I have heard many comments along the lines of 'Oh she's cut again. Why doesn't she just do it properly and kill herself.'
>
> Sandra

Another 'less deserving' category seems to be people with alcohol dependence. In a British study using case vignettes, consultant psychiatrists were asked to assess the influence of a past diagnosis of alcohol dependence on their views about what treatment they would recommend. Psychiatrists receiving the vignette with the diagnosis of alcohol dependence were more likely to rate the patient as difficult, annoying, less in need of admission, uncompliant, having a poor prognosis and more likely to be discharged from follow-up.[72]

A further group that appears to be less popular with general psychiatrists are people with a diagnosis of learning disabilities/mental handicap.[73, 74] The importance of such strong and rejecting prejudicial attitudes is that they can translate into discriminatory behaviour, for example inpatient unit staff or community mental health teams can set exclusion criteria for people with a diagnosis of personality disorder, so that it becomes a diagnosis of exclusion from care.[75–79]

If anything, service users report that some family physicians/general practitioners are even more often stigmatising than psychiatrists in responding unsympathetically to people with mental illnesses.[80–82] A series of focus groups in England asked service users about their experiences of stigma and about who should receive targeted educational sessions to reduce discrimination. The group most often mentioned (by about two-thirds of service users) was family doctors, closely followed by school children, employers and police.[83, 84] This view is justified by the findings of a national survey in Australia which showed that family doctors and psychiatrists had more pessimistic views about the outcomes for mental illnesses than psychologists and the general public.[85] The attitudes of psychiatric nurses were similar to those of psychiatrists, except that nurses were generally more positive about alternative and complementary approaches to treatment, such as vitamins, minerals and naturopathy.[86,87]

Negative attitudes can develop early. The findings of studies with medical students in several countries are far from reassuring.[88–91] In Croatia, for example, trainee doctors have been found to have stigmatising attitudes to mental illness, largely based upon fear and ignorance.[92] As we saw earlier, contact with people with mental illness is also linked with more favourable attitudes among medical students,[93,94] nursing,[95] or occupational therapy students[96] although enduring and positive changes in such attitudes may be difficult to achieve.[97–100]

Medical students also had clear preferences for particular categories of patients, and were less sympathetic toward those whom they believed to be undeserving of treatment because they were responsible for their condition, for example people with eating disorders.[101,102] One effect of these inaccurate and negative views by medical students about people with mental illness is that relatively few choose psychiatry as a career. There is evidence that psychiatry is attracting fewer medical graduates, with associated shortages of qualified doctors in some economically developed countries.[103] As a result there is a 'brain drain' of psychiatrists from less economically developed countries who move to richer countries, leaving their own countries even further depleted of staff.[104]

To return to the core concern of this book, the experience of discrimination by service users, then a new dimension emerges – dehumanization.[105] The core issues that occur time and again in service users' accounts are of being spoken to as if they were children, being excluded from important decisions and staff assuming the lack of capacity to be responsible for their own lives. Further recurrent themes from the perspective of service users are being given insufficient information about their condition and treatment options, and feeling that behind many encounters with psychiatric staff is the usually unspoken threat of coercive treatment.[106–109]

> Whilst I have had good experiences in the NHS, it being a microcosm of society, there is fear and prejudice there too. Overworked casualty staff have little energy left to treat self-harm with the sympathy and respect it deserves

and often it is just treated with contempt. I have been stitched without anaesthetic which feels like punishment and comments like 'You should be letting us treat patients who are really ill' are not uncommon. Treatment like this is dehumanizing and just increases the feeling of being stigmatised.

Sandra

Stigma against mental health staff

While of relatively less importance than the discrimination against people with a mental illness, mental health staff are also subjected to a form of 'stigma by association'.[110–112] As a psychiatrist myself I am very often astonished by what most people think that I do at work. Common views are that: psychiatrists 'have x-ray vision', can 'see into people's minds', read 'others people's thoughts', spend most of their time 'analysing' hypochondriacs who lie on couches, tend to be bearded (most psychiatrists in the UK are now women!) and are suspected of being somewhat eccentric if not mentally unbalanced themselves ('trick cyclists'). The limited work that has examined these curious views suggest that they largely stem from portrayals in the cinema.[113–115]

There may be also more sinister consequences of stigma for mental health staff and students, for example that they receive worse treatment if they themselves become mentally ill than members of the general public.[116–121]

I was an Approved Social Worker working for the local authority when I developed a mental illness. As I took a considerable amount of time off work, I was requested to have an assessment by the occupational doctor. Unfortunately, I was too unwell to attend an appointment and requested the doctor assess me at home. This request was refused and I was medically retired based on one psychiatric report on my mental illness. I have also been discriminated against because of my previous position as a social worker by people looking after my care. I was assessed for a day centre. I was accepted for the service. However, a couple of days later the day care provision stated that they discussed my case and decided that as I was a social worker, it would not be appropriate for me to attend day care, as my position may affect the other clients, despite the fact that I did not work in that local area. When I became very unwell, I was referred to a psychiatric unit in the community. Following an assessment, I was informed that I should be admitted providing I did not tell the other patients that I was a social worker. This put a great strain on me as other patients did ask my occupation and I had to lie. I have lost all my friends since the onset of my mental illness. My ex-colleagues at work have also ceased all contact with me. My family have been through a lot with me and my mental illness. They find it difficult to cope with me, which I understand. My relationship with my family has changed. They spend their time making sure I am taking my medication, observing my behaviour. I lost my career, my own flat, my car. Mental illness has destroyed my life.

Fiona

There are strong and deep currents running among professionals here. One aspect of what has been called the 'helper syndrome' is that those providing care feel that there is a categorical difference between themselves (as well individuals, examples of health) and those whom they treat (who are sick, weak and dependent).[122] To some extent one advantage of such beliefs is that they allow staff to cope with the emotionally demanding work they face. But on the other hand these views are dysfunctional when it comes to adjusting to mental illness when it affects colleagues. Interestingly these issues are not often discussed or written about.

Physical health care

> When I took an overdose, I was kept in A&E (emergency room) for the night. The staff were very rude to me, which has stopped me from going back there when I am in a crisis.
>
> Fiona

If staff attitudes are problematic within mental health services, is the situation any better when people with mental illness also need treatment for physical health problems? If anything, as Diana indicated at the beginning of this chapter, the situation may be even worse. There is strong evidence that people with a diagnosis of a mental illness, for example, have less access to primary health care,[123] and also receive inferior care for diabetes and heart attacks,[124–126] even though rates of physical illness and poor dental health among people with severe mentally illnesses are much higher than in the general population,[127–130] with especially high levels of cardiovascular disease, obesity, diabetes and HIV/AIDS.[131] This combination of high rates of physical illness and low rates of effective treatment leads to the fatal consequences of discrimination and neglect: people with all types of mental disorders have an increased risk of premature death.[132]

> The worst I have come across is medical people. I suffer badly from stomach problems. I have always had a sensitive stomach, i.e. stomach ulcers, bleeding stomach, and IBS (irritable bowel syndrome). But when I try to get help from my doctor, they say 'Oh it's your depression', or my phobia. I'm far from stupid and I'm well aware of the difference between IBS pain and what symptoms I get because of my phobia. I've even been told I'm anorexic and in denial. From the time doctors are aware of my mental problems, they talk at me, instead of to me, like I haven't a mind of my own.
>
> Eva

The parts of the general health system that seem to be most despised by many people with mental illness are the casualty (emergency room, accident and emergency) departments.[133] The same themes occur repeatedly in service users' accounts. The first issue is that people who attend after harming themselves very often feel deliberately punished by staff.

> This is very damaging, if you have to attend A&E (Accident and Emergency Department) after an incident of DSH (deliberate self-harm) and have been made to feel worthless, a waste of time etc. Consider what message this sends out. DSH is all about transferring the emotional into the physical. You feel SO bad about yourself that you cut yourself to the bone to feel alive, YOU burn yourself until you can smell your skin burning and your arm twitching. Why? You don't understand the pain that you are going through. You cannot talk to anyone about it because they don't understand. You get stuck in a spiral of despair, which as the years go on gets deeper and deeper. Your first involvement with psychiatric services is innocent enough. YOU really believe that they will be able to help, but you are still involved in the system years later. Again I question why?
>
> Martina

The second key theme that emerges about casualty departments is that people going there for help report that they are not treated with respect.

> In my experience it has been mostly health professionals who have been at fault when it comes to treating me with respect and dignity. Some of these are or were within the mental health service, but more often it was other health professionals. My experiences include the following incidents. (1) Talking to me in a derogatory manner, as if I was a child or wouldn't understand. This contrasted with how they spoke to my husband, who sometimes accompanied me to appointments. (2) They would say one thing at one appointment and then something else at the next, as if I would not remember what had been said the first time. (3) Not fully explaining to me what's going on with my treatment, apparently fearing that I would not be able to cope with the truth. Whilst that was possible, once I did find out the truth, difficulties in coping with it were exacerbated by a deep sense of betrayal. (4) After taking overdoses, overhearing the comments of nurses in A&E or on the ward, and in some cases these comments were said directly to me. They included: 'It's your own fault you're here' and (most hurtful of all) 'Don't you think we have better things to do, treating people with real problems.' On one occasion, I was so upset by these comments that I pulled out a drip and ran out of hospital. After my first overdose, my G P said it had 'Gone too far' for her. On another occasion, when I went to see her on a medical matter, she said abruptly 'What do you expect me to do about it?' Attitudes varied enormously depending on the perceived cause of the crisis (overdose). At first, when I was waiting to hear whether my cancer was in remission, doctors and nurses in A&E were highly supportive. Later, as soon as they knew that I was known to the mental health services, their attitude changed. It was as if they could relate to someone who had cancer but not to someone with mental health problems.
>
> Nadia

Choosing to stop contact with mental health services

Perhaps not surprisingly, the single biggest factor which leads to stopping contact with mental health services, according to a Danish study, is dissatisfaction with the care received.[134] When people with mental illness leave treatment before making full recovery, then their reasons for this may be especially revealing. Generally speaking it is people who are young, poor, single, uninsured, or who have more than one diagnosis who are more likely to stop contact with services,[134] even if they are still unwell when they take their own discharge.[135–138] Interestingly, dropout rates are higher for people who believe that psychiatric treatments are rarely effective, who are embarrassed to be seen by a mental health professional, or who are prescribed medication without any psychological treatment.[139] Surprisingly little has been written about why people stop attending appointments, from the point of view of service users themselves, either to understand what affects their satisfaction with care, or to find out how stigma and discrimination play a role in these treatment decisions, or to appreciate the mixed feelings many people with mental illness have about their harmful healers.[140–143]

> I hope to God I never get any serious mental health issues again, because I couldn't handle being treated like I'm nobody, and have no say in how I'm treated. When I used to go to see my psychiatrist, I'd see people in there, sobbing their hearts out because the council have told them to go away, and treated them like nothing, and they have had to come down to the centre to get their psychiatrist to help them with benefits, and its really horrible to see.
>
> Eva

References

1. Pinfold V, Thornicroft G, Huxley P, Farmer P. Active ingredients in anti-stigma programmes in mental health. *International Review of Psychiatry* 2005; 17; 123–131.
2. Cooper AE, Corrigan PW, Watson AC. Mental illness stigma and care-seeking. *J Nerv Ment Dis* 2003; 191(5):339–341.
3. Compton MT, Kaslow NJ, Walker EF. Observations on parent/family factors that may influence the duration of untreated psychosis among African-American first-episode schizophrenia-spectrum patients. *Schizophr Res* 2004; 68(2–3):373–385.
4. Johannessen JO, McGlashan TH, Larsen TK, Horneland M, Joa I, Mardal S *et al.* Early detection strategies for untreated first-episode psychosis. *Schizophr Res* 2001; 51(1):39–46.
5. Black K, Peters L, Rui Q, Milliken H, Whitehorn D, Kopala LC. Duration of untreated psychosis predicts treatment outcome in an early psychosis program. *Schizophr Res* 2001; 47(2–3):215–222.
6. Wang PS, Berglund P, Olfson M, Pincus HA, Wells KB, Kessler RC. Failure and delay in initial treatment contact after first onset of mental disorders in the National Comorbidity Survey Replication. *Arch Gen Psychiatry* 2005; 62(6): 603–613.

7. Wang PS, Lane M, Olfson M, Pincus HA, Wells KB, Kessler RC. Twelve-month use of mental health services in the United States: results from the National Comorbidity Survey Replication. *Arch Gen Psychiatry* 2005; 62(6):629–640.

8. Wang PS, Berglund PA, Kessler RC. Patterns and correlates of contacting clergy for mental disorders in the United States. *Health Serv Res* 2003; 38(2):647–673.

9. Angermeyer MC, Matschinger H, Riedel-Heller SG. Whom to ask for help in case of a mental disorder? Preferences of the lay public. *Soc Psychiatry Psychiatr Epidemiol* 1999; 34(4):202–210.

10. Simon GE, Fleck M, Lucas R, Bushnell DM. Prevalence and predictors of depression treatment in an international primary care study. *Am J Psychiatry* 2004; 161(9):1626–1634.

11. Narrow WE, Regier DA, Rae DS, Manderscheid RW, Locke BZ. Use of services by persons with mental and addictive disorders. Findings from the National Institute of Mental Health Epidemiologic Catchment Area Program. *Arch Gen Psychiatry* 1993; 50(2):95–107.

12. Regier DA, Narrow WE, Rae DS, Manderscheid RW, Locke BZ, Goodwin FK. The de facto US mental and addictive disorders service system. Epidemiologic catchment area prospective 1-year prevalence rates of disorders and services. *Arch Gen Psychiatry* 1993; 50(2):85–94.

13. Kessler RC, Demler O, Frank RG, Olfson M, Pincus HA, Walters EE *et al.* Prevalence and treatment of mental disorders, 1990 to 2003. *N Engl J Med* 2005; 352(24):2515–2523.

14. Mann CE, Himelein MJ. Factors associated with stigmatization of persons with mental illness. *Psychiatr Serv* 2004; 55(2):185–187.

15. Corrigan P. How stigma interferes with mental health care. *Am Psychol* 2004; 59(7):614–625.

16. Hines-Martin V, Malone M, Kim S, Brown-Piper A. Barriers to mental health care access in an African American population. *Issues Ment Health Nurs* 2003; 24(3):237–256.

17. Diala C, Muntaner C, Walrath C, Nickerson KJ, LaVeist TA, Leaf PJ. Racial differences in attitudes toward professional mental health care and in the use of services. *Am J Orthopsychiatry* 2000; 70(4):455–464.

18. Snowden LR. Barriers to effective mental health services for African Americans. *Ment Health Serv Res* 2001; 3(4):181–187.

19. Snowden LR. Bias in mental health assessment and intervention: theory and evidence. *Am J Public Health* 2003; 93(2):239–243.

20. Thornicroft G, Davies S, Leese M. Health service research and forensic psychiatry: a black and white case. *International Review of Psychiatry* 1999; 11:250–257.

21. Davis S, Ford M. A conceptual model of barriers to mental health services among African-Americans. *African-American Research Perspectives* 2004; 10:44–54.

22. Corrigan PW, Markowitz FE, Watson AC. Structural levels of mental illness stigma and discrimination. *Schizophr Bull* 2004; 30(3):481–491.

23. Swanson GM, Ward AJ. Recruiting minorities into clinical trials: toward a participant-friendly system. *J Natl Cancer Inst* 1995; 87(23):1747–1759.

24. Keating F, Robertson D. Fear, black people and mental illness. A vicious circle? *Health and Social Care in the Community* 2004; 12(5):439–447.

25. National Institute for Mental Health in England. *Inside Outside: Improving mental health services for black and minority ethnic communities in England.* London: Department of Health; 2003.

26. Hines-Martin V, Brown-Piper A, Kim S, Malone M. Enabling factors of mental health service use among African-Americans. *Arch Psychiatr Nurs* 2003; 17 (5):197–204.

27. Al-Krenawi A, Graham JR, Dean YZ, Eltaiba N. Cross-national study of attitudes towards seeking professional help: Jordan, United Arab Emirates (UAE) and Arabs in Israel. *Int J Soc Psychiatry* 2004; 50(2):102–114.

28. Hoge CW, Castro CA, Messer SC, McGurk D, Cotting DI, Koffman RL. Combat duty in Iraq and Afghanistan, mental health problems, and barriers to care. *N Engl J Med* 2004; 351(1):13–22.

29. Corrigan PW. *On the Stigma of Mental Illness: Practical strategies for research and social change*. Washington, DC: American Psychological Association; 2004.

30. Kessler RC, Berglund PA, Bruce ML, Koch JR, Laska EM, Leaf PJ *et al.* The prevalence and correlates of untreated serious mental illness. *Health Serv Res* 2001; 36(6 Pt 1):987–1007.

31. Link BG, Cullen FT, Struening EL, Shrout PE, Dohrenwend BP. A modified labeling theory approach in the area of mental disorders: An empirical assessment. *American Sociological Review* 1989; 54:100–123.

32. Hirschfeld RM, Keller MB, Panico S, Arons BS, Barlow D, Davidoff F *et al.* The National Depressive and Manic-Depressive Association consensus statement on the undertreatment of depression. *JAMA* 1997; 277(4):333–340.

33. Rost K, Smith GR, Taylor JL. Rural-urban differences in stigma and the use of care for depressive disorders. *J Rural Health* 1993; 9(1):57–62.

34. Hoyt DR, Conger RD, Valde JG, Weihs K. Psychological distress and help-seeking in rural America. *Am J Community Psychol* 1997; 25(4):449–470.

35. Fox JC, Blank M, Berman J, Rovnyak VG. Mental disorders and help-seeking in a rural impoverished population. *Int J Psychiatry Med* 1999; 29(2):181–195.

36. Smith LD, McGovern RJ, Peck PL. Factors contributing to the utilization of mental health services in a rural setting. *Psychol Rep* 2004; 95(2):435–442.

37. Costello EJ, Keeler GP, Angold A. Poverty, race/ethnicity, and psychiatric disorder: a study of rural children. *Am J Public Health* 2001; 91(9):1494–1498.

38. Angold A, Erkanli A, Farmer EM, Fairbank JA, Burns BJ, Keeler G *et al.* Psychiatric disorder, impairment, and service use in rural African-American and white youth. *Arch Gen Psychiatry* 2002; 59(10):893–901.

39. Gregoire A. The mental health of farmers. *Occup Med (Lond)* 2002; 52(8):471–476.

40. Hawton K, Fagg J, Simkin S, Harriss L, Malmberg A, Smith D. The geographical distribution of suicides in farmers in England and Wales. *Soc Psychiatry Psychiatr Epidemiol* 1999; 34(3):122–127.

41. Thomas HV, Lewis G, Thomas DR, Salmon RL, Chalmers RM, Coleman TJ *et al.* Mental health of British farmers. *Occup Environ Med* 2003; 60(3):181–185.

42. Voracek M, Fisher ML, Marusic A. The Finno-Ugrian suicide hypothesis: variation in European suicide rates by latitude and longitude. *Percept Mot Skills* 2003; 97(2):401–406.

43. Notkola VJ, Martikainen P, Leino PI. Time trends in mortality in forestry and construction workers in Finland 1970–85 and impact of adjustment for socioeconomic variables. *J Epidemiol Community Health* 1993; 47(3):186–191.

44. Li ZJ, Chen SY, Zhou J, Wu YQ. [The study of poisoning-suicide-attempted patients in emergency departments of 25 hospitals in China]. *Zhonghua Liu Xing Bing Xue Za Zhi* 2004; 25(4):285–287.

45. Page AN, Fragar LJ. Suicide in Australian farming, 1988–1997. *Aust N Z J Psychiatry* 2002; 36(1):81–85.

46. Sundar M. Suicide in farmers in India. *Br J Psychiatry* 1999; 175:585–586.

47. Goffman I. *Stigma: Notes on the management of spoiled identity.* Harmondsworth, Middlesex: Penguin Books; 1963.

48. Goffman I. *Asylums.* Harmondsworth: Pelican Books; 1968.

49. Gove WR, Fain T. The stigma of mental hospitalization. An attempt to evaluate its consequences. *Arch Gen Psychiatry* 1973; 28(4):494–500.

50. Bar-Levav R. The stigma of seeing a psychiatrist. *Am J Psychother* 1976; 30(3):473–482.

51. Sartorius N. Iatrogenic stigma of mental illness. *BMJ* 2002; 324(7352):1470–1471.

52. National Institute for Clinical Excellence (NICE). *Management of Depression in Primary and Secondary Care. Clinical Guideline 23.* London: National Institute for Clinical Excellence (NICE); 2004.

53. Benkert O, Graf-Morgenstern M, Hillert A, Sandmann J, Ehmig SC, Weissbecker H *et al.* Public opinion on psychotropic drugs: an analysis of the factors influencing acceptance or rejection. *J Nerv Ment Dis* 1997; 185(3):151–8.

54. Burti L, Mosher LR. Attitudes, values and beliefs of mental health workers. *Epidemiol Psichiatr Soc* 2003; 12(4):227–231.

55. Hugo M. Mental health professionals' attitudes towards people who have experienced a mental health disorder. *Journal of Psychiatric and Mental Health Nursing* 2001; 8:419–425.

56. Lau S. [How effective is community-based therapy of criminals? The effectiveness of community-related measures to prevent re-offending in criminals and mentally ill lawbreakers]. *Psychiatr Prax* 2003; 30(3):119–126.

57. Harding CM, Brooks GW, Ashikaga T, Strauss JS, Breier A. The Vermont longitudinal study of persons with severe mental illness, I: Methodology, study sample, and overall status 32 years later. *Am J Psychiatry* 1987; 144(6):718–726.

58. Harding CM, Brooks GW, Ashikaga T, Strauss JS, Breier A. The Vermont longitudinal study of persons with severe mental illness, II: Long-term outcome of subjects who retrospectively met DSM-III criteria for schizophrenia. *Am J Psychiatry* 1987; 144(6):727–735.

59. Ciompi L. Learning from outcome studies. Toward a comprehensive biological-psychosocial understanding of schizophrenia. *Schizophr Res* 1988; 1(6):373–384.

60. Murray MG, Steffen JJ. Attitudes of case managers toward people with serious mental illness. *Community Ment Health J* 1999; 35(6):505–14.

61. Camp DL, Finlay WM, Lyons E. Is low self-esteem an inevitable consequence of stigma? An example from women with chronic mental health problems. *Soc Sci Med* 2002; 55(5):823–834.

62. Lequesne ER, Hersh RG. Disclosure of a diagnosis of borderline personality disorder. *J Psychiatr Pract* 2004; 10(3):170–176.

63. Nehls N. Borderline personality disorder: gender stereotypes, stigma, and limited system of care. *Issues Ment Health Nurs* 1998; 19(2):97–112.

64. Markham D. Attitudes towards patients with a diagnosis of 'borderline personality disorder': social rejection and dangerousness. *Journal of Mental Health* 2005; 12:595–612.

65. Lewis G, Appleby L. Personality disorder: the patients psychiatrists dislike. *Br J Psychiatry* 1988; 153:44–49.

66. Gallop R, Lancee WJ, Garfinkel P. How nursing staff respond to the label 'borderline personality disorder'. *Hosp Community Psychiatry* 1989; 40(8):815–819.

67. Fraser K, Gallop R. Nurses' confirming/disconfirming responses to patients diagnosed with borderline personality disorder. *Arch Psychiatr Nurs* 1993; 7(6):336–341.

68. Davidson J. Contesting stigma and contested emotions: Personal experience and public perception of specific phobias. *Soc Sci Med* 2005; 61; 2155–2164.

69. Jason LA, Taylor RR, Plioplys S, Stepanek Z, Shlaes J. Evaluating attributions for an illness based upon the name: chronic fatigue syndrome, myalgic encephalopathy and Florence Nightingale disease. *Am J Community Psychol* 2002; 30(1): 133–148.

70. Asbring P, Narvanen AL. Women's experiences of stigma in relation to chronic fatigue syndrome and fibromyalgia. *Qual Health Res* 2002; 12(2):148–160.

71. MacLean G, Wessely S. Professional and popular views of chronic fatigue syndrome. *BMJ* 1994; 308(6931):776–777.

72. Farrell M, Lewis G. Discrimination on the grounds of diagnosis. *Br J Addict* 1990; 85(7):883–890.

73. Lennox N, Chaplin R. The psychiatric care of people with intellectual disabilities: the perceptions of consultant psychiatrists in Victoria. *Aust N Z J Psychiatry* 1996; 30(6):774–780.

74. Lennox N, Chaplin R. The psychiatric care of people with intellectual disabilities: the perceptions of trainee psychiatrists and psychiatric medical officers. *Aust N Z J Psychiatry* 1995; 29(4):632–637.

75. Department of Health. *Personality Disorder no Longer a Diagnosis of Exclusion: Policy implementation guidance for the development of services for people with personality disorder.* London: Department of Health; 2003.

76. Beales D. Continuing stigmatisation by psychiatrists. *Br J Psychiatry* 2001; 178:475.

77. Chaplin R. Psychiatrists can cause stigma too. *Br J Psychiatry* 2000; 177:467.

78. Corker E. Stigma and discrimination: the silent disease. *Int J Clin Pract* 2001; 55(2):138–140.

79. Corker E. Stigma caused by psychiatrists. *Br J Psychiatry* 2001; 178:379.

80. Broadhead WE. Misdiagnosis of depression. Physicians contribute to the stigmatization of mental illness. *Arch Fam Med* 1994; 3(4):319–320.

81. Hodges B, Inch C, Silver I. Improving the psychiatric knowledge, skills, and attitudes of primary care physicians, 1950–2000: a review. *Am J Psychiatry* 2001; 158(10):1579–1586.

82. Schlosberg A. Psychiatric stigma and mental health professionals (stigmatizers and destigmatizers). *Med Law* 1993; 12(3–5):409–416.

83. Pinfold V, Toulmin H, Thornicroft G, Huxley P, Farmer P, Graham T. Reducing psychiatric stigma and discrimination: evaluation of educational interventions in UK secondary schools. *Br J Psychiatry* 2003; 182:342–346.

84. Pinfold V, Huxley P, Thornicroft G, Farmer P, Toulmin H, Graham T. Reducing psychiatric stigma and discrimination – evaluating an educational intervention with the police force in England. *Soc Psychiatry Psychiatr Epidemiol* 2003; 38(6):337–344.

85. Jorm AF, Korten AE, Jacomb PA, Christensen H, Henderson S. Attitudes towards people with a mental disorder: a survey of the Australian public and health professionals. *Aust N Z J Psychiatry* 1999; 33(1):77–83.

86. Caldwell TM, Jorm AF. Mental health nurses' beliefs about interventions for schizophrenia and depression: a comparison with psychiatrists and the public. *Aust N Z J Psychiatry* 2000; 34(4):602–611.

87. Caldwell TM, Jorm AF. Mental health nurses' beliefs about likely outcomes for people with schizophrenia or depression: a comparison with the public and other healthcare professionals. *Aust N Z J Ment Health Nurs* 2001; 10(1):42–54.

88. Mukherjee R, Fialho A, Wijetunge A, Checinski K, Surgenor T. The stigmatisation of psychiatric illness: The attitudes of medical students and doctors in a London teaching hospital. *Psychiatr Bull* 2002; 26:178–181.

89. Mino Y, Yasuda N, Tsuda T, Shimodera S. Effects of a one-hour educational program on medical students' attitudes to mental illness. *Psychiatry Clin Neurosci* 2001; 55(5):501–507.

90. Mino Y, Yasuda N, Kanazawa S, Inoue S. Effects of medical education on attitudes towards mental illness among medical students: a five-year follow-up study. *Acta Med Okayama* 2000; 54(3):127–132.

91. Rodrigues CR. [Comparison of the attitudes of Brazilian and Spanish medical students towards mental disease]. *Actas Luso Esp Neurol Psiquiatr Cienc Afines* 1992; 20(1):30–41.

92. Filipcic I, Pavicic D, Filipcic A, Hotujac L, Begic D, Grubisin J *et al.* Attitudes of medical staff towards the psychiatric label 'schizophrenic patient' tested by an anti-stigma questionnaire. *Coll Antropol* 2003; 27(1):301–307.

93. Arikan K, Uysal O, Cetin G. Public awareness of the effectiveness of psychiatric treatment may reduce stigma. *Isr J Psychiatry Relat Sci* 1999; 36(2):95–99.

94. Arikan K, Uysal O. Emotional reactions to the mentally ill are positively influenced by personal acquaintance. *Isr J Psychiatry Relat Sci* 1999; 36(2):100–4.

95. Llerena A, Caceres M, Penas-LLedo E. Schizophrenia stigma among medical and nursing undergraduates. *Eur Psychiatry* 2002; 17(5):298.

96. Lyons M, Ziviani J. Stereotypes, stigma, and mental illness: learning from fieldwork experiences. *Am J Occup Ther* 1995; 49(10):1002–8.

97. Arkar H, Eker D. Influence of a 3-week psychiatric training programme on attitudes toward mental illness in medical students. *Soc Psychiatry Psychiatr Epidemiol* 1997; 32(3):171–176.

98. Roth D, Antony MM, Kerr KL, Downie F. Attitudes toward mental illness in medical students: does personal and professional experience with mental illness make a difference? *Med Educ* 2000; 34(3):234–6.

99. Sivakumar K, Wilkinson G, Toone BK, Greer S. Attitudes to psychiatry in doctors at the end of their first post-graduate year: two-year follow-up of a cohort of medical students. *Psychol Med* 1986; 16(2):457–460.

100. Sadow D, Ryder M, Webster D. Is education of health professionals encouraging stigma towards the mentally ill? *Journal of Mental Health* 2002; 11:657–665.

101. Fleming J, Szmukler GI. Attitudes of medical professionals towards patients with eating disorders. *Aust N Z J Psychiatry* 1992; 26(3):436–443.

102. Wiese HJ, Wilson JF, Jones RA, Neises M. Obesity stigma reduction in medical students. *Int J Obes Relat Metab Disord* 1992; 16(11):859–868.

103. Sierles FS, Taylor MA. Decline of U.S. medical student career choice of psychiatry and what to do about it. *Am J Psychiatry* 1995; 152(10):1416–1426.

104. Chikara F, Manley MR. Psychiatry in Zimbabwe. *Hosp Community Psychiatry* 1991; 42(9):943–947.

105. Corrigan P. *On the Stigma of Mental Illness.* Washington, DC: American Psychological Association; 2005.

106. Chamberlin J. User/consumer involvement in mental health service delivery. *Epidemiol Psichiatr Soc* 2005; 14; 10–14.

107. Chamberlin J. *On Our Own: Patient-controlled alternatives to the mental health system.* New York: McGraw-Hill; 1979.

108. Szmukler G, Appelbaum P. Treatment pressures, coercion and compulsion. In: Thornicroft G, Szmukler G, eds., *Textbook of Community Psychiatry*, pp. 529–544. Oxford: Oxford University Press; 2001.

109. Ucok A, Polat A, Sartorius N, Erkoc S, Atakli C. Attitudes of psychiatrists toward patients with schizophrenia. *Psychiatry Clin Neurosci* 2004; 58(1):89–91.

110. Lamontagne Y. The public image of psychiatrists. *Can J Psychiatry* 1990; 35(8):693–695.

111. Persaud R. Psychiatrists suffer from stigma too. *Psychiatr Bull* 2000; 24:284–285.

112. Fink PJ. Dealing with psychiatry's stigma. *Hosp Community Psychiatry* 1986; 37(8):814–818.

113. Gabbard GO, Gabbard K. Cinematic stereotypes contributing to the stigmatization of psychiatrists. In: Fink P, Tasman A, eds., *Stigma and Mental Illness*, pp. 113–126. Washington DC: American Psychiatric Press; 1992.

114. Clare A. Cinematic portrayals of psychiatrists. In: Crisp A, ed., *Every Family in the Land*, pp. 105–109. London: Royal Society of Medicine; 2004.

115. Byrne P. Imagining the nineties: mental illness stigma in contemporary cinema. In: Crisp AH, ed., *Every Family in the Land*, pp. 110–117. London: Royal Society of Medicine; 2004.

116. Repper J, Perkins R. *Social Inclusion and Recovery.* Edinburgh: Balliere Tindall; 2003.

117. Clark DC, Zeldow PB. Vicissitudes of depressed mood during four years of medical school. *JAMA* 1988; 260(17):2521–2528.

118. White R. Stigmatisation of mentally ill medical students. In: Crisp A, ed., *Every Family in the Land*, pp. 365–366. London: Royal Society of Medicine; 2004.

119. Lethem R. Mental illness in medical students and doctors: fitness to practice. In: Crisp A, ed., *Every Family in the Land*, 356–364. London: Royal Society of Medicine; 2004.

120. Fost N. Licensing boards and the stigma of mental illness. *JAMA* 1999; 281(7):606.

121. Chander K. Licensing boards and the stigma of mental illness. *JAMA* 1999; 281(7):606–607.

122. Gmel G. Help the helper-addiction research and the helper syndrome. *Addiction* 2004; 99(2):154–155.

123. Levinson MC, Druss BG, Dombrowski EA, Rosenheck RA. Barriers to primary medical care among patients at a community mental health center. *Psychiatr Serv* 2003; 54(8):1158–1160.

124. Desai MM, Rosenheck RA, Druss BG, Perlin JB. Mental disorders and quality of diabetes care in the veterans health administration. *Am J Psychiatry* 2002; 159(9):1584–1590.

125. Druss BG, Bradford WD, Rosenheck RA, Radford MJ, Krumholz HM. Quality of medical care and excess mortality in older patients with mental disorders. *Arch Gen Psychiatry* 2001; 58(6):565–572.

126. Druss BG. Cardiovascular procedures in patients with mental disorders. *JAMA* 2000; 283(24):3198–3199.

127. Jones DR, Macias C, Barreira PJ, Fisher WH, Hargreaves WA, Harding CM. Prevalence, severity, and co-occurrence of chronic physical health problems of persons with serious mental illness. *Psychiatr Serv* 2004; 55(11):1250–1257.

128. Phelan M, Stradins L, Morrison S. Physical health of people with severe mental illness. *BMJ* 2001; 322(7284):443–444.

129. McCreadie RG. Diet, smoking and cardiovascular risk in people with schizophrenia: descriptive study. *Br J Psychiatry* 2003; 183:534–539.

130. McCreadie RG, Stevens H, Henderson J, Hall D, McCaul R, Filik R *et al.* The dental health of people with schizophrenia. *Acta Psychiatr Scand* 2004; 110(4):306–310.

131. Rethink. *Running on Empty: Building momentum to improve wellbeing in severe mental illness.* London: Rethink; 2005.

132. Harris EC, Barraclough B. Excess mortality of mental disorder. *Br J Psychiatry* 1998; 173:11–53.

133. Mazeh D, Melamed Y, Barak Y. Emergency psychiatry: Treatment of referred psychiatric patients by general hospital emergency department physicians. *Psychiatr Serv* 2003; 54(9):1221–2, 1225.

134. Tehrani E, Krussel J, Borg L, Munk-Jorgensen P. Dropping out of psychiatric treatment: a prospective study of a first-admission cohort. *Acta Psychiatr Scand* 1996; 94(4):266–271.

135. Young AS, Grusky O, Jordan D, Belin TR. Routine outcome monitoring in a public mental health system: the impact of patients who leave care. *Psychiatr Serv* 2000; 51(1):85–91.

136. Killaspy H, Banerjee S, King M, Lloyd M. Prospective controlled study of psychiatric outpatient non-attendance. Characteristics and outcome. *Br J Psychiatry* 2000; 176:160–165.

137. Edlund MJ, Wang PS, Berglund PA, Katz SJ, Lin E, Kessler RC. Dropping out of mental health treatment: patterns and predictors among epidemiological survey respondents in the United States and Ontario. *Am J Psychiatry* 2002; 159(5):845–851.

138. Rossi A, Amaddeo F, Bisoffi G, Ruggeri M, Thornicroft G, Tansella M. Dropping out of care: inappropriate terminations of contact with community-based psychiatric services. *Br J Psychiatry* 2002; 181(4):331–338.

139. Edlund MJ, Wang PS, Berglund PA, Katz SJ, Lin E, Kessler RC. Dropping out of mental health treatment: patterns and predictors among epidemiological survey respondents in the United States and Ontario. *Am J Psychiatry* 2002; 159(5):845–51.

140. Parkman S, Davies S, Leese M, Phelan M, Thornicroft G. Ethnic differences in satisfaction with mental health services among representative people with psychosis in south London: PRiSM study 4. *Br J Psychiatry* 1997; 171:260–264.

141. Sirey JA, Meyers BS, Bruce ML, Alexopoulos GS, Perlick DA, Raue P. Predictors of antidepressant prescription and early use among depressed outpatients. *Am J Psychiatry* 1999; 156(5):690–696.

142. Sirey JA, Bruce ML, Alexopoulos GS, Perlick DA, Friedman SJ, Meyers BS. Stigma as a barrier to recovery: Perceived stigma and patient-rated severity of illness as predictors of antidepressant drug adherence. *Psychiatr Serv* 2001; 52(12):1615–20.

143. Sirey JA, Bruce ML, Alexopoulos GS, Perlick DA, Raue P, Friedman SJ *et al.* Perceived stigma as a predictor of treatment discontinuation in young and older outpatients with depression. *Am J Psychiatry* 2001; 158(3):479–481.

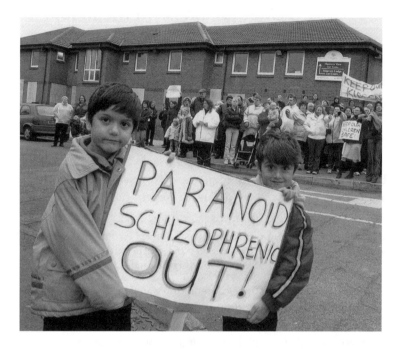

Child protestors outside the former Manvers Lodge Old Age People's Home in Highwoods Road, Mexborough, near Doncaster, Yorkshire, joining the protest against turning it into a rehabilitation unit for people with mental illness, 2004.
Courtesy of Sheffield Newspapers Ltd.

Chapter 6 Profiting from prejudice

Mental illness in the media

Fury over home for mentally ill. Residents draw up battle lines over plan for
rehabilitation unit ... Community campaigners are fighting plans to house
mental patients next to a Doncaster primary school ... Young protestors
Adam and Daniel Khan, aged six and five, join the protest (holding a placard
saying 'PARANOID SCHIZOPHRENIC OUT!').[1]

Our popular images of madness are both long-standing and remarkably
stable.[2] One of the best established patterns is to refer to people with mental
illnesses as the 'polar opposites'[3] of 'us'. In Western culture, for example,

[a] polar antiworld of human types has been developed, populated by the
Black, the Jew, the Gypsy, the madman among others ... its source lies in the
sense of distance between the perceiver and the perceived ... a distance
imposed by the perceiver based on the anxiety generated by his perception.[3]

This chapter will discuss these contemporary anxieties, and how they shape
the way mental illnesses are portrayed in films, in the broadcast and in the
print media.

Most people gather what they know about mental illnesses either from
personal contact with people with such conditions, or from the mass
media.[4, 5] Remarkably little is formally taught on mental disorders in any
part of the educational system.[6] Nevertheless, contact with people with mental
illness is common. A nationwide representative survey of almost 2000 people
in the UK asked 'Do you know someone with mental illness?', and 52 per cent
said yes. When the survey was repeated in 2003 the question was rephrased to
ask about seven specific diagnoses, and this time 77 per cent said that they
knew at least one person with a specific mental disorder.[7] But even when we
have direct personal contact with people with mental illness, the way we
interpret these experiences is heavily influenced by three things: our background *knowledge* of what these diagnoses mean, our *attitudes* on what
emotional reactions toward mentally ill people are socially acceptable, and
our understanding of what types of *behaviour* towards people with mental
illness are socially allowed. The main flows of information to us are through
the channels of the mass media,[8] so the content of these streams of information (on knowledge, attitudes and behaviour) are of the utmost importance.

Newspaper portrayals of mental illness

What information predominates in newspaper coverage about mental illness, and what messages does this convey? There is now strong and consistent evidence to help us answer this.[9] A careful evaluation of one month's stories about mental illness in newspapers throughout New Zealand found 600 items.[10] Most (94 per cent) were news items or editorials, and the remainder were letters, cartoons or advertisements. In results closely similar to an earlier Australian study,[11] more than half of all the items depicted the mentally ill person as dangerous,[10] and the key themes that emerged were danger to others (61 per cent), criminality (47 per cent), unpredictability (24 per cent) and danger to self (20 per cent). Most of these newspaper stories used undifferentiated terms such as 'psychiatric patient' or 'mentally ill'. The authors concluded that 'print media portrayals are negative, exaggerated and do not reflect the reality of most people with mental illness'.[10, 12]

'Maniac killed twin sisters.'
Front page headline, *London Evening Standard*, 18 April 2005
(England)

This New Zealand report found that fewer than five per cent of the articles were personal stories or in-depth accounts as told directly by the person concerned. By comparison, among the 29 personal accounts by people with mental illness the tables were turned: most (59 per cent) were positive stories, only seven per cent referred to a risk to others and none mentioned criminality.[10] Of all the items assessed, very few items (less than one per cent) quoted the person concerned in their own words. Where this did happen, the key themes were ordinariness, and overcoming adversity, particularly that associated with stigma. The authors of this study particularly emphasized that 'these speakers provided accessible and recognizably human self-portrayals. That finding intensifies our concern that most researchers appear to be unaware that these consumer voices are largely absent from mass media depictions of mental illnesses.'[13]

'Knife maniac freed to kill. Mental patient ran amok in the park.'
Front page headline, *Daily Mail*, 26 February 2005 (England)

In Canada very similar results have been found. The content of a random selection of items in eight major Canadian newspapers was compared with that of two specialized mental health publications which did not have a mass circulation.[14] The newspapers portrayed mental illness 'in a manner which could be described as essentially pejorative'. There was also an unexpected finding: the newspapers presented more favourable images for community-based mental health services than for traditional asylums.

A slightly different approach was taken in an investigation of nine national newspapers in the UK. All health-related items were identified, and the coverage of the mental health and physical health items was compared.[15] The authors tested their hypothesis that newspaper coverage of psychiatric issues would be more negative than for general medical topics. This was confirmed: 64 per cent of psychiatric stories were negative compared with 46 per cent of general medical pieces. There were also five times more articles about physical than about mental illnesses. Their analysis suggested that 'negative articles about medicine tended to describe *bad doctors*, whereas negative articles on psychiatry tended to describe *bad patients*'.[15] On the other hand, one stereotype was not supported: broadsheet ('quality') newspapers were about five times more likely to be critical of psychiatry than of medicine, the same as for the tabloid ('popular') newspapers. Another UK newspaper clipping survey produced comparable results, and also discovered that almost a half of tabloid stories covering mental illness included pejorative terms such as 'nutter' or 'looney'.[16]

> I grew up on a pre-war council estate in Wimbledon in the 1950s. Illness, other than a cold or flu, or illness afflicting the elderly like gout, etc., was hardly spoken about. Madness and mental illness happened in the tabloids all of the time, often to sex perverts and murderers. Those 'nutters' that were, rightly or wrongly, locked away from society.
>
> Paul

In the USA, over 3000 newspaper stories about mental illness in 2002 were categorized. Again they found that most often the stories focused on dangerousness and violence, often in front page stories (39 per cent), and less often did they refer to treatment (14 per cent) or to recovery (4 per cent). A substantial minority of items (20 per cent) referred to advocacy, such the shortage of investment in mental health care, the lack of good-quality housing, or the goal of insurance parity. Interestingly this systematic tendency to highlight violence above all other aspects of mental illness was described by the authors as 'structural discrimination',[17] which we shall return to in Chapters 9 and 11. They also concluded that there is a stunning lack of accurate information about mental illnesses in the public domain.

Such widespread ignorance was reinforced by another survey of US newspapers, which compared references to cancer and schizophrenia. Among nearly 2000 articles, cancer stories were used in a metaphorical (rather than literal) way in only 1 per cent of articles, compared with 28 per cent of articles about schizophrenia.[18]

Much less research has been conducted on magazines and popular periodicals than on newspapers. One such survey looked at articles about mental health which were indexed in the *Readers' Guide to Periodical Literature* in the

USA between 1965 and 1988. Over this period the number of articles about mental illness increased significantly, particularly those describing specific disorders, and the article headings tended to use less and less stigmatising terms.[4] When it came to schizophrenia, however, the picture was reversed. Such stories continued to focus most upon hallucinations and delusions. Only a few of these pieces were included in general circulation magazines, and misconceptions about schizophrenia were rarely addressed.[19]

'Violent, mad. So Docs set him free. New "Community Care" scandal.'
The Sun, 26 February 2005 (England)

In fact mental illness is often described as an undifferentiated term. Most magazine articles do not use particular diagnostic categories. An American report investigated how one specific condition, obsessive compulsive disorder, was reported in magazines over a fifteen year period.[20] About a third of the 107 articles found described this diagnosis directly and the reports were reasonably accurate. Most of the remaining articles were about 'obsessive compulsive behaviour' and focused on the 'stalking' of famous people by 'obsessed fans',[21] so that these stories assisted both understanding and misunderstanding at the same time.

Occasionally a well-publicized violent incident can be assessed for its impact on public opinion. A national survey on public attitudes to people with mental illness took place just before Michael Ryan killed 15 people in Hungerford in the British country of Berkshire. The survey was repeated, again with a national sample of almost 1000 members of the general public. On each occasion about a third agreed that mentally ill people are likely to be violent. When put the other way, there was a significant increase after the event in the number of people who agreed that people who commit horrific crimes are likely to be mentally ill. This difference had reduced again six months later. Notably, newspaper reports of these murders suggested that Michael Ryan was mentally ill, although no clear evidence of this was pre-sented. The conclusions of this study were that 'either the Hungerford mas-sacre, or the media account of it, strengthened the public view of extreme violence as a product of mental illness'.[22]

A German study looked at how two violent attacks by people with mental illness upon prominent politicians were reported in the newspapers, and their influence on public attitudes.[23] In a sequence of three public opinion surveys, the first was carried out before either attack, the second survey after the first incident, and the last survey after the second violent act. A clear-cut pattern emerged. The authors showed that over the two-year period there was significant deterioration in 'social distance' towards people with schizophrenia, but not towards those with depression. This included, for example, greater reluctance to let a room to a person with a diagnosis of schizophrenia, to help such a person find a job, or to let them marry into the family. Two years later there was some improvement in this aversion among the general public, but it had not returned to the baseline level. The main conclusion reached was: 'it is our contention that the relationship between the two violent attacks and the development in attitudes towards the schizophrenically ill is not only a temporal, but also a causal one'.[23]

Subsequent work developed this theme and showed that the largest-circulation German tabloid newspaper, called *BILD-Zeitung*, contained very little information on mental illnesses, which featured in fewer than 1 per cent of its articles.[24] Of these, most (51 per cent) referred to links between crime and mental illness, overshadowing by far the second most common category about new types of treatment (18 per cent of stories). The findings were stark: the repeated tendency of reporters and editors was to concentrate upon forensic cases, spectacular events, 'crime stories' and 'bad news'.[25] It concluded, 'there is no doubt about the media's crucial influence in the production of stereotypical images. This implies, however, that the media can also be a powerful vehicle for changing stigmatising representations of mental illness.'[24]

Despite this trend to negative coverage, most of these studies also indicate that a modest minority of press reports are reasonably accurate or do report positive aspects of mental illness. Commonly these are stories of celebrities who have experienced some form of mental illness. For example:

> Self-harm disclosure. Olympic winner Kelly Holmes tells of hidden scars. Double-gold winning Olympic athlete Dame Kelly Holmes has revealed how she slashed her body with scissors just a year before she triumphed at the Athens games.
>
> (*The Guardian*, 30 May 2005, England).
>
> Less often such stories will focus on human rights issues, such as Ashes amid dust tell of ignored lives, deaths. 3489 urns of mental patients in Oregon. The urns hold the ashes of mental patients who died here from the late 1880s to the mid 1970s. The remains were unclaimed by families who had long abandoned their relatives, both when they were alive and after they were dead.
>
> (*Chicago Tribune*, 18 March 2005, USA)

Less often still do newspaper stories include features about the personal experiences of people with mental illness and their families. One such report was published in Canada: 'Schizophrenia: two steps forward, one step back. As the realities become better understood, the stigma has lessened. But it hasn't disappeared. My first memory of my father is meeting him behind bars ...' (*Vancouver Sun*, 4 December. 2004). It is therefore misleading to think that there is a uniformly negative coverage of mental illness in the print media.

Evens so, taken together these findings do all point in the same direction: newspaper coverage of mental illness tends to be short of accurate and detailed content, emphasizes violence over all other aspects of mental illness, and reinforces prejudices against people with mental illness. In short, there is 'ample evidence for a distorted presentation of mentally ill people in newspapers'.[26]

> Newspapers label us all mad and dangerous, the only person I'm a danger to when ill is myself. But the stigma of the newspapers has me down as an axe murderer because of my illness. I've never even hurt a fly let alone another person.
>
> Maria

Television

Are the representations of mental illness on television any different from those in newspapers, and is their impact more or less? There have been several studies of these questions, although only in more economically developed countries. They present compelling evidence. In one of the most detailed of these evaluations, the Glasgow Media Group in Scotland analysed one month's output for national and local television, the press and magazines, including all content from factual news through to cartoons.[27] Altogether 570 items were found, of which 85 per cent were non-fictional. Among all the extracts, those which reported harm to others were by far the most common (66 per cent), followed by treatment/advice/recovery (18 per cent), harm to self (12 per cent), comic images (2 per cent) and criticisms of accepted definitions of mental illness (2 per cent). Fictional representations were slightly different from the overall pattern, more often including comic images (16 per cent) and less often mentioning self-harm (7 per cent), but still paying most attention to harm to others (60 per cent). The authors summarized by saying that 'the bulk of media content situates mental illness in a context of violence and harm ... such representations can clearly affect audiences'.[27]

Such a predominant concern with violence is found repeatedly in such studies. A content analysis of prime-time television in the USA concluded that mentally ill characters were nearly 10 times more violent than the general population of television characters, and 10 to 20 times more violent (during a two week sample) than the mentally ill in the US population (over the course of an entire year). The mentally ill on television were also judged to have a negative impact on society.[28]

A German national survey interviewed over 5000 members of the general public, asking about attitudes towards people with mental illness, and about 'consumption' of television and newspapers. Greater social distance (a wish to avoid contact with mentally ill people) was found for people who watched more television, were older, had a lower level of education, and who had less direct personal contact with people with mental illness.[29]

There is a predictable uniformity to the television images of mental illness across different countries.[30] In the US 73 per cent of peak-time television characters with mental illness were shown as violent individuals.[31,32] Almost identically, in prime-time television dramas in New Zealand three quarters of the mentally ill characters were portrayed as physically violent, as well as 'simple or lacking in comprehension and appearing lost, unpredictable, un-productive, asocial, vulnerable, dangerous to self or others because of incompetent behaviours, untrustworthy, and social outcasts.'[33]

Overall it seems that the pattern we saw in newspaper coverage, that between a half and three-quarters of all items about mental illness focus solely on violence, is repeated in television programmes. Does this matter? Do the general public distinguish 'media stories' from their understanding of the reality of mental illness, often based upon direct contact with people with mental illness?

Television pictures of what mental illnesses are, and what they mean, are important, because this medium is the main sources of information about mental illness for most people. Work in the USA found that 87 per cent of people said that television was one of their main sources of information, compared with 51 per cent from friends and 29 per cent from medical professionals.[34] What happens when media imagery and personal experience of people with mental illness do not coincide? Very little has been written about this, but one study unexpectedly found that the media images would predominate over a person's own direct experience.[35] Television therefore does matter.

Films

Are films also significant? In the most complete assessment of how 'madness' is portrayed in films, many hundreds of productions over a decade were carefully analysed.[36] The author of this compendium came to the conclusion that:

> Media portrayals are inaccurate. They depict people with mental illness as different, dangerous and laughable. They misuse or casually use psychiatric terms. Media depictions of mental illness ... do have important and wide-ranging consequences for the lives of those with mental illness and for the ways people act towards others with psychiatric disorders. People learn about mental illnesses from what they see and hear in the mass media.[36]

The study went on to see whether watching such films had any impact on behaviour, and found that people who had seen a film showing a violent person with a mental illness were later more likely to speak of their concerns about mentally ill people and to be less in favour of community care, compared with people who had seen a control film unrelated to mental illness.[37]

To take one particular example, German researchers looked at the impact of watching the film *The White Noise*. The synopsis of the film is:

> The White Noise of the title refers to a phenomenon known as EVP (Electronic Voice Phenomena). Listen carefully, believers will tell you, and in amidst the white noise of a detuned radio you might hear voices … and in amidst the white noise of a detuned television, you might see faces. These, they'll tell you, are the voices and faces of the dead.

A film audience were assessed for their attitudes towards people with schizophrenia before and after watching the film. Predictably, after seeing the film negative stereotypes were reinforced and social distance was increased.[38]

As we found with newspapers and television, although the imagery used in films is predominantly focused on violence, other themes do also enter the frame.[39] Another examination of film themes identified several common patterns that conformed to one of the following stereotypes: 'rebellious free spirit, homicidal maniac, seductress, enlightened member of society, narcissistic parasite, and zoo specimen'.[40] As with the other media, there are exceptions. While 'psychokiller' is the dominant character, minor parts are also played by roles showing 'humour', 'indulgence and pretence', and 'the poor things'.[41] To sum up what is known about the content and the impact of films, the message is essentially the same as what we saw earlier about newspapers and television: a spotlight upon violence and, almost offstage, small roles for treatment and care[42] and for human rights issues.[43]

Images of mental health staff

If people with mental illness fare poorly in their media portrayals, do mental health staff do any better? One reviewer puts the essence of the psychiatrist as portrayed in the media in this way:

> omnipotent and useless, progressive and reactionary, compassionate and destructive, perceptive and blind … the psychiatrist as manipulator, as priest, as pervert, as lecher, as stricken, tortured soul … the public's perception of the psychiatrist is formed at second hand.[44]

As a psychiatrist myself, all this seems a long way from the often mundane practice of most psychiatrists![45]

Even if we are subjected to mistaken identity, are we respected as authoritative sources of information by journalists? The evidence here is also dire. In Auckland, New Zealand lay members of the public were compared with psychiatrists as sources for news stories. Tellingly, people with mental illness themselves were not treated as credible sources of information about their own conditions.[46] The results were that the depictions of mental illness were primarily those of the journalists, using 'relatively standard, predictable narratives, discourses and preferred images … the stories rely on commonsense understandings about mental illness as unpredictable and violent as the basis for a preferred or obvious reading'.[46] In other words the stories were deliberately designed to be consistent with (and so to reinforce) pre-existing popular 'common-sense' views of mental illness. The psychiatrists' more postive reports made little difference to the overall negative slant of these stories. What of nurses? Despite the prominence and romanticization of general nurses in the broadcast media, mental health nurses are notably absent from the public eye, except when they misuse their position of professional trust.[47–50] *'Mental illness is seen in such a negative way that it should be a four-letter word with all the connotations they conjure up'* (Maria).

Children's programmes

If adults are usually offered information by the print and broadcast media that conforms with their existing and negative views,[51] are children spared such a diet? The research group in Auckland have also examined these questions. They analysed all children's television programmes during a typical week on two national channels. They found 128 episodes of 46 programmes, of which 60 per cent were produced in the USA.[52] Interestingly, almost a half (46 per cent) of all the episodes contained some reference to mental illness, especially in cartoons. They found that the vocabulary used was *'predominantly negative … fundamentally disrespectful. The characters were typically losing control, constantly engaged in illogical and irrational actions',* and were *'stereotypically and blatantly negative, and served as objects of amusement, derision or fear'.*[52]

Evaluations of children's programmes shown in the USA have produced almost identical results. They also discovered that images and references to mental illnesses were very common in the children's media, were largely negative, and portrayed characters with mental illness as unattractive, violent and criminal. These images were 'typically used to disparage and ridicule'.[53] References were especially common in children's films, two thirds of which had characters with features of mental illness, and most of these (67 per cent) depicted them as violent.[54]

More specifically, a Canadian study looked at Disney animated films for children and found that this trend was even more exaggerated: 85 per cent contained verbal references to mental illness and they were mainly used to 'set apart and denigrate' the characters.[55] It therefore appears that the stereotypes used in children's television programmes are essentially the same as in adult-orientated productions, but, if anything, the links made between mental illness and violence are even more common in programmes made for children.

> Everybody has a right to an opinion but nobody in this world has a right to judge. Nobody. Now why, because people have mental health problems, are they nutters? You know the names we are called, and we don't get help. We don't get the help that the others with no mental health history get. We really don't.
>
> Sandra

Why do the media trade in stereotypes?

As we shall see in Chapter 7, the extent to which public concerns and media representations about mental illness highlight violence far exceeds the real level of risk posed by mentally ill people. So why do the media trade in stereotypes? To pursue this question the Glasgow Media Group in Scotland conducted detailed interviews with 15 senior production staff including executive producers, story-editors, script editors, and writers for factual and fictional television programmes in the UK.[56] The results were particularly revealing. The researcher found that:

> What we ultimately see on our television screens is the outcome of a complex negotiation process ... Every representation of mental illness is, therefore, a product based on input from a number of individuals throughout the broadcast hierarchy ... the key factor which underpins all of these concerns is the need to attract and maintain audiences.

Most programmes see their remit as focusing firmly upon entertainment rather than education.[57] News and features emphasize the newsworthy rather than the worthy. The 'news values' that guide the selection of content include: novelty, universality, topicality, impact and controversy. These values shape editor's snap decisions about what is news and what is not. News production is now done continuously and with no time for reflection. Stereotypes are therefore enormously useful and they short-circuit the need to spend time understanding a topic. They simply follow a rapid tried and tested formula which is known to work commercially. Since the media largely consist of commercial businesses, there are powerful incentives to roll out the clichés and to play to the prejudices of their audience - and very few disincentives.[17] Since most news editors know no more about mental illness than the average member of the public, perhaps it should come as no surprise that people with mental illness get a raw deal from the media.

In terms of editorial judgement, the need for perceived realism is constantly balanced against the needs of the audience, as perceived by the programme producers. Therefore the key guiding values are 'entertainment and acceptability to audiences'.[56] Paradoxically, evidence can be seen in this context as contaminating, and writers may prefer to rely on the 'psychological truth' of a situation or to 'go for the truth of the feelings'.[56] One way to present such truths is to concentrate the storyline so as to extract the maximum possible drama, including key dramatic 'televisual' moments, along with their resolutions, and in doing so to maintain audience tension and pleasure.

More specifically in relation to mental illness, an important question is 'who speaks?' As we saw earlier in considering newspapers, direct statements by people with mental illnesses are relatively rare on television, and spokespersons when they do appear are likely to have less disabling types of mental illness. It is uncommon, for example, to see a person with a diagnosis of schizophrenia, whether well or unwell, discussing the condition in his or her own words in a television programme.[58] More often a voice-over paraphrases their comments. This is consistent with the tendency for people with mental illness, when not shown as violent predators,[59] to be allocated to the category of 'helpless victim'. The simplified allocation to a single stereotypical category is far more common that the portrayal of complexity. Further, this raises 'ethical questions about the effect of featuring people in a way which makes them feel that TV was interested in them only when they were behaving "oddly" '.[56]

In other words, although the subjects of programmes seek to advance their own message and agenda, 'journalists organise their materials to present the appearance of objectivity, while giving priority to newsworthy elements understood to attract readers ... which are conflict and deviance'.[46] The active use of stereotypes of mental illness is therefore common in such journalistic practices and reflects the production values that such decisions are based upon. Given time pressure, conflicting material is avoided in the name of economy. The third key feature that allows stereotypes to persist is the mixing of authority and opinion, for example through editorialized voice-overs, to avoid the direct speech of those portrayed offering any dissonant messages to the main common-sense themes.[46] Although in a sense 'stigmatization depends on an audience whose members sit in judgement of a person or group of persons',[60] in fact this judgement has already been made by those creating the programme. The audience role is simply silent confirmation.

> A lack of understanding is what lies beneath stigma. Stigma will always exist by the very nature of the make up of society. No one can eradicate it completely. But does this mean that we should not try? It should not be the case that people have to shelter themselves from the stigma of society. I choose not to expose myself to it, and make myself more vulnerable. I welcome those who stand up and be

counted, warts and all, and who are proud of who they are. It takes a lot of courage to do this and makes the world a far more interesting place.

Martina

The techniques used in television, for example, to directly and indirectly convey such common-sense themes are carefully coordinated. A New Zealand team, for example, analysed a prime-time television drama to dissect the production methods used. Nine devices were identified: appearance, music and sound effects, lighting, language, inter-cutting, jump-cutting, point-of-view shots, horror story conventions, and so-called 'intertextuality' (using references to other programmes or films, such as images or sounds from *Psycho*). Together, all of these pointed unambiguously to the dangerousness of people receiving care in the community for a mental illness. As we shall see in Chapter 7, these both conveyed an apparently factual message of danger linked to mental illness, and closely intertwined with this was a layer of emotional meaning, intended to produce fear and anxiety in the viewer.[61] This suggests that those wishing to use television to promote different representations of mental illness need to have a sophisticated understanding of how the production techniques can be harnessed to produce the intended reactions in the viewer.

I think people are frightened by 'the mind illness' whereas 'physical illness' is there to be seen.

Linda

Do media representations of mental illnesses matter?

Even if we agree that how mental illnesses are shown in the print and broadcast media are partial, dramatic and unfavourable, does this really matter? Since up to three quarters of us know someone with a mental illness, can we not distinguish reality from what we see in the cinema and from what we read in the newspapers?

It seems that media representations do matter and do play an active part in shaping and sustaining what mental illness means in our cultures.[36] This is, first of all, because such meanings persist.[23] In the newspaper coverage of the Hungerford killings referred to earlier in this chapter, for example, more hostile public views about mental illness were evident six months after these events,[22] and the same trend has been found after other such events.[62,37]

To an extraordinary extent many members of the public are able to mimic stories about mental illness which mirror what they have seen in the mass media. The Glasgow Media Group showed this in a remarkable exercise. Focus groups, which were representative of the general population, were organised in the West of Scotland. Within groups of two or three people, members were asked to write a news report (after being given only its headline) or the dialogue for a fictional programme, such as a soap opera.[63] This was deliberately designed as a group exercise in which ideas can be expressed in an informal way. Individuals were subsequently interviewed in detail about the themes which emerged. The stories and dialogue which they produced bore an uncanny resemblance to actual news reports and paralleled 'exactly the demonology of popular media', reproducing 'the phrasing of the tabloids with apparent ease'.[63] They found that the way real news stories were understood was by referring to elements derived from fictional sources, particularly dramatic and widely seen feature films. In this way fiction was used to interpret facts.

Nevertheless the findings of the more detailed interviews also suggested that these processes are neither simple nor straightforward. About a quarter of those involved, for example, said that the news stories they had seen made them both more fearful *and* more sympathetic towards mentally ill people.[63] The authors concluded that although television may be watched by individuals alone, nevertheless television-viewing should be seen as a communal activity because the meanings of programmes depended upon collective discussion. Such meanings are designed, for some programmes, to 'exploit deep anxieties about security, the unknown and the unpredictable in what is seen as a very frightening world'.[63] The Glasgow Media Group drew clear conclusions about the significance of their findings: 'we can see the media as a crucial variable, not merely for reinforcement, but as a powerful influence in the development of beliefs, attitudes and emotional response in this key area of social life'.

So media images do matter.[64, 65] They are a part of the everyday experience of all who read newspapers, listen to radio, or watch television or films. They are one of most potent forces in what we shall consider in Chapter 11 as 'structural discrimination' against people with mental illness.[17, 66]

References

1. Kessen D. Fury over home for mentally ill. *The Star (Sheffield and Doncaster)* 2004; 11 November:4.
2. Roback AA, Kiernan T. *Pictorial History of Psychology and Psychiatry.* New York: Philosophical Library; 1969.
3. Gilman SL. *Seeing the Insane.* Wiley: New York; 1982.
4. Wahl OF, Kaye AL. Mental illness topics in popular periodicals. *Community Ment Health J* 1992; 28(1):21–28.
5. Borinstein AB. Public attitudes toward persons with mental illness. *Health Aff (Millwood)* 1992; 11(3):186–196.

6. Pinfold V, Toulmin H, Thornicroft G, Huxley P, Farmer P, Graham T. Reducing psychiatric stigma and discrimination: evaluation of educational interventions in UK secondary schools. *Br J Psychiatry* 2003; 182:342–346.

7. Crisp A, Gelder MG, Goddard E, Meltzer H. Stigmatization of people with mental illnesses: a follow-up study within the Changing Minds campaign of the Royal College of Psychiatrists. *World Psychiatry* 2005; 4:106–113.

8. Philo G. *Media and Mental Distress.* London: Longman; 1996.

9. Nunnally JC. *Popular Conceptions of Mental Health.* New York: Holt, Rinehart &Winston; 1961.

10. Coverdale J, Nairn R, Claasen D. Depictions of mental illness in print media: a prospective national sample. *Aust N Z J Psychiatry* 2002; 36(5):697–700.

11. Williams M, Taylor J. Mental illness: Media perpetuation of stigma. *Contemporary Nurse* 1995; 4:41–46.

12. Nairn R, Coverdale J, Claasen D. From source material to news story in New Zealand print media: a prospective study of the stigmatizing processes in depicting mental illness. *Aust N Z J Psychiatry* 2001; 35(5):654–659.

13. Nairn RG, Coverdale JH. People never see us living well: an appraisal of the personal stories about mental illness in a prospective print media sample. *Aust N Z J Psychiatry* 2005; 39(4):281–287.

14. Day DM, Page S. Portrayal of mental illness in Canadian newspapers. *Can J Psychiatry* 1986; 31(9):813–817.

15. Lawrie SM. Newspaper coverage of psychiatric and physical illness. *Psychiatr Bull* 2000; 24:104–106.

16. Ward G. *Mental Health and the National Press.* London: Health Education Authority; 1997.

17. Corrigan PW, Watson AC, Gracia G, Slopen N, Rasinski K, Hall LL. Newspaper stories as measures of structural stigma. *Psychiatr Serv* 2005; 56(5):551–556.

18. Duckworth K, Halpern JH, Schutt RK, Gillespie C. Use of schizophrenia as a metaphor in US newspapers. *Psychiatr Serv* 2003; 54(10):1402–1404.

19. Wahl OF, Borostovik L, Rieppi R. Schizophrenia in popular periodicals. *Community Ment Health J* 1995; 31(3):239–248.

20. Wahl OF. Obsessive-compulsive disorder in popular magazines. *Community Ment Health J* 2000; 36(3):307–312.

21. Wahl OF. Obsessive-compulsive disorder in popular magazines. *Community Ment Health J* 2000; 36(3):307–312.

22. Appleby L, Wessely S. Public attitudes to mental illness: the influence of the Hungerford massacre. *Med Sci Law* 1988; 28(4):291–295.

23. Angermeyer MC, Matschinger H. The effect of violent attacks by schizophrenic persons on the attitude of the public towards the mentally ill. *Soc Sci Med* 1996; 43(12):1721–1728.

24. Angermeyer MC, Schulze B. Reinforcing stereotypes: how the focus on forensic cases in news reporting may influence public attitudes towards the mentally ill. *Int J Law Psychiatry* 2001; 24(4–5):469–486.

25. Steadman HJ, Cocozza JJ. Public perceptions of the criminally insane. *Hosp Community Psychiatry* 1978; 29(7):457–459.

26. Angermeyer MC, Dietrich S, Pott D, Matschinger H. Media consumption and desire for social distance towards people with schizophrenia. *Eur Psychiatry* 2005; 20(3):246–250.

27. Philo G, McLaughlin G, Henderson L. Media content. In: Philo G, ed., *Media and Mental Distress,* pp. 45–81. London: Longman; 1996.

28. Diefenbach DL. The portrayal of mental illness on prime-time television. *Journal of Community Psychology* 1998;(3):289–302.

29. Angermeyer MC, Dietrich S, Pott D, Matschinger H. Media consumption and desire for social distance towards people with schizophrenia. *Eur Psychiatry* 2005; 20(3):246–250.

30. Rose D. Television, madness and community care. *Journal of Community and Applied Social Psychology* 1998; 8(213):228.

31. Gerbner G. *Media Stereotypes of Mental Illness, their Role in Promoting Stigma, and Advocacy Efforts to Overcome such Stereotypes and Stigma.* Bethesda, Maryland: Centre for Mental Health Services, US Department of Health and Human Services; 1990.

32. Signorielli N. The stigma of mental illness on television. *Journal of Broadcasting and Electronic Media* 1989; 33:325–331.

33. Wilson C, Nairn R, Coverdale J, Panapa A. Mental illness depictions in prime-time drama: identifying the discursive resources. *Aust N Z J Psychiatry* 1999; 33(2):232–239.

34. Yankelovich D. *Public Attitudes Toward People With Chronic Mental Illness: Final report.* Princeton, New Jersey: Robert Wood Johnson Foundation; 1990.

35. Philo G, Henderson L, McLaughlin G. *Mass Media Representation of Mental Health/Illness.* Report for the Health Education Board for Scotland. Glasgow: Glasgow University; 1993.

36. Wahl O. *Media Madness.* New Brunswick, New Jersey: Rutgers University Press; 1995.

37. Wahl OF, Lefkowits JY. Impact of a television film on attitudes toward mental illness. *Am J Community Psychol* 1989; 17(4):521–528.

38. Baumann A, Zaeske H, Gaebel W. [The image of people with mental illness in movies: effects on beliefs, attitudes and social distance, considering as example the movie 'The white noise']. *Psychiatr Prax* 2003; 30(7):372–378.

39. Hyler SE. DSM-III at the cinema: madness in the movies. *Compr Psychiatry* 1988; 29(2):195–206.

40. Hyler SE, Gabbard GO, Schneider I. Homicidal maniacs and narcissistic parasites: stigmatization of mentally ill persons in the movies. *Hosp Community Psychiatry* 1991; 42(10):1044–1048.

41. Byrne.P. Imagining the nineties: mental illness stigma in contemporary cinema. In: Crisp AH, ed., *Every Family in the Land*, pp. 110–117. London: Royal Society of Medicine; 2004.

42. Berlin FS, Malin HM. Media distortion of the public's perception of recidivism and psychiatric rehabilitation. *Am J Psychiatry* 1991; 148(11):1572–1576.

43. Sayce L. *From Psychiatric Patient to Citizen. Overcoming discrimination and social exclusion.* Basingstoke: Palgrave; 2000.

44. Clare A. Cinematic portrayals of psychiatrists. In: Crisp A, ed., *Every Family in the Land*, pp. 105–109. London: Royal Society of Medicine; 2004.

45. Schneider I. The theory and practice of movie psychiatry. *Am J Psychiatry* 1987; 144:996–1002.

46. Nairn R. Does the use of psychiatrists as sources of information improve media depictions of mental illness? A pilot study. *Aust N Z J Psychiatry* 1999; 33:583–589.

47. Case 7: breach of confidentiality. Psychiatric nurse talks about a client to a newspaper and radio. *Br J Nurs* 1999; 8(12):767.

48. Castledine G. Professional misconduct case studies. Case 17: Respecting the dignity of patients. Nurse who showed a video film containing dubious material. *Br J Nurs* 1999; 8(22):1482.

49. Castledine G. Nurse who made a video of herself mocking patients. *Br J Nurs* 2002; 11(12):798.

50. Kalisch PA, Kalisch BJ. Psychiatric nurses and the press: a troubled relationship. *Perspect Psychiatr Care* 1984; 22(1):5–15.

51. Cutcliffe JR, Hannigan B. Mass media, 'monsters' and mental health clients: the need for increased lobbying. *J Psychiatr Ment Health Nurs* 2001; 8(4):315–321.

52. Wilson C, Nairn R, Coverdale J, Panapa A. How mental illness is portrayed in children's television. A prospective study. *Br J Psychiatry* 2000; 176:440–443.

53. Wahl OF. Depictions of mental illness in children's media. *Journal of Mental Health* 2003; 12(3):249–258.

54. Wahl O. Mental illness depiction in children's films. *Journal of Community Psychology* 2003;(31):553–560.

55. Lawson A, Fouts G. Mental illness in Disney animated films. *Can J Psychiatry* 2004; 49(5):310–314.

56. Henderson L. Selling suffering: mental illness and media values. In: Philo G, ed., *Media and Mental Distress*, pp. 18–36. London: Longman; 1996.

57. Sieff EF. Media frames of mental illnesses: the potential impact of negative frames. *Journal of Mental Health* 2003; 12(3):259–269.

58. Nairn RG, Coverdale JH. People never see us living well: an appraisal of the personal stories about mental illness in a prospective print media sample. *Aust N Z J Psychiatry* 2005; 39(4):281–287.

59. Crepaz-Keay D. A sense of perspective: the media and the Boyd Inquiry. In: Philo G, ed., *Media and Mental Distress*, pp. 37–44. London: Longman; 1996.

60. Falk G. *Stigma: How We Treat Outsiders.* New York: Prometheus Books; 2001.

61. Wilson C, Nairn R, Coverdale J, Panapa A. Constructing mental illness as dangerous: a pilot study. *Aust N Z J Psychiatry* 1999; 33(2):240–247.

62. Hallam A. Media influences on mental health policy: long-term effects of the Clunis and Silcock cases. *International Review of Psychiatry* 2002; 14:26–33.

63. Philo G. The media and public belief. In: Philo G, ed., *Media and Mental Distress*, pp. 82–103. London: Longman; 1996.

64. McKeown M, Clancy B. Media influence on societal perceptions of mental illness. *Mental Health Nursing* 1995; 15(2):10–12.

65. Secker J, Platt S. Why media images matter. In: Philo G, ed., *Media and Mental Distress*, pp. 1–17. London: Longman; 1996.

66. Corrigan PW, Markowitz FE, Watson AC. Structural levels of mental illness stigma and discrimination. *Schizophr Bull* 2004; 30(3):481–491.

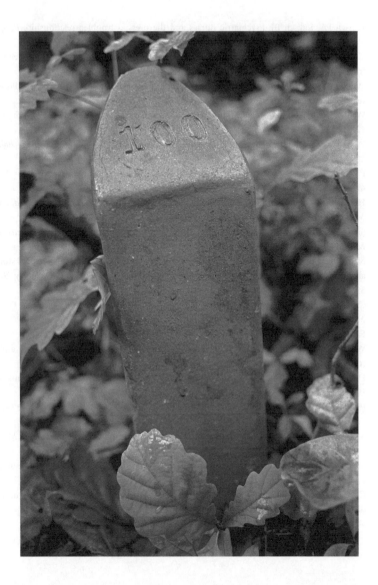

Unmarked pauper's gravestone, Warlingham Park Hospital, UK, 2001.
© Paul Treacy

Chapter 7 Danger or disinformation

The facts about violence and mental illness

What is my crime?

What have I done?

What crime have I committed?

I am ill, that is my crime, and oh what a crime, a mental illness.

Depression, borderline personality disorder, you pick the label.

I lived contentedly enough in my little flat, never bothering anyone,

Never bothered by anyone until now,

Horror of horrors, a forensic hostel for people with mental health problems is planned a few minutes walk away from where I live.

That is when the horror started.

The neighbourhood is in uproar.

The papers tell of this paedophile centre for murderers.

All of a sudden, my little haven becomes a hell.

Dog mess is pushed through my letterbox, closely followed by paint stripper being thrown over the door.

All of a sudden, my flat stands out from the rest of the road.

I can repair the damage to the property, but I cannot repair the damage done to my sense of safety, of belonging to a community.

I have been living here for seven years never harming anyone.

I had the occasional spell in hospital that kept me away from home for a while.

Once the news of the proposed hostel was made known.

I become a leper, no longer welcome in a local shop I have used for years.

My crime, they knew I had spent time in a psychiatric hospital, and therefore I must be grouped with the supposed paedophiles that were meant to be coming to live amongst the community.

I have never committed a crime, never hurt a fly.

All at once, I am no longer welcome in my home.

Who says stigma is dead?

Just because I have a mental health problem.

Even though it has not been a problem for others until now.

I am now shunned.
My life made even more difficult to live.

Suicide becomes an even more attractive proposition.
I have known depression over the years but now it is no longer just a danger within.
Now I have dangers outside.
What will happen next?
I have stopped coming home late at night; make sure I am home early.
I no longer feel safe, need to see who is around me.
Will I be attacked just for living in the community with a mental illness?

Just think on, depending on what report you read one in four people will experience mental health problems in their lives.
Will you be one of them?
Will you still be able to live where you do in safety?

Oh, there is the uproar about the community's safety from people with mental health problems.
But what about our safety from the community, and their lynch mobs.
Who needs protecting from whom?'

Maria

As we saw in the last chapter, by far the strongest defining feature of mental illnesses, according to its popular portrayals in the mass media, is the link with violence.[1] Are these concerns justified? Is there a kernel of truth in these worries?[2] Do such fears exaggerate or underestimate the real level of risk posed by people with mental illness, compared with the risks from people without such conditions? Should policy-makers and the producers of media orientate themselves to the 'real' facts of such risks, rather to perceived risks, or are both important? How far do popular concerns reflect real danger or real disinformation? These are the questions that we shall consider in this chapter.

While exaggerated claims reinforce popular stereotypes, superficial denials of any risk, unless founded on hard facts, provide a public disservice,[3] and will fail to find widespread credibility. Although it is clear that people with mental illnesses are at least as likely to be the victims as the perpetrators of crime, including violent crime,[4] the focus of this chapter is upon the latter as this is key to discrimination.[5–10] Fortunately there is no lack of evidence to summarise on this topic: rather the problem is to cut through the many thousands of papers and books written on the subject to find the essential facts.[11]

Until recently it was common to hear that, as a whole category, people with mental illnesses were no more violent than anyone else.[12] In 1987 the official

American Psychiatric Association classification of mental disorders stated, 'Although violent acts performed by people with [schizophrenia] often attract public attention, whether their frequency is actually greater than in the general population is not known.'[13] Indeed such a view was based at that time on the available scientific literature:

> An exhaustive search of the epidemiological literature, including correspondence with the leading researchers in the field, has revealed no study of the prevalence of true mental disorder in the general population that has inquired whether the individuals identified as mentally ill were ever arrested for, or admit to ever having committed, criminal acts.'[14]

This view is less common now that more recent studies have begun to paint a more detailed picture. Such research is complex, and we need to tread with care.[11] First, it is more accurate to record actual violent events rather than officially registered crimes, which tend to be underestimate violence. Second, research should consider all the characteristics of those who are violent (for example their age, and alcohol and drug use) and not simply attribute all offences to mental illness alone. Third, we need to distinguish carefully between having a history of mental illness, as against experiencing psychiatric symptoms at the time of a violent act. Fourth, such research needs to consider whether wider social changes, such as unemployment rates,[15] or changes in the patterns of mental healthcare, have any bearing on rates of violence. Fifth, we need to distinguish relative risks (how much more often people with a particular condition may commit violent acts than those without this condition), from absolute risks (the actual number of such incidents or events).[16–19] Indeed, such absolute risks vary between countries and regions, and this strongly suggests that factors other than illness have an impact on rates of crime committed by people with mental illness. Finally, it is not good enough simply to describe 'the mentally ill' (we would not report violence by 'the physically ill'). Rather we need to be much more detailed in understanding the nature of the symptoms and problems faced by people who are violent, and to compare these groups fairly with others of similar social background.[20] For example we know that at least half of all people with a mental illness receive no treatment, and people who are violent and mentally ill are more likely to be treated. Therefore studies of people with treated mental illness will show artificially high rates of violence compared with rates for all people with a mental illness, whether treated or not.[21] Such challenges means that information about violence and mental illness needs to be interpreted with great care.[22,23] With these caveats in mind, we shall now consider the evidence about violence in relation to the main type of adult mental illness.

Psychotic disorders

Schizophrenia is a relatively uncommon condition, affecting about one person in 400 at any one time. Nevertheless, such is the fascination of this condition that far more has been written about schizophrenia and stigma than about all other types of mental illness put together, and this is also true in relation to the literature on violence. These questions have been approached from a range of different perspectives. One study reviewed rates of violent behaviour committed by people with a diagnosis of schizophrenia in seven countries, and found that for men rates were between 3.9–8.0 times higher than for the general population, and were 4.3–4.4 times higher for women.[17] For the wider category of 'major mental disorders', which includes other psychotic conditions, the increased rates were 4.2–4.5 for men and 8.7–27.4 for women.

Such elevated rates of violence by people with a diagnosis of schizophrenia have been found in many different countries. In the Australian state of Victoria, for example, criminal convictions for people with this diagnosis were examined over a 25-year period,[24] compared with people in the general community who were similar for age, gender and residential neighbourhood. Among the people with mental illness, convictions were more common (21.6 per cent versus 7.8 per cent), as were convictions for violent offences (8.2 per cent vs. 1.8 per cent). Substance use increased among people with schizophrenia from 8.3 per cent in 1975 to 26.1 per cent in 1995. This was important because higher conviction rates were found for patients with substance use than without (68.1 per cent vs. 11.7 per cent). Even so, the increase in the frequency of convictions was similar among service users and among the comparison group.[24]

Similar results were found in a large Danish study.[25] Among all people born between 1944–1947, when schizophrenia, bipolar disorder and organic brain syndromes were combined, criminal violence was higher for this group than for people never admitted for psychiatric treatment: 2.0–8.8 times higher for men and 3.9–23.2 times higher for women. These higher rates were explained in part by demographic factors (such as neighbourhood of residence) or by substance use, rather than by the type of mental illness.[25]

In Austria a long-term study, also over 25 years, examined the association between psychotic disorders, major depression and homicide.[26] Again offence rates were elevated for the mentally ill group, with a sixfold greater likelihood of committing homicide for men with a diagnosis of schizophrenia, and an eighteen times higher rate for women. As we saw earlier, the rates were increased even more among people with schizophrenia and with alcohol misuse.[27]

A different approach is to ask the question: what proportion of homicides are committed by people with a clear diagnosis of schizophrenia?[28] A review of the evidence gathered over the last 30 years found the following.[29] Across eight economically developed countries worldwide between 6–15 per cent of all homicides were committed by people with a clear diagnosis of schizophrenia, while a more recent review concluded that the range is between 5–10 per cent.[26, 28, 30, 31] In Finland, for example,[32] compared with the general population, the risk of being convicted of homicide was calculated to be 8 times higher for men and 6.5 times higher for women with a diagnosis of schizophrenia.

Looked at from the opposite direction, a study in Germany showed that individuals with a diagnosis of schizophrenia were between 13–17 times more likely to commit or attempt homicide than people without this diagnosis, and that there had been no change in these rates over a 30 year period.[29] Somewhat more modestly, a large national survey of people with a diagnosis of schizophrenia found that 3.6 per cent had committed seriously violent acts, and that this was most closely associated with psychotic symptoms such as persecutory ideas, depression, childhood conduct problems and having been the victim of violence.[33]

There is some imprecision in these figures as they compare studies that are carried out in different ways. For example, the definitions of crimes vary to some extent between countries, the health and criminal justice systems are dissimilar, mental illness categories change over time, and details of the crimes (for example whether a homicide was combined with a suicide) are often missing. Nevertheless, the overall picture shows a clear pattern. For example a national study in Germany concluded that people with a diagnosis of schizophrenia are three times more likely to kill than people without this condition.[34,35] Another study from the same country concluded that the rate is 13–17 times higher, and an overview suggested that the increased homicide rate for men is somewhere in between, about seven times higher.[23] It therefore seems likely that the truth lies somewhere in this range. The available information suggest that men with a diagnosis of schizophrenia are 3–7 times more likely to commit violent acts than men without this condition, but there is less adequate information available for women.[23]

Is violence becoming more common among people with schizophrenia? Probably not. Few studies have examined this question, but a careful review from the Czech Republic looked at rates of violence over the last 50 years. Most people with a diagnosis of schizophrenia were not found to be violent, although rates of violence were higher for men (42 per cent) than for women (33 per cent). There were no clear changes in these rates since 1949.[36]

As there is a clear increased risk of violence by people with a diagnosis of schizophrenia compared with members of the general population, does this amount to a substantial threat to public health? Here we need to distinguish between risks which are *relatively* increased, as against the *actual* number of violent incidents (that is the *absolute* number events, sometimes called the 'population attributable fraction'). Schizophrenia is relatively rare, affecting about one person in 200 each year and about one person in 100 over the course of a lifetime.[37, 38] Looked at in this way the evidence suggests that the overall percentage of violent acts which are committed by people with schizophrenia is about 10 per cent.[39] Contrary to popular belief, family members and friends are far more often the victims of such violence than are strangers.[40–42]

Bipolar disorder

Like schizophrenia, bipolar disorder affects about one in every 200 people:[43,44] unlike schizophrenia, very little is written about its associations with violence.[45–47] In part this is a technical issue as the condition is often lumped together with 'affective disorders', or with 'major mental illness' (often because the number of events is small), and so is difficult to disentangle from other categories of mental illness. But in part this also reflects how much the popular and scientific imagination has been focussed upon violence and schizophrenia, to the exclusion of almost all other conditions.

To summarize the evidence that is available, in the United States two large national surveys have been conducted which provide useful information.[48, 49] Among people who do not have a mental disorder, about two per cent are violent in any year, and also about two per cent are violent over the course of their lifetime. By comparison, every year about 11–16 per cent of people with bipolar disorder are violent on at least one occasion. Similarly, over the course of their lifetime violent acts are committed by about 12 per cent of people with bipolar disorder.[11] Overall this diagnosis confers a risk of behaving violently about nine times higher than for people with no mental disorder (although such figures may include contact with the police for reasons not related to violence),[50] and these risks are a particular concern to many family members.[51, 52]

In relation to homicide the findings are less clear-cut. An Austrian study found no greater risk of committing homicide for people with bipolar disorder,[26] while work in the USA showed that manic symptoms were associated with 'homicidality'.[53,54] Given this lack of evidence it seems fair to provisionally conclude that people who have bipolar disorder seem to have a 5–9 times higher risk of acting violently towards others while they have symptoms of the disorder, but that there is no clear increased risk of committing homicide.

Depression

Depression is a broad category which ranges from the common-sense meaning of feeling 'down', 'sad' or 'blue' through to severely disabling types of mental illness, which can include psychotic symptoms.[55] Its relationship to violence has been largely overlooked.[56–58] Most of this research refers to 'clinical depression', meaning symptoms of depression sufficiently severe to need treatment, although such cases are often grouped together with people with a diagnosis of bipolar disorder as 'major affective disorders'.[59] In the two large surveys in the USA referred to earlier, about nine per cent of people with a diagnosis of dysthymia (a long-term type of mild depression) reported being violent in the previous year, while seven per cent of those with 'major depression' (moderately or severely disabling depression) said that they had been violent or had police contact for some other reason in the previous year, compared with two per cent among those with no psychiatric diagnosis. This suggests that rates of violence may be about four times higher among people with current or recent depression.[60] On the other hand, these surveys also asked about previous diagnoses. For people who had at some time in their lives been diagnosed with depression, but had not had the condition in the last year, the rates of violence were one per cent, that is half the rate of those who had never been given a psychiatric diagnosis.[60]

For homicides we see the reverse picture of schizophrenia, namely a relatively low relative risk, but a relatively large actual contribution to violent events, because depression is much more common than schizophrenia.[61] A national inquiry into homicides in the UK, for example, identified 718 homicides over an 18-month period. Full records were available for 500 cases and among these 71 of the perpetrators were found to have features of mental illness at the time of the homicide (14 per cent of the total), of whom 48 (10 per cent) had symptoms of depression. Slightly more (11 per cent) had been given a diagnosis of an affective disorder at some time in their lives.[62]

A particular type of case, which is more often documented, concerns homicide-suicides in which the perpetrator of a homicide commits suicide soon after. A series of studies suggest that depression is relatively common, both among the victims and the perpetrators of these homicides.[63–68] The most wide-ranging review of this topic study found that 2–3 homicide-suicides occurs every year for every one million person-years and account for approximately 1000 to 1500 deaths yearly in the United States. The annual number of these tragic events is fairly constant across industrialized countries and has not significantly changed over recent decades. The main perpetrators are young males with intense sexual jealousy, depressed mothers, or despairing elderly men with ailing spouses. The principal victims are female sexual partners or other family members, usually young children, and clinical depression is relatively common among perpetrators.[69]

Anxiety-related disorders

Perhaps surprisingly, there is evidence that rates of violence are raised in some types of anxiety-related disorder. Surveys in the USA, for example, suggest higher rates of violence for people who have been diagnosed as having agoraphobia (two times higher), or post-traumatic stress disorder (PTSD, also two times higher), but no increased risk of violence for people with simple phobias, social phobias, generalized anxiety disorder, or panic disorder.[60] Among people with no psychiatric condition about two per cent are violent in any year. By comparison, having symptoms of an anxiety-related disorder within the last year is associated with a modest increase in the risk of violence (or police contact for other reasons) for the following conditions: simple phobia (5.0–5.8 per cent), social phobia (7.7 per cent), agoraphobia (7.8 per cent), generalized anxiety disorder (6.4 per cent), panic disorder (8.4 per cent) and PTSD (7.5 per cent).[60,70] There is no strong evidence that people with anxiety-related disorders have an increased risk of committing homicide.[32]

Drug and alcohol use

The opposite is the case for people with alcohol or drug use or dependence, where rates of committing violent crimes including homicide are substantially increased. In Sweden people discharged from hospital with a diagnosis of substance misuse, for example, were studied to track their offending behaviour. Of all violent crimes, 16.1 per cent were committed by people with alcohol misuse and 11.6 per cent by those with drug misuse.[71] Over half of those with drug misuse who were violent were using two or more drugs at the time of the incident. An international review from seven different countries came to a similar conclusion. Compared with members of the general population with a similar social background, men with 'substance use disorder' were 9–15 times more likely to behave violently, and this risk was 15–55 times higher among women.[72] Such violence appears to be particularly targeted towards family members and friends.[73]

Again much of the strongest information comes from large-scale surveys in the USA. One such study, for example, found that people with alcohol or drug misuse were more than twice as likely as those with a diagnosis of schizophrenia to report being violent.[74,75] According to a later survey, there were higher rates of violent behaviour by people who have ever had periods of alcohol misuse (four times higher) or drug abuse (five times higher), compared with people who had never had a psychiatric disorder.[60]

When it comes to current substance misuse the picture is still worse. For people with alcohol use in the previous year, 9–25 per cent report violent behaviour, and for those with current or recent drug misuse the figures rise again with 20–35 per cent reporting violent behaviour. As an illustration of this point, a large study in New Zealand identified about 1000 individuals who were born between April 1972 and March 1973. Particular groups were more likely to be violent: those with alcohol dependence (1.9 times higher), marijuana dependence (3.8 times higher), and 'schizophrenia-spectrum disorder' (2.5 time higher). People with at least one of these three disorders constituted one-fifth of the sample, but they accounted for about a half of all violent crimes committed.[76]

Despite some contrary results,[36] taken together these findings point to the same conclusion: drug or alcohol misuse are strong predictors of violence, are more closely associated with violence than are psychotic disorders, and play a part in contributing to at least one quarter of all violent incidents.

How does substance misuse contribute towards violence? This is not well understood. A recent study throughout the USA found that drug and alcohol use did clearly contribute towards minor acts of violence by people with mental illness, but was less implicated for severe violence, where other factors such as younger age, psychotic symptoms, depression, childhood conduct problems and recent victimization were stronger predictors.[33]

Personality disorder

The types of mental health problem which are called personality disorders remain controversial.[77, 78] Even so, they are remarkably common and together affect 20–30 per cent of the population in any year.[79] The American diagnostic system, described in the *Diagnostic and Statistical Manual* (DSM) recognises ten types of personality disorder,[80] while the World Health Organisation system, the International Classification of Disease (ICD) describes nine, largely overlapping, types.[81]

Concerning violence and homicide, most research concerns itself with one of these categories, which is called either antisocial (DSM) or dissocial (ICD) personality disorder. One international review found that violent behaviour is 7–19 times higher for men with any diagnosis of personality disorder, and 12–50 times more common for women with these diagnoses.[72] The same appears to be true for homicide. A large Finnish study found that antisocial personality disorder increases the risk for committing homicide tenfold in men and over 50-fold in women.[32]

Some caution is needed here in interpreting these findings as criminal behaviour to a substantial extent overlaps with the definition of antisocial personality disorder (ASPD). The US diagnostic system (DSM-IV-TR), states that ASPD is a pervasive pattern of disregard for and violation of the rights of others occurring since age 15 years, as indicated by three (or more) of the following:

- failure to conform to social norms with respect to lawful behaviours as indicated by repeatedly performing acts that are grounds for arrest;
- deceitfulness, as indicated by repeated lying, use of aliases, or conning others for personal profit or pleasure;
- impulsivity or failure to plan ahead;
- irritability and aggressiveness, as indicated by repeated physical fights or assaults;
- reckless disregard for safety of self or others;
- consistent irresponsibility, as indicated by repeated failure to sustain steady work or honour financial obligations;
- lack of remorse, as indicated by being indifferent to or rationalizing having hurt, mistreated, or stolen from another.[80]

It is therefore hardly surprising that individuals who meet these criteria form a large proportion of those who commit crimes and who serve prison sentences. In Sweden, for example one study examined the psychiatric diagnoses of all 2005 individuals convicted of homicide or attempted homicide between 1988 and 2001. Where records were available over half (54 per cent) of those convicted met criteria for personality disorder.[82] Seen from another angle, how many of those in prison have previously had contact with psychiatric services? A study in Victoria, Australia looked into this question and found that 25 per cent of those convicted in the courts had prior psychiatric contact, and that personality disorder and substance misuse accounted for most of these cases.[31] It is therefore clear that people with personality disorders (especially antisocial personality disorder) commit a large proportion of the total number of violent offences, and commit far more of these offences than do people with psychotic disorders.[31, 83]

Comorbidity

So far we have considered diagnostic groups one at a time. In the real world, however, people often meet the criteria for more than one condition, so called 'comorbidity'. In fact only about a half (55 per cent) of all people with a mental illness have one disorder alone, according to a national US survey, while a quarter (22 per cent) had two diagnosable conditions, and a further quarter

(23 per cent) had three or more different problems at the same time. Those with the greatest degree of disability more often have comorbid conditions.[84] Such overlapping conditions are especially important when it comes to the links between comorbid mental illnesses and violence, where the evidence is now overwhelming. There are three potentially crucial elements: psychotic illness, antisocial personality disorder, and alcohol/drug misuse.

Among Canadian prisoners sentenced for severe offences, for example, it emerged that people with both 'major mental disorders' (psychotic conditions) and with antisocial personality disorders more often began their criminal activities in childhood, and had more convictions than those with psychotic conditions alone.[85] Very similar findings were apparent in a study of men in prison in the UK.[86] Among a group of people with schizophrenia, about a quarter (28 per cent) were identified as also meeting the criteria for a personality disorder, and this group were more likely to behave violently than those with schizophrenia alone.[87]

Quite often such abnormal personality features are clear from childhood or adolescence, when they are called 'conduct disorders'.[88, 89] Overall it is clear that among people with psychotic disorders, the minority who also meet the criteria for antisocial personality disorder are much more likely to commit violent acts. Indeed there is emerging evidence that there may be a common genetic basis for conduct disorder in childhood and for substance misuse and antisocial behaviour in adulthood.[86, 89, 90]

A second comorbidity is especially important: people who both have a psychotic disorder and who misuse alcohol/drugs. This is not uncommon. Several studies suggest that in more economically developed countries between one-third and two-thirds of people with psychotic conditions also have substance misuse, sometimes called 'dual diagnosis'.[91–94] Such concurrent problems increase the chance of being convicted of a crime and behaving violently.[95] There is further evidence from the USA that rates of violence are especially high among for people with dual diagnosis who do not take their medication as recommended.[96, 97] In fact it appears from research in both Switzerland and the USA that among people with psychotic conditions, substance misuse doubles the probability of having a criminal record.[98–100]

Research from many countries confirms these findings. A review of work in seven nations showed that people with a diagnosis of schizophrenia were seven times more likely than those with no mental illness to be convicted of homicide. By comparison people with both a psychotic illness and alcoholism were seventeen times more likely to be convicted of homicide.[30]

The role of alcohol or drug use therefore appears to be a stronger predictor for violence than does having a diagnosis of a severe mental illness. Context is also important. One American study, which followed up people discharged from acute psychiatric inpatient units, found no difference between rates of violence among the discharged patients who did or did not have substance misuse. Nevertheless, rates of violence for both groups (and indeed for the local population as a whole) were very high in this greatly impoverished neighbourhood in Pittsburgh.

This suggests that for this group with dual diagnosis it was both substance misuse and the nature of the neighbourhood which acted to increase the risk of violence.[73] More specifically, the rate of substance misuse was twice as high among people with mental illness than in the community group (32 per cent vs. 18 per cent). So substance misuse is more likely to affect people with mental illnesses, and when it does, it acts as a more potent risk factor for violence than it does for people who are not mentally ill. At the same time it seems likely that there are other issues, for example intellectual disability, or social and cultural factors in poor neighbourhoods, which can further increase the risk of violence.[73, 101, 102]

The picture that therefore emerges strongly suggests that there is an interaction between these three key ingredients (psychotic disorder, antisocial personality disorder and substance misuse).[24, 33] Their combination is greater than the sum of their parts. For example, when multiple diagnoses were considered in two large national psychiatric surveys, a history of violent or criminal behaviour was found in about 2 per cent of those with no recent psychiatric diagnosis, about 6 per cent of people with one condition, 8–18 per cent of those with two disorders and in 12–24 per cent of people with three or more conditions.[60]

There seems to be little doubt that the most potent combination of conditions is psychotic disorder, antisocial personality disorder and alcohol/drug misuse, which together very substantially escalate the risk of violent behaviour. At the same time it needs to be recognised that such a combination applies to a relatively small fraction of the one in 200 people who have a psychotic disorder, and that they also contribute to a relatively small proportion of all violent crimes.[101, 103] We also need to appreciate the additional influences of familial risk factors[88] and the social environment (such as having been a victim of violence).[104]

Community care

Those unconvinced about the wisdom of developing community-based mental health services have claimed that this policy, by closing beds in long-stay hospitals and transferring people to residential facilities in the community, places the public at risk. Is there any foundation in fact for these fears? In short, no. The evidence suggests the opposite and several studies indicate that community based care can in fact prevent violence.[105–108]

In the Australian state of Victoria, for example, patterns of offending among people with a diagnosis of schizophrenia were tracked over a 20-year period, before and after deinstitutionalization. Such patients did tend to commit more crimes as time went on, in line with overall population trends, and those with additional substance misuse accounted for a disproportionately large proportion of the offences. Overall, hospital closure did not contribute to additional recorded offences.[109] A further analysis of violent crimes came to the same conclusion,[24] as did a similar study in Germany.[29]

Among over 500 long-stay patients discharged to nursing homes and social care homes in north London, when the two local psychiatric hospitals were closed, rates of criminal convictions were very low.[110] In New Zealand a study of hospital closure conducted between 1970–2000 found that the proportion of all homicides which were committed by people known to be 'mentally abnormal' declined from 20 to 5 per cent.[111] A less dramatic result came from an English study which showed that while the annual number of homicides in the general population more than tripled between 1957 and 1995, there was little fluctuation in the numbers of people with a mental illness committing homicide, and that this represented a three per cent annual decline in their contribution to the total number of such offences.[112] Nevertheless again we need to proceed cautiously, because where the sample of offenders is defined by court judgements of 'insanity', then this can underestimate the occurrence of offending by people with mental illness.

A more particular concern is so-called 'stranger homicides', where the perpetrator is unknown to the victim. In the UK this is relatively uncommon and occurs in 22 per cent of all homicides. Perpetrators of such crimes are less likely to have mental illness than for other types of homicide.[113] Further, only about three per cent of all violent offences are attributable to people with mental disorder.[114] It is therefore clear that there is no good evidence that the policy to develop community care has led to a greater risk of violence to the public.

The consequences of assuming dangerousness

Some types of mental disorder do therefore confer a higher likelihood of a person behaving violently, and other conditions do not. Nevertheless, as we saw in Chapter 6 on the media, *all* mental illnesses are usually assumed, by both the general public and by policy-makers, to be closely associated with violence, even if this assumption is not factually based. What are the consequences of assuming dangerousness, and are they realistic and fair, or are they disproportionate and discriminatory?

One consequence is that popular opinions are used to support repressive mental health policies. Those members of the public who believe that people with mental illness pose a risk of violence are also more likely to favour compulsory treatment in community settings. In the USA data from the General Social Survey found that 60 per cent of the population believe that people with schizophrenia are likely to commit violent acts toward others. Nearly 50 per cent say they favour laws to force persons with schizophrenia to visit a clinic or doctor, while 42 per cent support legally forcing people with this diagnosis to take prescription medication.[1]

Measures to allow compulsory community treatment are increasingly common.[115] While most countries have laws which allow compulsory treatment in hospital,[116] relatively few have legal powers to require people with mental illness to comply with treatment recommendations while living outside hospital.[117, 118] Such community treatment orders (also know as 'involuntary outpatient commitment') remain controversial, and have so far been found to have little consistent effect upon patient outcomes or risk-reduction.[119–126] The extension of such compulsory powers outside hospital, without clear-cut evidence of any benefit, has both been supported by family members in some studies,[120–122,127–130] and has also been described as discriminatory by consumer groups.[131–135]

Based upon beliefs that people with mental illness do pose a risk to the public, most countries have enacted separate legislation to specify the conditions under which people with mental illnesses can be treated without their consent or against their stated preferences.[136–138] For other conditions that may lead to threatening or dangerous behaviour, for example epilepsy, the central question is whether the person concerned has the mental capacity to make valid judgements and decisions and to act in his or her best interests.[139] In most jurisdictions the conditions under which people with mental illness can be compulsorily detained and treated do not refer to that person's capacity or competence, but rather to the presence or history of mental illness, and the results of an assessment of the degree of risk posed to themselves or to others. Measures which apply only to people who pose such risks by virtue of mental, but not physical, disorders can themselves be seen as discriminatory.[140, 141]

It is becoming common in many countries to implement methods of risk assessment in routine clinical care.[142] These procedures are applied, for example, to all people assessed or treated by specialist mental health services, whatever the individual characteristics of each person.[143, 144] Again we see that the assumption of dangerousness is applied to the whole category of people with any type of mental illness, whether or not this is justified by the evidence. In fact such systems of risk prediction tend to be very imprecise. One review of this field asked the question: how accurately can we predict which people with mental illness are likely to be violent in the future? The answer is: with relatively little precision. For every six people identified at high risk of committing a violent act in the future, in the short-term or in the long-term, only one would in fact go on to commit such an act.[145] At present mental health staff are rather inaccurate in predicting the future in terms of violence committed by people with mental illness, and therefore in identifying who should receive targeted clinical or environmental interventions.[146]

Putting risk in proportion

From this discussion it is apparent that this is a complex field where the evidence is clear on some points and opaque on others. It is possible to draw the following conclusions. It is misleading to speak of violence or danger in relation to 'the mentally ill', just as it would be in relation to 'the physically ill'. Whether or not there is any additional risk depends upon the type of diagnosis,[60] the nature and severity of the symptoms present,[147] whether the person is receiving treatment and care,[96] if there is a past history of violence by an individual,[148] the co-occurrence of antisocial personality disorder and substance misuse and the social, economic and cultural context in which an individual lives.[149–152] The social environment may be particularly important as it is striking that in many countries where people with schizophrenia do not live with their families,[153] they tend to congregate in areas which are the most deprived, socially disorganized and which have the highest rates of crime.[154] Alongside the risks they may pose to others, they also experience higher rates of victimization themselves.[155]

Mental disorders have been described as producing a 'modest association between having a mental illness and an increased propensity to violence',[147] or, expressed differently, 'violent and criminal acts directly attributable to mental illness account only for a very small proportion of such acts in the society'.[156] The strength of this link is less than the association between alcohol or drugs and violence. Of all violent incidents, far more are connected to alcohol or drugs than are attributable to mental illnesses, while the mental disorder about which there is most popular concern, schizophrenia, is also one of the least common of mental illnesses.

The best evidence on how to minimize these risks suggests that good treatment and care reduces the likelihood of harm to others. In studies of

718 homicides in the UK, for example, about one in seven perpetrators (14 per cent) had symptoms of mental illness at the time of the event.[41] The same proportion (14 per cent) had previously had contact with psychiatric services at some time, and half (8 per cent) had received treatment in the previous year. At the time of the homicide 60 were not receiving any treatment and only 15 were in contact with intensive support.[41] Further, we need specific interventions that target specific problems such as aggressive behaviour, substance misuse or antisocial attitudes.[157] These and similar findings worldwide suggest that targeting intensive treatment towards such prioritized groups is at present the approach most strongly supported by the available evidence.[147, 158] Nevertheless there are also other protective factors besides treatment. Social support, for example contact with family and friends, is generally protective, although this is a complex relationship and in a minority of people with mental illness social contact may actually increase risk in some patients with more severe psychiatric disturbance.[159]

In general we can say that violence is rare among people with psychiatric disorders, but when serious violence does occur, it carries a very high human and social cost. The likelihood that some people with mental illnesses will assault others is a small but real risk that needs to be addressed by mental health staff, service users and care-givers. These are difficult risks to manage because such violent acts are not only rare but are complex behaviours that are very difficult to predict.[145] Some of the most significant risk factors for violence, such as poverty and victimization, are less amenable to conventional mental health service interventions. Even so, both violence, and the perception of violence, impose significant limitations in the move to normalize mental health services within the community. Mental health service users, professionals and researchers have to walk a fine line in this area because by focusing on violence and trying to understand its causes, they run the risk of simply reinforcing the harmful stigma they seek to reduce.[160]

It is therefore misleading to deny that people with particular types of mental illness do have a higher risk of harming other people.[97, 161] At the same time it is clear that the contribution of people with psychotic conditions (about whom there is most concern, as we saw in Chapter 6 on the media) towards all violent acts is relatively small,[162,163] and that the degree of preoccupation with 'violence and mental illness' by the print and broadcast media,[164] which is real in its consequences,[165,166] is both disproportionate and discriminatory.

References

1. Pescosolido BA, Monahan J, Link BG, Stueve A, Kikuzawa S. The public's view of the competence, dangerousness, and need for legal coercion of persons with mental health problems. *Am J Public Health* 1999; 89(9):1339–45.

2. Corrigan PW, Watson AC, Ottati V. From whence comes mental illness stigma? *Int J Soc Psychiatry* 2003; 49(2):142–157.

3. Torrey EF. Stigma and violence. *Psychiatr Serv* 2002; 53(9):1179.

4. Teplin LA, McClelland GM, Abram KM, Weiner DA. Crime victimization in adults with severe mental illness: comparison with the National Crime Victimization Survey. *Arch Gen Psychiatry* 2005; 62(8):911–921.

5. Walsh E, Moran P, Scott C, McKenzie K, Burns T, Creed F *et al.* Prevalence of violent victimisation in severe mental illness. *Br J Psychiatry* 2003; 183:233–238.

6. Hiday VA, Swartz MS, Swanson JW, Borum R, Wagner HR. Criminal victimization of persons with severe mental illness. *Psychiatr Serv* 1999; 50(1):62–68.

7. Daniels K. Intimate partner violence and depression: a deadly comorbidity. *J Psychosoc Nurs Ment Health Serv* 2005; 43(1):44–51.

8. Lipsky S, Caetano R, Field CA, Bazargan S. The role of alcohol use and depression in intimate partner violence among black and Hispanic patients in an urban emergency department. *Am J Drug Alcohol Abuse* 2005; 31(2):225–242.

9. Nixon RD, Resick PA, Nishith P. An exploration of comorbid depression among female victims of intimate partner violence with posttraumatic stress disorder. *J Affect Disord* 2004; 82(2):315–320.

10. Fergusson DM, Swain-Campbell NR, Horwood LJ. Does sexual violence contribute to elevated rates of anxiety and depression in females? *Psychol Med* 2002; 32(6):991–996.

11. Corrigan P.W., Cooper AE. Mental illness and dangerousness: fact or misperception, and implications for stigma. In: Corrigan PW, ed., *On the Stigma of Mental Illness*, pp. 165–180. Washington DC: American Psychological Association; 2005.

12. Stuart H. Violence and mental illness: an overview. *World Psychiatry* 2003; 2:121–124.

13. American Psychiatric Association. *Diagnostic and Statistical Manual*, 3rd Edition (Revised) (DSM-III-R). Washington DC: American Psychiatric Association; 1987.

14. Monahan J, Steadman HJ. Crime and mental disorder: An epidemiological approach. In: Morris N, Tonry M, eds., *Crimes and Justice: An annual review of research, Vol. 3* pp. 145–189. Chicago: University of Chicago Press; 1983.

15. Catalano R, Dooley D, Novaco RW, Wilson G, Hough R. Using ECA survey data to examine the effect of job layoffs on violent behavior. *Hosp Community Psychiatry* 1993; 44(9):874–879.

16. Arboleda-Florez J. Mental illness and violence: an epidemiological appraisal of the evidence. *Can J Psychiatry* 1998; 43(10):989–996.

17. Angermeyer MC. Schizophrenia and violence. *Acta Psychiatr Scand Suppl* 2000;(407):63–67.

18. Angermeyer MC, Cooper B, Link BG. Mental disorder and violence: results of epidemiological studies in the era of de-institutionalization. *Soc Psychiatry Psychiatr Epidemiol* 1998; 33 Suppl. 1:S1–S6.

19. Wessely S. The epidemiology of crime, violence and schizophrenia. *Br J Psychiatry Suppl* 1997;(32):8–11.

20. Hodgins S. Epidemiological investigations of the associations between major mental disorders and crime: methodological limitations and validity of the conclusions. *Soc Psychiatry Psychiatr Epidemiol* 1998; 33 Suppl. 1:S29–S37.

21. Wang PS, Lane M, Olfson M, Pincus HA, Wells KB, Kessler RC. Twelve-month use of mental health services in the United States: results from the National Comorbidity Survey Replication. *Arch Gen Psychiatry* 2005; 62(6):629–640.

22. Hodgins S. Epidemiological investigations of the associations between major mental disorders and crime: methodological limitations and validity of the conclusions. *Soc Psychiatry Psychiatr Epidemiol* 1998; 33 Suppl. 1:S29–S37.

23. Eronen M, Angermeyer MC, Schulze B. The psychiatric epidemiology of violent behaviour. *Soc Psychiatry Psychiatr Epidemiol* 1998; 33 Suppl. 1:S13–S23.

24. Wallace C, Mullen PE, Burgess P. Criminal offending in schizophrenia over a 25-year period marked by deinstitutionalization and increasing prevalence of comorbid substance use disorders. *Am J Psychiatry* 2004; 161(4):716–727.

25. Brennan PA, Mednick SA, Hodgins S. Major mental disorders and criminal violence in a Danish birth cohort. *Arch Gen Psychiatry* 2000; 57(5):494–500.

26. Schanda H, Knecht G, Schreinzer D, Stompe T, Ortwein-Swoboda G, Waldhoer T. Homicide and major mental disorders: a 25-year study. *Acta Psychiatr Scand* 2004; 110(2):98–107.

27. Shaw J, Hunt IM, Flynn S, Meehan J, Robinson J, Bickly H, *et al.* Rates of mental disorder in people convicted of homicide. National clinical survey. *Br J Psychiatry* 2006; 188: 143–147.

28. Mullen P. Facing up to our responsibilities. *Psychiatr Bull* 2005; 29:248–249.

29. Erb M, Hodgins S, Freese R, Muller-Isberner R, Jockel D. Homicide and schizophrenia: maybe treatment does have a preventive effect. *Crim Behav Ment Health* 2001; 11(1):6–26.

30. Eronen M, Tiihonen J, Hakola P. Schizophrenia and homicidal behavior. *Schizophr Bull* 1996; 22(1):83–89.

31. Wallace C, Mullen P, Burgess P, Palmer S, Ruschena D, Browne C. Serious criminal offending and mental disorder. Case linkage study. *Br J Psychiatry* 1998; 172:477–484.

32. Eronen M, Hakola P, Tiihonen J. Mental disorders and homicidal behavior in Finland. *Arch Gen Psychiatry* 1996; 53(6):497–501.

33. Swanson JW, Swartz MS, Van Dorn RA, Elbogen EB, Wagner HR, Rosenheck RA *et al.* A national study of violent behavior in persons with schizophrenia. *Archives of General Psychiatry* 2005; (in press).

34. Haefner H, Boeker W. *Crimes of Violence by Mentally Abnormal Offenders. A psychiatric and epidemiological study in the Federal German Republic.* Cambridge: Cambridge University Press; 1982.

35. Wessely S, Taylor PJ. Madness and crime: criminology versus psychiatry. *Criminal Behaviour and Mental Health* 1991; 1:193–228.

36. Vevera J, Hubbard A, Vesely A, Papezova H. Violent behaviour in schizophrenia. Retrospective study of four independent samples from Prague, 1949 to 2000. *Br J Psychiatry* 2005; 187:426–430.

37. Kendler KS, Gallagher TJ, Abelson JM, Kessler RC. Lifetime prevalence, demographic risk factors, and diagnostic validity of nonaffective psychosis as assessed in a US community sample. The National Comorbidity Survey. *Arch Gen Psychiatry* 1996; 53(11):1022–1031.

38. Jenkins R, Bebbington P, Brugha TS, Farrell M, Lewis G, Meltzer H. British psychiatric morbidity survey. *Br J Psychiatry* 1998; 173:4–7.

39. Walsh E, Buchanan A, Fahy T. Violence and schizophrenia: examining the evidence. *Br J Psychiatry* 2002; 180:490–495.

40. Estroff SE, Swanson JW, Lachicotte WS, Swartz M, Bolduc M. Risk reconsidered: targets of violence in the social networks of people with serious psychiatric disorders. *Soc Psychiatry Psychiatr Epidemiol* 1998; 33 Suppl. 1:S95–101.

41. Shaw J, Appleby L, Amos T, McDonnell R, Harris C, McCann K *et al.* Mental disorder and clinical care in people convicted of homicide: national clinical survey. *BMJ* 1999; 318(7193):1240–1244.

42. Simpson AI, McKenna B, Moskowitz A, Skipworth J, Barry-Walsh J. Homicide and mental illness in New Zealand, 1970–2000. *Br J Psychiatry* 2004; 185:394–398.

43. Kessler RC, Rubinow DR, Holmes C, Abelson JM, Zhao S. The epidemiology of DSM-III-R bipolar I disorder in a general population survey. *Psychol Med* 1997; 27(5):1079–1089.

44. Mitchell PB, Slade T, Andrews G. Twelve-month prevalence and disability of DSM-IV bipolar disorder in an Australian general population survey. *Psychol Med* 2004; 34(5):777–785.

45. Feldmann TB. Bipolar disorder and violence. *Psychiatr Q* 2001; 72(2):119–129.

46. Simon RI. Clinical risk management of the rapid-cycling bipolar patient. *Harv Rev Psychiatry* 1997; 4(5):245–254.

47. Yesavage JA. Bipolar illness: correlates of dangerous inpatient behaviour. *Br J Psychiatry* 1983; 143:554–557.

48. Kessler RC, McGonagle KA, Zhao S, Nelson CB, Hughes M, Eshleman S *et al.* Lifetime and 12-month prevalence of DSM-III-R psychiatric disorders in the United States. Results from the National Comorbidity Survey. *Arch Gen Psychiatry* 1994; 51(1):8–19.

49. Regier DA, Myers JK, Kramer M, Robins LN, Blazer DG, Hough RL *et al.* The NIMH Epidemiologic Catchment Area program. Historical context, major objectives, and study population characteristics. *Arch Gen Psychiatry* 1984; 41 (10):934–941.

50. Corrigan PW, Watson AC. Findings from the National Comorbidity Survey on the frequency of violent behavior in individuals with psychiatric disorders. *Psychiatry Res* 2005; 136(2–3):153–162.

51. Swanson JW, Holzer CE, III, Ganju VK, Jono RT. Violence and psychiatric disorder in the community: evidence from the Epidemiologic Catchment Area surveys. *Hosp Community Psychiatry* 1990; 41(7):761–770.

52. Dore G, Romans SE. Impact of bipolar affective disorder on family and partners. *J Affect Disord* 2001; 67(1–3):147–158.

53. Pera SB, Dailliet A. Homicide by mentally ill: clinical and criminological analysis. *Encephale* 2005; 31 (5 Pt 1): 539–549.

54. Schwartz RC, Reynolds CA, Austin JF, Petersen S. Homicidality in schizophrenia: a replication study. *Am J Orthopsychiatry* 2003; 73(1):74–77.

55. Goldberg D, Goodyer I. *Genesis of Common Mental Disorders.* London: Brunner-Routledge; 2005.

56. Rosenbaum M, Bennett B. Homicide and depression. *Am J Psychiatry* 1986; 143(3):367–370.

57. Malmquist CP. Depression and homicidal violence. *Int J Law Psychiatry* 1995; 18(2):145–162.

58. Collins P, White T. Depression, homicide and diminished responsibility: new Scottish directions. *Med Sci Law* 2003; 43(3):195–202.

59. Hodgins S, Lapalme M, Toupin J. Criminal activities and substance use of patients with major affective disorders and schizophrenia: a 2-year follow-up. *J Affect Disord* 1999; 55(2–3):187–202.

60. Corrigan P.W., Watson A. Findings from the National Comorbidity Survey on the frequency of violent behaviour in individuals with psychiatric disorders. *Psychiatry Research* 2005; 136 (2–3): 153–162.

61. Barraclough B, Harris EC. Suicide preceded by murder: the epidemiology of homicide-suicide in England and Wales 1988–92. *Psychol Med* 2002; 32(4): 577–584.

62. Shaw J, Appleby L, Amos T, McDonnell R, Harris C, McCann K *et al.* Mental disorder and clinical care in people convicted of homicide: national clinical survey. *BMJ* 1999; 318(7193):1240–1244.

63. Rosenbaum M. The role of depression in couples involved in murder-suicide and homicide. *Am J Psychiatry* 1990; 147(8):1036–1039.

64. Chan CY, Beh SL, Broadhurst RG. Homicide-suicide in Hong Kong, 1989–1998. *Forensic Sci Int* 2004; 140(2–3):261–267.

65. Koh KG, Gwee KP, Chan YH. Psychiatric aspects of homicide in Singapore: a five-year review (1997–2001). *Singapore Med J* 2006; 47 (4): 297–304.

66. Malphurs JE, Cohen D. A statewide case-control study of spousal homicide-suicide in older persons. *Am J Geriatr Psychiatry* 2005; 13(3):211–217.

67. Malphurs JE, Eisdorfer C, Cohen D. A comparison of antecedents of homicide-suicide and suicide in older married men. *Am J Geriatr Psychiatry* 2001; 9(1):49–57.

68. Malphurs JE, Cohen D. A statewide case-control study of spousal homicide-suicide in older persons. *Am J Geriatr Psychiatry* 2005; 13(3):211–217.

69. Marzuk PM, Tardiff K, Hirsch CS. The epidemiology of murder-suicide. *JAMA* 1992; 267(23):3179–3183.

70. Swanson JW, Holzer CE, III, Ganju VK, Jono RT. Violence and psychiatric disorder in the community: evidence from the Epidemiologic Catchment Area surveys. *Hosp Community Psychiatry* 1990; 41(7):761–770.

71. Grann M, Fazel S. Substance misuse and violent crime: Swedish population study. *BMJ* 2004; 328(7450):1233–1234.

72. Angermeyer MC. Schizophrenia and violence. *Acta Psychiatr Scand Suppl* 2000;(407):63–67.

73. Steadman HJ, Mulvey EP, Monahan J, Robbins PC, Appelbaum PS, Grisso T *et al.* Violence by people discharged from acute psychiatric inpatient facilities and by others in the same neighborhoods. *Arch Gen Psychiatry* 1998; 55(5):393–401.

74. Swanson JW, Holzer CE, III, Ganju VK, Jono RT. Violence and psychiatric disorder in the community: evidence from the Epidemiologic Catchment Area surveys. *Hosp Community Psychiatry* 1990; 41(7):761–770.

75. Swanson J. Alcohol abuse, mental disorder, and violent behavior: An epidemiologic inquiry. *Alcohol Health and Research World* 1993; 17(2):123–132.

76. Arseneault L, Moffitt TE, Caspi A, Taylor PJ, Silva PA. Mental disorders and violence in a total birth cohort: results from the Dunedin Study. *Arch Gen Psychiatry* 2000; 57(10):979–986.

77. Lewis G, Appleby L. Personality disorder: the patients psychiatrists dislike. *Br J Psychiatry* 1988; 153:44–49.

78. Department of Health. *Personality Disorder no Longer a Diagnosis of Exclusion: Policy implementation guidance for the development of services for people with personality disorder.* London: Department of Health; 2003.

79. Moran P, Jenkins R, Tylee A, Blizard R, Mann A. The prevalence of personality disorder among UK primary care attenders. *Acta Psychiatr Scand* 2000; 102(1):52–57.

80. American Psychiatric Association. *Diagnostic and Statistical Manual of Mental Disorders: DSM-IV-TR:* 4th Edition Text Revision. Washington DC: American Psychiatric Publishing Inc; 2000.

81. World Health Organisation. *ICD 10: the International Classification of Mental and Behavioural Disorders: Clinical Descriptions and Diagnostic Guidelines.* Geneva: World Health Organisation; 1992.

82. Fazel S, Grann M. Psychiatric morbidity among homicide offenders: a Swedish population study. *Am J Psychiatry* 2004; 161(11):2129–2131.

83. Hodgins S, Mednick SA, Brennan PA, Schulsinger F, Engberg M. Mental disorder and crime. Evidence from a Danish birth cohort. *Arch Gen Psychiatry* 1996; 53(6):489–496.

84. Kessler RC, Chiu WT, Demler O, Merikangas KR, Walters EE. Prevalence, severity, and comorbidity of 12–month DSM-IV disorders in the National Comorbidity Survey Replication. *Arch Gen Psychiatry* 2005; 62(6):617–627.

85. Hodgins S, Cote G. Major mental disorder and antisocial personality disorder: a criminal combination. *Bull Am Acad Psychiatry Law* 1993; 21(2):155–160.

86. Moran P, Hodgins S. The correlates of comorbid antisocial personality disorder in schizophrenia. *Schizophr Bull* 2004; 30(4):791–802.

87. Moran P, Walsh E, Tyrer P, Burns T, Creed F, Fahy T. Impact of comorbid personality disorder on violence in psychosis: report from the UK700 trial. *Br J Psychiatry* 2003; 182:129–134.

88. Kim-Cohen J, Caspi A, Moffitt TE, Harrington H, Milne BJ, Poulton R. Prior juvenile diagnoses in adults with mental disorder: developmental follow-back of a prospective-longitudinal cohort. *Arch Gen Psychiatry* 2003; 60(7):709–717.

89. Hodgins S, Tiihonen J, Ross D. The consequences of conduct disorder for males who develop schizophrenia: associations with criminality, aggressive behavior, substance use, and psychiatric services. *Schizophr Res*; 78; 323–335.

90. Naudts K, Hodgins S. Neurobiological correlates of violent behavior among persons with schizophrenia. *Schizophr Bull*; 2006–not yet published.

91. Wright S, Gournay K, Glorney E, Thornicroft G. Dual diagnosis in the suburbs: prevalence, need, and in-patient service use. *Soc Psychiatry Psychiatr Epidemiol* 2000; 35(7):297–304.

92. Weaver T, Madden P, Charles V, Stimson G, Renton A, Tyrer P *et al.* Comorbidity of substance misuse and mental illness in community mental health and substance misuse services. *Br J Psychiatry* 2003; 183:304–313.

93. Lehman AF, Myers CP, Corty E. Assessment and classification of patients with psychiatric and substance abuse syndromes. *Psychiatr Serv* 2000; 51(9):1119–1125.

94. Cuffel BJ. Comorbid substance use disorder: prevalence, patterns of use, and course. *New Dir Ment Health Serv* 1996;(70):93–105.

95. Scott H, Johnson S, Menezes P, Thornicroft G, Marshall J, Bindman J *et al.* Substance misuse and risk of aggression and offending among the severely mentally ill. *Br J Psychiatry* 1998; 172:345–350.

96. Swartz MS, Swanson JW, Hiday VA, Borum R, Wagner HR, Burns BJ. Violence and severe mental illness: the effects of substance abuse and nonadherence to medication. *Am J Psychiatry* 1998; 155(2):226–231.

97. Torrey EF. Violent behavior by individuals with serious mental illness. *Hosp Community Psychiatry* 1994; 45(7):653–662.

98. Modestin J, Wuermle O. Criminality in men with major mental disorder with and without comorbid substance abuse. *Psychiatry Clin Neurosci* 2005; 59(1):25–29.

99. Swanson JW, Holzer CE, III, Ganju VK, Jono RT. Violence and psychiatric disorder in the community: evidence from the Epidemiologic Catchment Area surveys. *Hosp Community Psychiatry* 1990; 41(7):761–770.

100. Swartz MS, Swanson JW, Hiday VA, Borum R, Wagner R, Burns BJ. Taking the wrong drugs: the role of substance abuse and medication noncompliance in violence among severely mentally ill individuals. *Soc Psychiatry Psychiatr Epidemiol* 1998; 33 Suppl 1:S75–S80.

101. Walsh E, Gilvarry C, Samele C, Harvey K, Manley C, Tattan T *et al.* Predicting violence in schizophrenia: a prospective study. *Schizophr Res* 2004; 67(2–3):247–252.

102. Hodgins S. Mental disorder, intellectual deficiency, and crime. Evidence from a birth cohort. *Arch Gen Psychiatry* 1992; 49(6):476–483.

103. Walsh E, Buchanan A, Fahy T. Violence and schizophrenia: examining the evidence. *Br J Psychiatry* 2002; 180:490–495.

104. Swanson JW, Swartz MS, Essock SM, Osher FC, Wagner HR, Goodman LA *et al.* The social-environmental context of violent behavior in persons treated for severe mental illness. *Am J Public Health* 2002; 92(9):1523–1531.

105. Swanson J, Estroff S, Swartz M, Borum R, Lachicotte W, Zimmer C *et al.* Violence and severe mental disorder in clinical and community populations: the effects of psychotic symptoms, comorbidity, and lack of treatment. *Psychiatry* 1997; 60(1):1–22.

106. Swanson JW, Swartz MS, Elbogen EB. Effectiveness of atypical antipsychotic medications in reducing violent behavior among persons with schizophrenia in community-based treatment. *Schizophr Bull* 2004; 30(1):3–20.

107. Swanson JW, Swartz MS, Borum R, Hiday VA, Wagner HR, Burns BJ. Involuntary outpatient commitment and reduction of violent behaviour in persons with severe mental illness. *Br J Psychiatry* 2000; 176:324–331.

108. Monahan J, Steadman HJ, Silver E, Appelbaum PS, Robbins PC, Mulvey EP *et al. Rethinking Risk Assessment: The MacArthur Study of Mental Disorder and Violence.* Oxford: Oxford University Press; 2001.

109. Mullen PE, Burgess P, Wallace C, Palmer S, Ruschena D. Community care and criminal offending in schizophrenia. *Lancet* 2000; 355(9204):614–617.

110. Trieman N, Leff J, Glover G. Outcome of long stay psychiatric patients resettled in the community: prospective cohort study. *BMJ* 1999; 319(7201):13–16.

111. Simpson AI, McKenna B, Moskowitz A, Skipworth J, Barry-Walsh J. Homicide and mental illness in New Zealand, 1970–2000. *Br J Psychiatry* 2004; 185:394–398.

112. Taylor PJ, Gunn J. Homicides by people with mental illness: myth and reality. *Br J Psychiatry* 1999; 174:9–14.

113. Shaw J, Amos T, Hunt IM, Flynn S, Turnbull P, Kapur N *et al.* Mental illness in people who kill strangers: longitudinal study and national clinical survey. *BMJ* 2004; 328(7442):734–737.

114. Swanson JW. Mental disorder, substance abuse, and community violence: An epidemiological approach. In: Monahan J, Steadman HJ, eds., *Violence and Mental Disorder,* pp. 101–136. Chicago: University of Chicago Press; 1994.

115. Torrey EF, Zdanowicz M. Outpatient commitment: what, why, and for whom. *Psychiatr Serv* 2001; 52(3):337–341.

116. World Health Organisation. *WHO Resource Book on Mental Health, Human Rights and Legislation.* Geneva: World Health Organisation; 2005.

117. Salize HJ, Dressing H. Epidemiology of involuntary placement of mentally ill people across the European Union. *Br J Psychiatry* 2004; 184:163–168.

118. Dressing H, Salize HJ. Compulsory admission of mentally ill patients in European Union Member States. *Soc Psychiatry Psychiatr Epidemiol* 2004; 39(10):797–803.

119. Ridgely MS, Borum R, Petrila J. *The Effectiveness of Involuntary Outpatient Treatment.* Santa Monica, California: RAND Corporation.; 2001.

120. Kisely S, Campbell L, Preston N. *Compulsory community and involuntary outpatient treatment for people with severe mental disorders.* Cochrane Database Syst Rev 2005; 3:CD004408.

121. Kisely SR, Xiao J, Preston NJ. Impact of compulsory community treatment on admission rates: survival analysis using linked mental health and offender databases. *Br J Psychiatry* 2004; 184:432–438.

122. Preston NJ, Kisely S, Xiao J. Assessing the outcome of compulsory psychiatric treatment in the community: epidemiological study in Western Australia. *BMJ* 2002; 324(7348):1244.

123. Gray JE, O'Reilly RL. Canadian compulsory community treatment laws: recent reforms. *Int J Law Psychiatry* 2005; 28(1):13–22.

124. McIvor R. The community treatment order: clinical and ethical issues. *Aust N Z J Psychiatry* 1998; 32(2):223–228.

125. Swartz MS, Swanson JW. Involuntary outpatient commitment, community treatment orders, and assisted outpatient treatment: what's in the data? *Can J Psychiatry* 2004; 49(9):585–591.

126. Swartz MS, Swanson JW, Wagner HR, Burns BJ, Hiday VA, Borum R. Can involuntary outpatient commitment reduce hospital recidivism?: Findings from a randomized trial with severely mentally ill individuals. *Am J Psychiatry* 1999; 156(12):1968–1975.

127. McFarland BH, Faulkner LR, Bloom JD, Hallaux R, Bray JD. Family members' opinions about civil commitment. *Hosp Community Psychiatry* 1990; 41 (5):537–540.

128. Adams NH, Hafner RJ. Attitudes of psychiatric patients and their relatives to involuntary treatment. *Aust N Z J Psychiatry* 1991; 25(2):231–237.

129. Draine J. Conceptualizing services research on outpatient commitment. *J Ment Health Adm* 1997; 24(3):306–315.

130. Swartz MS, Swanson JW, Wagner HR, Hannon MJ, Burns BJ, Shumway M. Assessment of four stakeholder groups' preferences concerning outpatient commitment for persons with schizophrenia. *Am J Psychiatry* 2003; 160 (6):1139–1146.

131. Borum R, Swartz M, Riley S, Swanson J, Hiday VA, Wagner R. Consumer perceptions of involuntary outpatient commitment. *Psychiatr Serv* 1999; 50(11):1489–1491.

132. Greenberg D, Mazar J, Brom D, Barer YC. Involuntary outpatient commitment: a naturalistic study of its use and a consumer survey at one community mental health center in Israel. *Med Law* 2005; 24(1):95–110.

133. Chamberlin J. User/consumer involvement in mental health service delivery. *Epidemiol Psychiatr Soc* 2005.

134. Repper J, Perkins R. *Social Inclusion and Recovery*. Edinburgh: Balliere Tindall; 2003.

135. Swartz MS, Wagner HR, Swanson JW, Elbogen EB. Consumers' perceptions of the fairness and effectiveness of mandated community treatment and related pressures. *Psychiatr Serv* 2004; 55(7):780–785.

136. Bean P. *Mental Disorder and Legal Control*. Cambridge: Cambridge University Press; 1986.

137. Fennell P. *Treatment Without Consent*. London: Routledge; 1996.

138. Szmukler G, Appelbaum P. Treatment pressures, coercion and compulsion. In: Thornicroft G, Szmukler G, eds., *Textbook of Community Psychiatry*, pp. 529–544. Oxford: Oxford University Press; 2001.

139. Szmukler G. Double standard on capacity and consent? *Am J Psychiatry* 2001; 158(1):148–149.

140. Bindman J, Maingay S, Szmukler G. The Human Rights Act and mental health legislation. *Br J Psychiatry* 2003; 182:91–94.

141. Szmukler G, Holloway F. Reform of the Mental Health Act. Health or safety? *Br J Psychiatry* 2000; 177:196–200.

142. Watts D, Bindman J, Slade M, Holloway F, Rosen A, Thornicroft G. Clinical assessment of risk decision support (CARDS): The development and evaluation of a feasible violence risk assessment for routine psychiatric practice. *Journal of Mental Health* 2004; 13:569–581.

143. Monahan J, Steadman HJ, Robbins PC, Appelbaum P, Banks S, Grisso T *et al.* An actuarial model of violence risk assessment for persons with mental disorders. *Psychiatr Serv* 2005; 56(7):810–815.

144. Munro E, Rumgay J. Role of risk assessment in reducing homicides by people with mental illness. *Br J Psychiatry* 2000; 176:116–120.

145. Buchanan A, Leese M. Detention of people with dangerous severe personality disorders: a systematic review. *Lancet* 2001; 358(9297):1955–1959.

146. Hodgins S, Muller-Isberner R. Preventing crime by people with schizophrenic disorders: the role of psychiatric services. *Br J Psychiatry* 2004; 185:245–250.

147. Mullen PE. A reassessment of the link between mental disorder and violent behaviour, and its implications for clinical practice. *Aust N Z J Psychiatry* 1997; 31(1):3–11.

148. Humphreys MS, Johnstone EC, Macmillan JF, Taylor PJ. Dangerous behaviour preceding first admissions for schizophrenia. *Br J Psychiatry* 1992; 161:501–505.

149. Fitzpatrick KM, Piko BF, Wright DR, LaGory M. Depressive symptomatology, exposure to violence, and the role of social capital among African-American adolescents. *Am J Orthopsychiatry* 2005; 75(2):262–274.

150. Wessely SC, Castle D, Douglas AJ, Taylor PJ. The criminal careers of incident cases of schizophrenia. *Psychol Med* 1994; 24(2):483–502.

151. Silver E, Mulvey EP, Swanson JW. Neighborhood structural characteristics and mental disorder: Faris and Dunham revisited. *Soc Sci Med* 2002; 55(8):1457–1470.

152. Stueve A, Link BG. Violence and psychiatric disorders: results from an epidemiological study of young adults in Israel. *Psychiatr Q* 1997; 68(4):327–342.

153. Thornicroft G, Tansella M, Becker T, Knapp M, Leese M, Schene A *et al.* The personal impact of schizophrenia in Europe. *Schizophr Res* 2004; 69(2–3):125–132.

154. Dear M, Wolch J. *Landscapes of Despair.* Princeton, New Jersey: Princeton University Press; 1992.

155. Logdberg B, Nilsson LL, Levander MT, Levander S. Schizophrenia, neighbourhood, and crime. *Acta Psychiatr Scand* 2004; 110(2):92–97.

156. Modestin J. Criminal and violent behavior in schizophrenic patients: an overview. *Psychiatry Clin Neurosci* 1998; 52(6):547–554.

157. Hodgins S, Muller-Isberner R. Preventing crime by people with schizophrenic disorders: the role of psychiatric services. *Br J Psychiatry* 2004; 185:245–250.

158. Hodgins S, Muller-Isberner R. Preventing crime by people with schizophrenic disorders: the role of psychiatric services. *Br J Psychiatry* 2004; 185:245–250.

159. Swanson J, Swartz M, Estroff S, Borum R, Wagner R, Hiday V. Psychiatric impairment, social contact, and violent behavior: evidence from a study of outpatient-committed persons with severe mental disorder. *Soc Psychiatry Psychiatr Epidemiol* 1998; 33 Suppl 1:S86–S94.

160. Swanson JW. Personal communication. 2005.

161. Gregory RS, Satterfield TA. Beyond perception: the experience of risk and stigma in community contexts. *Risk Anal* 2002; 22(2):347–358.

162. Stuart HL, Arboleda-Florez JE. A public health perspective on violent offenses among persons with mental illness. *Psychiatr Serv* 2001; 52(5):654–659.

163. Monahan J, Arnold J. Violence by people with mental illness: a consensus statement by advocates and researchers. *Psychiatric Rehabilitation Journal* 1996; 19:67–70.

164. Ryan T. Perceived risks associated with mental illness: beyond homicide and suicide. *Soc Sci Med* 1998; 46(2):287–297.

165. Link BG, Monahan J, Stueve A, Cullen FT. Real in their consequences: a sociological approach to understanding the association between psychotic symptoms and violence. *American Sociological Review* 1999; 64:316–332.

166. Perlick DA, Rosenheck RA, Clarkin JF, Sirey JA, Salahi J, Struening EL *et al.* Stigma as a barrier to recovery: Adverse effects of perceived stigma on social adaptation of persons diagnosed with bipolar affective disorder. *Psychiatr Serv* 2001; 52(12):1627–32.

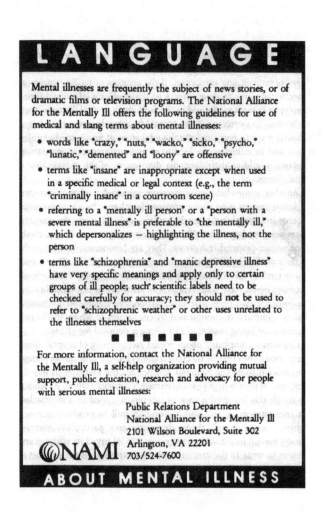

Newspaper advertisement by National Alliance for the Mentally Ill, USA.

Chapter 8 'Why Try?'

Self-stigmatisation and anticipated discrimination

Leroy is a 39 year old man who lives in England. His parents migrated from Jamaica 50 years ago, and then started their family. After school Leroy worked in manual and factory jobs until his early 30s, when he began to feel suspicious of other people and this eventually led to his compulsory admission to hospital. He was brought by the police, using handcuffs, to hospital for an emergency assessment, but he feels that he was treated respectfully, and he now thinks that what they did was necessary, 'They probably thought I was mad or would do something.' He has been under the care of the local mental health services for the last seven years. He has regular appointments at a local mental health centre, but thinks that staff stopped visiting him at home after he was given a diagnosis of paranoid schizophrenia, 'Maybe they're afraid I might attack them.'

His mental health problems have important consequences for him. He believes that since becoming unwell the staff from his local housing organisation visit him less often. 'I mean nobody comes round to see me from the housing association because of that.' Many of his links with the local community have been severed. 'Well, my neighbours don't speak to me. I just think it's because they know, they know something is wrong ... they gossip.' One neighbour nearby used to talk to him often but then changed her behaviour, 'She sees me on the street. She doesn't say 'Hi', and she just keeps on going.' His social life has also been devastated by the consequences of his mental illness. About friends he says, 'Well the fact is that I don't have them anymore, because they disappeared. I think because they knew I was mentally ill. They were asking about the pills that I was taking stuff like that.' His three best friends simply stopped contacting him.

He had enjoyed a close relationship with his girlfriend over many years. This stopped suddenly. After he was admitted to psychiatric hospital for the first time she finished the relationship. 'Well the person I was friendly with, she ended it ... stopped completely. We were friends for like seven years. We didn't have an argument.' Since he was discharged from hospital Leroy has no longer tried to find a new girlfriend, 'No, well I when came here I stopped. I stopped dating.' The reason is that he expects that any new girlfriend would find out about his mental illness and then reject him. 'I think about the fear that they find out eventually. I don't want to sit through that again.' He feels that even if he decided not to tell a new girlfriend about his mental illness, that sooner or later his guard would drop and that he would mention it somehow. 'Once you get close to someone you start talking. You might talk about where you are going … or else what pills you take.' He cannot completely conceal his psychiatric treatment. 'For example if they come to my house or I go to their house … they might see the pills and ask what it's for … and I think they would worry.'

Having been rejected and emotionally hurt once before he wants to avoid this ever happening again. He also feels that there is no point in applying for any jobs, because he expects that all his applications would fail. 'People like me can't work.' But there have also been some advantages from having a diagnosis of mental illness. A few years ago, when he was well, he decided to stop paying rent on his apartment. Eventually he was evicted, but he was quickly rehoused because of his diagnosis. 'Well when I was homeless, I mean I think that it was an advantage, because when I was homeless that's how I got my flat.'

The decision of Leroy, and of many others in his position, to conclude: 'Why try?' is the subject of this chapter. Sometimes this attitude is a result of painful experiences which people with mental illnesses want to avoid repeating. At other times such choices do not come *after* such experiences of rejection, but in *anticipation* of failure. This complex set of expectations, actions, reactions, inhibitions, avoidance, loss of confidence, and social withdrawal is sometimes called 'self-stigma'.[1-6]

The impact of personal experience

Some experiences by people with mental illnesses are so traumatic that they feel a need to completely stop doing what had previously been a very important aspect of their lives. For example, some people will stop applying for jobs or trying to form new relationships. This suggests that such encounters were particularly hurtful, distressing, embarrassing or humiliating. What is known about the nature and intensity of such experiences, as described directly by people with mental illness?

> I once made a list of everything I could think of that I'd done that was notably embarrassing or problematic when I was high, and there were about 35 items, every one affecting a person I knew and the relationship I have with them. I found that after depression people are generally just happy to 'have you back' whereas after mania everything seems to have changed, been damaged somehow. I think that I scared a number of people to death with the sort of things

that I talked about and the sort of mind games that I tried to get people to play. Then, when the dust settles, you have to hold your head up and return back to normal. There's an intense embarrassment about everything, and worse than that, the feeling that you are now 'branded' mentally ill for life, and that you are facing stigma from all directions.

Robert

The 'voice' of people who have (or who have had) mental illness comes closer to centre-stage, but this is a very recent development.[7] Although there are some accounts from as early as the fifteenth century of the experience of people with mental illness,[8] it is especially within the last 30 years that the user/survivor/consumer movement has become a significant force.[9] Despite this, oddly enough, the voice of service users is not strongly represented in the literature on stigma,[10–13] even though service users are increasingly asserting their point of view in terms of mental health policy, service planning, and treatment provision and research.[14–18] What are the key messages?

Control emerged as the core issue in one study carried in England. Over 30 service users with enduring mental health problems were interviewed in detail about their lives and about the impact of their conditions.[19] They said that their main goal was to 'enhance, sustain, and take control of their mental health'. One aspect they emphasized was developing therapeutic relationships with professionals based upon 'communication, trust, and continuity.' But they also reported frequent experiences of social isolation, economic deprivation, and stigmatisation.

Legally speaking, control is only formally taken away while service users are subjected to compulsory legal powers, usually during periods of involuntary admission to hospital. In practice the question of control is much more fluid. A series of recent studies in North America and Europe have shown that even while inpatients are technically admitted on a 'voluntary' basis, most understand that they are not fully free to stay or leave as they wish. There is an implied, and sometimes an explicit, threat that if they try to take their discharge against medical advice, they will be legally detained.[20–29] For professional staff, this is a difficult point to accept, as they work from day to day trying to do their best for the people they treat. But the evidence is clear that many of those receiving such treatment find that the basis of this 'therapeutic' relationship (blending care, concern and threat) is at best a mixed blessing, and at worst a dishonest amalgam of both help and control.[17, 30, 31]

A second core concern for service users is the need to be treated, in clinical and in human terms, with respect. One service user in London has written that 'respect for mad people has been a long time coming'.[32] He reflects upon what he felt were the disrespectful celebrations of the 750th anniversary of the founding of one of Britain's oldest psychiatric institutions, the Bethlem

Royal Hospital, 'We saw it as a commemoration service versus a celebration service: a time to remember the unmarked graves; those who had taken their own lives; and those who were victims of people who were ill.'[32] He describes very clearly the consequences for him of having a diagnosis of mental illness:

> When I lost my job at London Transport, I lost my friends and my social life too. I entered social isolation, became a social 'leper' at the most vulnerable time of my life. The irony was that when I needed friends they were nowhere to be found.[32]

As we saw in Chapter 5, contact with mental health services, whatever the intentions of staff, can be experienced by users as disrespectful. A national survey in Britain of over 500 people who had been admitted to psychiatric hospital, for example, found that the views of service users were not taken fully seriously by staff. The study conducted a review of the literature on service user views and concluded that: (i) service users' views were disregarded by researchers if they did not coincide with those of mental health professionals, (ii) there was a clear sense in the research that patients are continually irrational and so cannot give a valid opinion, (iii) service users and relatives were assumed to share the same interests (and if they do not, then family views predominated), and (iv) that some credence was given to the service user's view only as long as it coincides with the expert's view.[17]

The third theme that emerges from service users' description of their experiences – particularly of service contact – is that of powerlessness. A leading service user advocate has expressed this in the following way.

> Because of the inherent power differential between psychiatrists and people who have been diagnosed with serious mental illness, it is not at all surprising that users continue to have a very difficult time in getting their voices heard at all, let alone in making real and substantial changes in the conditions of their lives.[14]

This power differential has a long and painful history. Involuntary commitment is rarely acknowledged by professionals to be one fundamental element underlying mental health services. Yet it forms the backdrop to many discussions of user involvement ... 'so long as users can be subjected to involuntary interventions in supposedly voluntary services, the power differential is a real and overwhelming obstacle to any kind of real equality in decision-making.'[14]

There can be a tendency for the negative views of service users to be published more often than positive reactions, because these are what stick in the memory. So how common are such forms of discriminatory treatment? Detailed interviews with over 70 service users with diagnoses of psychotic disorders in Maryland found that 'almost all participants reported some stigma experiences'.[33] Similarly lengthy discussions with people in London, with a wider range of diagnoses, found that the majority had experienced verbal abuse, physical abuse, loss of social contacts, patronizing attitudes or direct discrimination against them.[34] The British survey mentioned earlier[17] asked over 500 former inpatients which aspects of their life had been most damaged by their mental health problems. The answers were especially revealing: self-confidence (82 per cent), family relationships (74 per cent), hopes for the future (71 per cent), work (62 per cent), relationships with friends (59 per cent) and their financial situation (58 per cent). So profoundly negative experiences of this type do not seem to be the exception, but the rule.[35–37]

Such negative reactions from other people appear to be easy to start but hard to stop. Once they have been established, they also seem to be largely separate from the severity of the mental illness, or the degree of recovery. In a sense once a person has been designated as a 'mental patient' then this is a largely indelible label. One study in New York City, for example, talked with over 80 men who had been given diagnoses of both psychotic illness and substance abuse,[38] and found that even a year after starting treatment, when most of their symptoms had substantially improved, there was still a 'relatively strong and enduring effect of stigma on well-being ... stigma continues to complicate the lives of the stigmatised even as treatment improves their symptoms and functioning'. The authors concluded that professionals 'must address stigma as a separate and important factor in its own right'.[38]

> But it's always in my mind now, that unless you keep explaining your mental problems, people treat you like a leper and assume all kinds of things. I am not as open and friendly anymore, and feel awkward around people now, because I don't want to have to feel like I did at my friend's house, and don't want to keep justifying everything.
>
> Eva

The force of expectations

So far we have considered the reactions of people with mental illness after they have felt discriminated against. But is direct discrimination necessary before people learn that they are the targets of stigmatisation? Almost certainly not. There is now strong evidence that people with a diagnosis of mental illness expect to be discriminated against, whether or not this happens in fact, and that these expectations can themselves be profoundly disabling.[39]

> We tell ourselves that we believe in this or that, but where do these beliefs come from? It is human nature that we are influenced by other people's experiences

and beliefs. I have permanent reminders of my mental illness and live with this everyday and indeed will for the rest of my life. I give myself a hard enough time without having to deal with the discrimination that exists in society.

Martina

This distinction is sometimes referred to as the difference between *enacted* and *felt* stigma. 'Enacted stigma' refers to episodes or events of discrimination against people who are considered unacceptable, while 'felt stigma' includes the experience of shame of having a condition, and the fear of encountering enacted stigma.[40,41] In the previous sections and chapters we have seen that enacted stigma experiences are very common and have potent consequences. What do we know about felt stigma?

A large study from eastern Germany compared what it called 'concrete stigmatisation' (enacted stigma) with 'subjective stigmatisation' (felt stigma) by interviewing over 200 people who either had a diagnosis of schizophrenia or depression. Most expected negative reactions from employers, even if they had not had this experience. Interestingly, those living in small towns more often expected discrimination than those in cities, even though both had actually experienced stigmatisation at a similar rate.[42]

Another way to look at this anticipation of being subjected to discrimination is to refer to it as 'stigma consciousness'.[43] A research group in Texas has developed a way to measure this using this questionnaire, and made an important discovery: that people who do expect to be discriminated against are less likely to take opportunities to challenge or reject stereotypes about their condition.[43] In other words, those who expect discrimination are more likely to accept it when it does occur: a self-fulfilling cycle.

Another view is that these thoughts and feelings should be described as 'internalized stigma', in parallel with 'internalized' racism[44] (see Chapter 9 for a more detailed discussion of focusing upon discrimination rather than stigma). Evidence for such anticipated stigma comes from many sources. Interviews with over 500 people with mental health problems in Greece found that fewer than a half had sought help, and the most common reason for this was to avoid stigma. This feeling was stronger in towns and villages than in the cities.[45] This may be a common pattern. As we saw in Chapter 1, the fear of adverse reactions from others seems to be greater in rural than in urban areas.[46] In the USA delays of over 10 years in seeking help have been found for some types of mental illness, again linked in part to the fear of stigma.[47] In Austria most people in one survey said that they would not advise a friend or family member with a mental illness to see a psychiatrist.[48] In New York State depressed people with lower levels of 'perceived stigma' were more likely to accept the treatment recommendations of their doctors.[49,50]

In a fascinating and important study at Columbia University in Manhattan, five groups were asked if they thought that people with a diagnosis of mental illness were devalued. The groups were: people with a recent diagnosis of mental illness; longer-term psychiatric patients; local residents who had previously been treated for mental illness; local community members who had features of mental illness, but who had not received treatment; and residents who were well and who had never been treated for a mental illness.[51]

The results were stark and surprising: all groups had strong views that people with mental illness are devalued, and there were few differences between these five groups. The degree of devaluation was not related to the severity of the condition. The researchers found that

> Acquiring the status of mental patient can imply grave consequences for people's beliefs about their standing in the community ... It is likely that those who fear rejection most have been depleted both internally and externally by their experience.[51]

More positively the study did suggest that as time passed, after a period of treatment, so expectations of rejection did gradually subside. This work is important because there has been an active debate on whether labelling 'caused' mental illness or not.[52] This study produced strong evidence that powerful and negative consequences followed the psychiatric diagnostic labels, whatever the primary cause of the condition.[53]

Although this work was carried out at a time when mental health care in the USA was largely hospital-based, there is little evidence that such social rejection is any milder now that community care become more widespread in many countries. A recent national survey in the USA included over 1300 people with diagnoses of mental illness, and 100 were invited for more detailed interviews. Most people said that they were:

- worried that others would see them unfavourably
- had come across messages in the mass media that were hurtful or offensive
- had avoided telling others about their condition
- had been treated by others as less competent; had been shunned or avoided
- had been advised to lower their expectations in life.[54]

In a similar vein, about 100 people with disabling psychiatric conditions, who were under the care of an assertive community treatment team, were interviewed in Ottawa, Canada. Despite their residence in the community, and the intensive support they received, most of these people believed that others did reject them. This view substantially damaged their sense of belonging to their local community.[55]

Not all the evidence is so relentlessly pessimistic. A comparison of the views of people with mental illnesses and the general public in Austria found that the former had more positive views when asked whether 'most people' think that people with a diagnosis of mental illness are: less intelligent, less trustworthy, personal failures, thought less of by others, or taken less seriously. Even so, the majority of people in both groups agreed with all of these statements.[56]

What all this adds up to is that before people with mental health problems receive treatment, and even before they experience any clear-cut discrimination against them, they very commonly expect to be treated in a discriminatory way, and that these expectations themselves shape their own behaviour.

So ideas have powerful consequences for behaviour, for example in making many people reluctant to seek help. At the same time, as we saw earlier in this chapter, the experience of being on the receiving end of actual discriminatory behaviour serves to reinforce such expectations. Indeed there is some suggestion that anticipated discrimination is more common than actual discrimination. A study in upstate New York found that among over 600 people in contact with mental health self-help groups, or in outpatient treatment, over two-thirds (72 per cent) said that they expected to be devalued and discriminated against, while only about half could recall actual events of discrimination.[57] We can begin to see a pattern emerging: a series of vicious circles which reinforce each other, adding layers of disadvantage.[58]

> I have a friend who is very stigmatising when he talks about people with mental illness. For this reason I hide my problem. I know that if he knew about me he would break up our friendship.
>
> Alexandros

The consequences of anticipated and actual discrimination

So far we have seen that both actual discriminatory events and the expectation of discrimination are common experiences for many people with mental illness. What are the consequences? First, there are important emotional implications of self-stigma. Careful interviews with people with diagnoses of psychotic conditions from throughout the USA have found that almost all (95 per cent) felt a lasting personal impact from their experiences of stigma. Most commonly these were: anger (33 per cent), emotional hurt (28 per cent), sadness and depression (18 per cent), or discouragement and disappointment (17 per cent).[59] Over a half said that their self-esteem or self-confidence had suffered as a consequence, about a third found that they had avoided social contact more than before, and a quarter reported that they were now less likely to make an application for a job.

> My life was already shamed with my disability, for which I hold no one to fault. I learned to live with who I am.
>
> Linda

In particular relation to self-stigmatisation, a common reaction is feelings of shame.[60, 61] Shame refers to the feelings of humiliation or distress caused by an awareness of 'wrong or foolish behaviour'.[62] Shame stems in part from how far a person feels guilty of some moral failing or weakness.[63] It is as if there is an unwritten rule of correct moral conduct that has been broken, for which the person deserves to be punished. The emotional impact may be profound. The sense that there has been a failure, *by the individual*, can be overwhelming. Such feelings can overwhelm a person with mental illness even in the absence of actively blaming behaviour by others.[64–66] We shall return to this moral dimension in more detail in Chapter 9. For the present it is enough to note that shame reflects an important self-judgement made by people who believe that they have broken some unwritten code about what it means to be a full member of society.[67]

Perhaps unsurprisingly, this potent cocktail of emotional reactions to stigma and discrimination includes feelings of hopelessness or depression.[68] The upstate New York study mentioned earlier, for example, found that people who reported high levels of anticipated or actual stigma were also worse off in terms of depression, self-esteem, life satisfaction and employment.[69]

A parallel study was coordinated in primary care settings in California and asked over 1000 people with a diagnosis of depression about stigma, employment, health insurance and friendships. Two-thirds of these people expected to have to face discrimination in the workplace, and this was substantially higher than the anticipated discrimination against people with hypertension or diabetes.[70]

Again we can see a set of circular processes start and then gain momentum. People with stronger expectations or experiences of discrimination were more depressed and had lower self-esteem. But at the same time 'mentally ill persons may expect and experience rejection at least in part because they think less of themselves, have limited social opportunities and resources, and because of the severity of their illness.'[69] But the precise causal sequence of events is not yet understood.

Yet another of these self-sustaining, destructive loops concerns who knows what. A landmark study in the USA over thirty years ago showed that if a person with mental illness *believed* that the person they were meeting knew about their illness, then the behaviour of the former deteriorated,[71] whether or not the other person did in fact know about the diagnosis. In other words, the expectation that another person will react in a discriminatory way can itself trigger behaviour in the person with mental illness which then does produce a stigmatising reaction.

These self-fulfilling patterns have also been described in relation to depression following racial discrimination, where tolerance or confrontation have been examined as potentially effective responses.[72] In mental health, as we shall see in more detail in Chapter 10, it seems to be true that a focus on self-confidence and self-esteem may be one way to break out of these destructive and self-destructive cycles.[73, 74]

It is striking that the emotional dimension of stigma is one that has only recently become recognised by researchers. An influential model of stigma developed by researchers in New York[75] has been recently modified to add in a stage describing the emotional reactions of service users to their stigma experiences.[76] Going a step further, research in Washington DC has examined some physiological aspects of emotional reactions in stigma. The researchers asked the study group to imagine meeting with other people, who were labelled as either having or not having schizophrenia. Eyebrow muscle tension, palm skin conductance and heart rate were measured and they showed higher levels of arousal among students who had more stigmatising attitudes towards people with mental illness. The findings suggest that one reason why people avoid individuals with mental illness may be to avoid the accompanying unpleasant feelings of physiological arousal.[77]

> The next time that you call someone strange, 'nutter, psycho, weirdo', silently or not, consider what it would be like to be in their shoes. Try and empathize. One day you might be in a similar position. How would you want society to treat you then? I used to be extremely sensitive when I hear people I know use these words like those above. Everyone is entitled to his or her beliefs and opinions, but how to challenge those when you believe that they are wrong is an area that needs further work. We don't realize how damaging the language we use can be sometimes. I questioned someone that I knew about this, asking them if they thought the same about me as I myself have mental health problems. The response was 'No, you are different.' I ask myself, why is it different? They know me, have grown up with me, and have seen how I have been affected by my life experiences. Apply this to a stranger and where is the difference? Ignorance is not bliss it is just ignorance.
>
> Martina

These are not straightforward processes to understand. At the same time we cannot simplify the complex ways that people react to being offered a diagnosis of mental illness.[78] A service user group in Wales has identified several common emotional reactions to having such a diagnosis: shame, terror, isolation, grief, 'mistake' and anger.[79] A further ingredient in this mix of feelings may be alienation, or feeling separate from society. A research group in San Francisco established that, among people with 'severe' mental illness, about a third had high levels of internalized stigma. They went on to describe internalized stigma as consisting of three components: alienation, stereotype endorsement and social withdrawal. All three of these components were associated with higher rates of depression, while only alienation predicted lower levels of self-esteem. The authors concluded that 'the finding that alienation further reduces morale speaks to the difficulty of pulling oneself out of this type of vicious cycle without assistance'.[80] 'Nobody knows what it feels like, nobody' (Robert).

For all of these reasons, avoidance is a path to which many people are drawn. Avoidance of going back to work, avoidance of applying for a job, avoidance of close relationships.[81] In short: 'Why try?'.[82, 83]

Such resignation can mean restricting social contacts to other people with similar conditions, who may be more tolerant of the diagnosis than the general public.[84, 85] Social withdrawal, for some people with mental illness, can be seen as a deliberate and active choice, to minimize the unpleasant consequences of contact with others who do not understand.[12, 86–88] As we saw earlier, this may be an avoidance of situations which have *already* been experienced as discriminatory, or avoidance of situations which are *expected* to be stigmatising.[89] The net effect is the same: degrees of social isolation and marginalization.

> I have suffered with depression since the age of 15 on a yearly basis. Often I have heard comments either said to me or about people with depression as 'lazy'. I was constantly tired and at low periods I would take to my bed and isolate myself from the outside/world.
>
> Tania

Identity

> I can't have schizophrenia because I'm not a violent person.
>
> Leroy

A very important consequence of all these processes is that some people with mental illness come to see this not as one feature of their lives, but as the *defining* aspect of their core identity,[90] sometimes called a 'master status'.[91] This is encouraged by the common use in medical and research writings of terms such as 'schizophrenics', or 'depressives', whereas it would be unacceptable to refer to people with heart disease as 'cardiacs'. This progression from seeing oneself as having a particular condition (along with many other characteristics and attributes), to being *essentially* identified by the disorder is a crucial step as these labels confer a lower social value on people to whom they stick,[91–94] both in that person's own eyes, and in the estimation of others,

There are varying degrees of mental illness and no one is immune. It can happen to anybody. I'm a very down-to-earth, jokey kind of person, and I wouldn't be violent to anyone. They liked me before they knew about my mental health problems. So what has changed? I'm still me, and if they had bothered to ask, the main reason I see a psychiatrist is because of a phobia.

Eva

Here again we see a two-way process. Not only do others tend to attach a lower social value to those whom they know have a diagnosis of mental illness, but also people with a diagnosis of mental illness can perform worse when their diagnosis is revealed to others, or if they believe this to be true. In a series of studies, students with a history of psychiatric treatment were asked to undertake tests of intellectual performance. In some of the tests, their diagnosis was known to others in the group. In other tests their medical history was concealed. The results showed that the students who revealed their psychiatric history did worse on the reasoning test than those who concealed their mental health status.[95]

The issue of stigma against mental illness sometimes feels like the worst part about it. I find that nearly every day I find myself lying or dodging questions to cover up my history of manic depression in an attempt to avoid the stigma that I perceive I'd encounter otherwise. I tend to explore what people think of it 'under cover' when I get the chance. For example, if I've just met someone who is talking about a person they know who had a mental illness, I won't let on that I have suffered, but instead I'll try to find out what they genuinely think about it. I do this because I need to know who is prejudiced and to keep in touch with what people think generally.

Robert

Many, subtle factors are operating at the same time in situations like this. Studies in the USA, for example, have suggested that black college students more often blamed low test scores to prejudiced marking by white examiners than white students blamed low marks on biased marking by black staff.[96] Similarly, self-esteem was particularly damaged for black students who were given low marks:

Self-esteem of Black students following positive and negative feedback depended both on the collective representations about prejudice that they brought with them to the situation, and on subtle features of the situation ... whereas the White students came to this situation with no collective representations about prejudice against their group.[96]

This raises the important implication that modifications to such 'collective representations' held by people with mental illness (for example to blame experiences of rejection on discrimination by others) may be protective against depression.

Societal beliefs reinforce personal beliefs. So not only are you the victim of society beliefs but also your own personal beliefs.

Martina

What is known about the effects of internalized or self-stigma therefore suggests that these are learned, and are both culturally and situationally specific.

One interesting example of this is the link between having a diagnosis of eating disorder and self-esteem. While eating disorders are sometimes described in relation to low self-esteem,[97–99] there are also studies which show that people who are overweight show few or no differences in self-esteem compared with those of normal weight.[100] Another example refers to African-Americans, where there is clear evidence of widespread discrimination,[101] yet where the available evidence indicates that if anything levels of self-esteem are higher among African-Americans than among Americans of European descent.[102] This also suggests that the relationships between core ingredients of stigma and discrimination are not fixed, and vary according to their social and cultural context.

In short, the social identity of people with mental illness can be influenced by the person's own sense of what it means to have a mental illness, by the expected discriminatory reactions of others, by the actual reactions of other combinations of these factors that can lead to material poverty,[84] social marginalization[103] and reduced social participation.[104] The evidence discussed in this chapter leads to the following conclusions: first, it suggests that the experience of mental illness may depend upon the mix of several factors at the same time; second, it is possible that an intervention for one particular aspect (for example for control,[105] self-esteem,[106] or acceptance, rejection[107] or denial[108] of the diagnosis) may have consequences in other domains (for example in employment); third, it raises the possibility that such experiences may vary in different places or at different times, and so be changeable.[109,110] We shall see how such positive changes can be achieved in Chapters 10 and 11.

References

1. Corrigan P.W., Watson AC. The paradox of self-stigma and mental illness. *Clinical Psychology: Science and Practice* 2002; 9:35–53.
2. Gallo KM. First person account: self-stigmatization. *Schizophr Bull* 1994; 20(2):407–410.
3. Sibicky M, Dovidio JF. Stigma of psychological therapy: stereotypes, interpersonal reactions, and the self-fulfilling prophecy. *Journal of Counseling Psychology* 2005; 33:148–154.
4. Yen CF, Chen CC, Lee Y, Tang TC, Yen JY, Ko CH. Self-stigma and its correlates among outpatients with depressive disorders. *Psychiatr Serv* 2005; 56(5):599–601.
5. Rusch N, Angermeyer MC, Corrigan PW. [The stigma of mental illness: concepts, forms, and consequences]. *Psychiatr Prax* 2005; 32(5):221–232.

6. Ritsher JB, Phelan JC. Internalized stigma predicts erosion of morale among psychiatric outpatients. *Psychiatry Res* 2004; 129(3):257–265.

7. Crossley ML, Crossley N. 'Patient' voices, social movements and the habitus; how psychiatric survivors 'speak out'. *Soc Sci Med* 2001; 52(10):1477–1489.

8. Peterson D. *A Mad People's History of Madness*. Pittsburgh, Pennsylvania: University of Pittsburgh Press; 1982.

9. Chamberlin J. *On Our Own: Patient-controlled alternatives to the mental health system*. New York: McGraw-Hill; 1979.

10. Schulze B, Angermeyer MC. Subjective experiences of stigma. A focus group study of schizophrenic patients, their relatives and mental health professionals. *Soc Sci Med* 2003; 56(2):299–312.

11. March DT. Personal accounts of consumer/survivors: insights and implications. *Journal of Clinical Psychology* 2000; 56(11):1447–1457.

12. Angell B, Cooke A, Kovac K. First-person accounts of stigma. In: Corrigan PW, ed., *On the Stigma of Mental Illness*, pp. 69–98. Washington, DC: American Psychological Association; 2005.

13. Bassman R. Agents, not objects: our fights to be. *J Clin Psychol* 2000; 56(11):1395–1411.

14. Chamberlin J. User/consumer involvement in mental health service delivery. *Epidemiol Psychiatr Soc* 2005.

15. Trivedi P, Wykes T. From passive subjects to equal partners: qualitative review of user involvement in research. *British Journal of Psychiatry* 2002; 181:468–472.

16. Thornicroft G, Rose D, Huxley P, Dale G, Wykes T. What are the research priorities of mental health service users? *Journal of Mental Health* 2002; 11:1–5.

17. Rogers A, Pilgrim D, Lacey R. *Experiencing Psychiatry. Users Views of Services*. London: MIND; 1993.

18. Bassman R. Consumers/survivors/ex-patients as change facilitators. *New Dir Ment Health Serv* 2000;(88):93–102.

19. Kai J, Crosland A. Perspectives of people with enduring mental ill health from a community-based qualitative study. *Br J Gen Pract* 2001; 51(470):730–6.

20. Bindman J, Reid Y, Szmukler G, Tiller J, Thornicroft G, Leese M. Perceived coercion at admission to psychiatric hospital and engagement with follow-up A cohort study. *Soc Psychiatry Psychiatr Epidemiol* 2005; 40(2):160–166.

21. Bonnie RJ, Monahan J. From coercion to contract: reframing the debate on mandated community treatment for people with mental disorders. *Law Hum Behav* 2005; 29; 485–503.

22. Cascardi M, Poythress NG. Correlates of perceived coercion during psychiatric hospital admission. *Int J Law Psychiatry* 1997; 20(4):445–458.

23. Gardner W, Hoge SK, Bennett N, Roth LH, Lidz CW, Monahan J *et al*. Two scales for measuring patients' perceptions for coercion during mental hospital admission. *Behav Sci Law* 1993; 11(3):307–321.

24. Hiday VA, Swartz MS, Swanson J, Wagner HR. Patient perceptions of coercion in mental hospital admission. *Int J Law Psychiatry* 1997; 20(2):227–241.

25. Monahan J, Hoge SK, Lidz C, Roth LH, Bennett N, Gardner W *et al*. Coercion and commitment: understanding involuntary mental hospital admission. *Int J Law Psychiatry* 1995; 18(3):249–263.

26. Swanson JW, Tepper MC, Backlar P, Swartz MS. Psychiatric advance directives: an alternative to coercive treatment? *Psychiatry* 2000; 63(2):160–172.

27. Szmukler G, Appelbaum P. Treatment pressures, coercion and compulsion. In: Thornicroft G, Szmukler G, eds., *Textbook of Community Psychiatry*, pp. 529–544. Oxford: Oxford University Press; 2001.

28. Monahan J, Redlich AD, Swanson J, Robbins PC, Appelbaum PS, Petrila J *et al.* Use of leverage to improve adherence to psychiatric treatment in the community. *Psychiatr Serv* 2005; 56(1):37–44.

29. Ivar IK, Hoyer G, Sexton H, Gronli OK. Perceived coercion among patients admitted to acute wards in Norway. *Nord J Psychiatry* 2002; 56(6):433–439.

30. Bean P. *Mental Disorder and Legal Control.* Cambridge: Cambridge University Press; 1986.

31. Fennell P. *Treatment Without Consent: Law, psychiatry and the treatment of mentally disordered people since 1845.* London: Routledge; 1995.

32. Shaughnessy P. Not in my back yard. Stigma from a personal perspective. In: Mason T, Carlisle C, Watkins C, Whitehead E, eds., *Stigma and Social Exclusion in Healthcare*, pp. 181–189. London: Routledge; 2001.

33. Dickerson FB, Sommerville J, Origoni AE, Ringel NB, Parente F. Experiences of stigma among outpatients with schizophrenia. *Schizophr Bull* 2002; 28(1):143–55.

34. Dinos S, Stevens S, Serfaty M, Weich S, King M. Stigma: the feelings and experiences of 46 people with mental illness. Qualitative study. *Br J Psychiatry* 2004; 184:176–181.

35. Jamison KR. Stigma of manic depression: a psychologist's experience. *Lancet* 1998; 352(9133):1053.

36. Poulin C, Masse R. [From deinstitutionalization to social rejection: the point of view of ex-psychiatric patients]. *Sante Ment Que* 1994; 19(1):175–194.

37. Corrigan P.W., Watson AC. Understanding the impact of stigma on people with mental illness. *World Psychiatry* 2002; 1:16–20.

38. Link BG, Struening EL, Rahav M, Phelan JC, Nuttbrock L. On stigma and its consequences: evidence from a longitudinal study of men with dual diagnoses of mental illness and substance abuse. *J Health Soc Behav* 1997; 38(2):177–190.

39. Rusch N, Angermeyer MC, Corrigan PW. [The stigma of mental illness: concepts, forms, and consequences.]. *Psychiatr Prax* 2005; 32(5):221–232.

40. Scrambler G, Hopkins A. Generating a model of epileptic stigma: the role of qualitative analysis. *Social Science and Medicine* 1990; 30(11):1187–1194.

41. Jacoby A. Felt versus enacted stigma: a concept revisited. Evidence from a study of people with epilepsy in remission. *Soc Sci Med* 1994; 38(2):269–274.

42. Angermeyer MC, Beck M, Dietrich S, Holzinger A. The stigma of mental illness: patients' anticipations and experiences. *Int J Soc Psychiatry* 2004; 50(2):153–162.

43. Pinel EC. Stigma consciousness: the psychological legacy of social stereotypes. *J Pers Soc Psychol* 1999; 76(1):114–128.

44. Ritsher JB, Otilingam PG, Grajales M. Internalized stigma of mental illness: psychometric properties of a new measure. *Psychiatry Res* 2003; 121(1):31–49.

45. Madianos MG, Madianou D, Stefanis CN. Help-seeking behaviour for psychiatric disorder from physicians or psychiatrists in Greece. *Soc Psychiatry Psychiatr Epidemiol* 1993; 28(6):285–291.

46. Rost K, Smith GR, Taylor JL. Rural-urban differences in stigma and the use of care for depressive disorders. *J Rural Health* 1993; 9(1):57–62.

47. Olfson M, Kessler RC, Berglund PA, Lin E. Psychiatric disorder onset and first treatment contact in the United States and Ontario. *Am J Psychiatry* 1998; 155(10):1415–1422.

48. Freidl M, Lang T, Scherer M. How psychiatric patients perceive the public's stereotype of mental illness. *Soc Psychiatry Psychiatr Epidemiol* 2003; 38(5):269–75.

49. Struening EL, Perlick DA, Link BG, Hellman F, Herman D, Sirey JA. Stigma as a barrier to recovery: The extent to which caregivers believe most people devalue consumers and their families. *Psychiatr Serv* 2001; 52(12):1633–1638.

50. Sirey JA, Bruce ML, Alexopoulos GS, Perlick DA, Friedman SJ, Meyers BS. Stigma as a barrier to recovery: perceived stigma and patient-rated severity of illness as predictors of antidepressant drug adherence. *Psychiatr Serv* 2001; 52(12):1615–20.

51. Link BG. Understanding labeling effects in the area of mental disorders: an assessment of the effects of expectations of rejection. *American Sociological Review* 1987; 52:96–112.

52. Scheff TJ. Shame in the labeling of mental illness. In: Gilbert P, Andrews B, eds., *Shame: Interpersonal behavior, psychopathology, and culture*, pp. 191–205. New York: Oxford; 1998.

53. Link BG, Cullen FT, Struening EL, Shrout PE, Dohrenwend BP. A modified labeling theory approach in the area of mental disorders: An empirical assessment. *American Sociological Review* 1989; 54:100–123.

54. Wahl OF. Mental health consumers' experience of stigma. *Schizophr Bull* 1999; 25(3):467–478.

55. Prince PN, Prince CR. Perceived stigma and community integration among clients of assertive community treatment. *Psychiatr Rehabil J* 2002; 25(4):323–331.

56. Freidl M, Lang T, Scherer M. How psychiatric patients perceive the public's stereotype of mental illness. *Soc Psychiatry Psychiatr Epidemiol* 2003; 38(5):269–275.

57. Markowitz FE. The effects of stigma on the psychological well-being and life satisfaction of persons with mental illness. *J Health Soc Behav* 1998; 39(4):335–347.

58. Sartorius N, Schulze H. *Reducing the Stigma of Mental Illness. A report from the Global Programme Against Stigma of the World Psychiatric Association.* Cambridge: Cambridge University Press; 2005.

59. Wahl OF. Mental health consumers' experience of stigma. *Schizophr Bull* 1999; 25(3):467–478.

60. Chapple A, Ziebland S, McPherson A. Stigma, shame, and blame experienced by patients with lung cancer: qualitative study. *BMJ* 2004; 328(7454):1470.

61. Corrigan P, Lundin R. *Don't Call Me Nuts.* Tinley Par, Illinois: Recovery Press; 2001.

62. Soanes C, Stevenson A. *Concise Oxford English Dictionary*, 11th edn. Oxford: Oxford University Press; 2003.

63. Wolpert L. Stigma of depression – a personal view. *Br Med Bull* 2001; 57:221–224.

64. Crisp A, Gelder MG, Goddard E, Meltzer H. Stigmatization of people with mental illnesses: a follow-up study within the Changing Minds campaign of the Royal College of Psychiatrists. *World Psychiatry* 2005; 4:106–113.

65. Oliver M, Barnes C. *Disabled People and Social Policy.* London: Longman; 1998.

66. Sayce L. *From Psychiatric Patient to Citizen. Overcoming Discrimination and Social Exclusion.* Basingstoke: Palgrave; 2000.

67. Morone JA. Enemies of the people: the moral dimension to public health. *Journal of Health Politics, Policy and Law* 1997; 22(4):993–1020.

68. Carroll A, Pantelis C, Harvey C. Insight and hopelessness in forensic patients with schizophrenia. *Aust N Z J Psychiatry* 2004; 38(3):169–173.

69. Markowitz FE. The effects of stigma on the psychological well-being and life satisfaction of persons with mental illness. *J Health Soc Behav* 1998; 39(4):335–47.

70. Roeloffs C, Sherbourne C, Unutzer J, Fink A, Tang L, Wells KB. Stigma and depression among primary care patients. *Gen Hosp Psychiatry* 2003; 25(5):311–315.

71. Farina A, Gliha D, Boudreau LA, Allen JG, Sherman M. Mental illness and the impact of believing others know about it. *J Abnorm Psychol* 1971; 77(1):1–5.

72. Noh S, Beiser M, Kaspar V, Hou F, Rummens J. Perceived racial discrimination, depression, and coping: a study of Southeast Asian refugees in Canada. *J Health Soc Behav* 1999; 40(3):193–207.

73. Corrigan PW, Calabrese JD. Strategies for assessing and diminishing self-stigma. In: Corrigan PW, ed., *On the Stigma of Mental Illness. Practical strategies for research and social change*, pp. 239–256. Washington DC: American Psychological Association; 2005.

74. Markowitz FE. Modeling processes in recovery from mental illness: relationships between symptoms, life satisfaction, and self-concept. *J Health Soc Behav* 2001; 42(1):64–79.

75. Link BG, Phelan JC. Conceptualizing stigma. *Annual Review of Sociology* 2001; 27:363–385.

76. Link BG, Yang LH, Phelan JC, Collins PY. Measuring mental illness stigma. *Schizophr Bull* 2004; 30(3):511–541.

77. Graves RE, Cassisi JE, Penn DL. Psychophysiological evaluation of stigma towards schizophrenia. *Schizophr Res* 2005; 76(2–3):317–327.

78. Hayward P, Bright JA. Stigma and mental illness: a review and critique. *Journal of Mental Health* 1997; 6(4):345–354.

79. O'Donoghue D. *Breaking Down Barriers. The stigma of mental illness: a user's point of view.* Aberystwyth: US, the All Wales User Network; 1994.

80. Ritsher JB, Phelan JC. Internalized stigma predicts erosion of morale among psychiatric outpatients. *Psychiatry Res* 2004; 129(3):257–265.

81. Asbring P, Narvanen AL. Women's experiences of stigma in relation to chronic fatigue syndrome and fibromyalgia. *Qual Health Res* 2002; 12(2):148–160.

82. Corrigan PW. Don't call me nuts: an international perspective on the stigma of mental illness. *Acta Psychiatr Scand* 2004; 109(6):403–404.

83. Evans S, Huxley P. Adaptation, response-shift and quality of life ratings in mentally well and unwell groups. *Qual Life Res* 2005; 14(7):1719–1732.

84. Estroff S. *Making it Crazy: Ethnography of psychiatric clients in an American community.* Berkeley, California: University of California Press; 1981.

85. Tait L, Birchwood M, Trower P. Adapting to the challenge of psychosis: personal resilience and the use of sealing-over (avoidant) coping strategies. *Br J Psychiatry* 2004; 185:410–415.

86. Dittmann J, Schuttler R. Disease consciousness and coping strategies of patients with schizophrenic psychosis. *Acta Psychiatrica Scandinavica* 1990;(4):318–322.

87. Angell B. Contexts of social relationship development among assertive community treatment clients. *Ment Health Serv Res* 2003; 5(1):13–25.

88. Wing JK, Brown G. *Institutionalism and Schizophrenia.* Cambridge: Cambridge University Press; 1970.

89. Stengler-Wenzke K, Angermeyer MC, Matschinger H. [Depression and stigma]. *Psychiatr Prax* 2000; 27(7):330–335.

90. Corrigan P.W. Dealing with stigma through personal disclosure. In: Corrigan PW, ed., *On the Stigma of Mental Illness. Practical strategies for research and social change*, pp. 257–280. Washington DC: American Psychological Press; 2005.

91. Smart L, Wegner D. The hidden costs of hidden stigma. In: Heatherton TF, Kleck RE, Hebl MR, Hull JG, eds., *The Social Psychology of Stigma*, pp. 220–242. New York: Guilford; 2000.

92. Dovidio J, Major B, Crocker J. Stigma: introduction and overview. In: Heatherton TF, Kleck RE, Hebl MR, Hull JG, eds., *The Social Psychology of Stigma*, pp. 1–28. New York: Guilford Press; 2000.

93. Smart L, Wegner DM. Covering up what can't be seen: concealable stigma and mental control. *J Pers Soc Psychol* 1999; 77(3):474–486.

94. Biernat M, Dovidio J. Stigma and stereotypes. In: Heatherton TF, Kleck RE, Hebl MR, Hull JG, eds, *The Social Psychology of Stigma*, pp. 88–125. New York: Guildford; 2000.

95. Quinn DM, Kahng SK, Crocker J. Discreditable: stigma effects of revealing a mental illness history on test performance. *Pers Soc Psychol Bull* 2004; 30(7):803–815.

96. Crocker J, Quinn DM. Social stigma and the self: meanings, situations, and self-esteem. In: Heatherton TF, Kleck RE, Hebl MR, Hull JG, eds., *The Social Psychology of Stigma*, pp. 153–183. New York: Guilford; 2000.

97. Steinberg BE, Shaw RJ. Bulimia as a disturbance of narcissism: self-esteem and the capacity to self-soothe. *Addict Behav* 1997; 22(5):699–710.

98. Geller J, Zaitsoff SL, Srikameswaran S. Beyond shape and weight: exploring the relationship between nonbody determinants of self-esteem and eating disorder symptoms in adolescent females. *Int J Eat Disord* 2002; 32(3):344–351.

99. Polivy J, Herman CP. Causes of eating disorders. *Annu Rev Psychol* 2002; 53:187–213.

100. Miller CT, Downey KT. A meta-analysis of heavyweight and self-esteem. *Personality and Social Psychology Review* 1999; 3:68–84.

101. Williams DR. Race, socioeconomic status, and health. The added effects of racism and discrimination. *Ann N Y Acad Sci* 1999; 896:173–188.

102. Gray-Little B, Hafdahl AR. Factors influencing racial comparisons of self-esteem: a quantitative review. *Psychol Bull* 2000; 126(1):26–54.

103. Dear M, Wolch J. *Landscapes of Despair*. Princeton, New Jersey: Princeton University Press; 1992.

104. Social Exclusion Unit. *Mental Health and Social Exclusion*. London: Office of the Deputy Prime Minister; 2004.

105. Fogarty JS. Reactance theory and patient noncompliance. *Soc Sci Med* 1997; 45(8):1277–1288.

106. Link BG, Struening EL, Neese-Todd S, Asmussen S, Phelan JC. Stigma as a barrier to recovery: The consequences of stigma for the self-esteem of people with mental illnesses. *Psychiatr Serv* 2001; 52(12):1621–6.

107. Camp DL, Finlay WM, Lyons E. Is low self-esteem an inevitable consequence of stigma? An example from women with chronic mental health problems. *Soc Sci Med* 2002; 55(5):823–834.

108. Pyne JM, Bean D, Sullivan G. Characteristics of patients with schizophrenia who do not believe they are mentally ill. *J Nerv Ment Dis* 2001; 189(3):146–153.

109. Estroff SE, Penn DL, Toporek JR. From stigma to discrimination: an analysis of community efforts to reduce the negative consequences of having a psychiatric disorder and label. *Schizophr Bull* 2004; 30(3):493–509.

110. Corrigan P. *On the Stigma of Mental Illness*. Washington, DC: American Psychological Association; 2005.

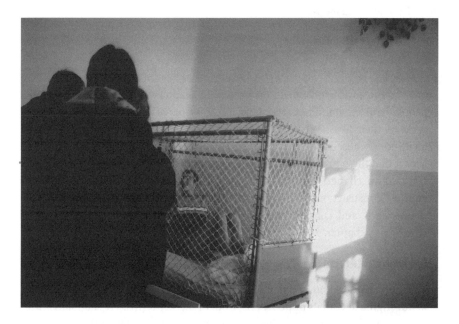

Cage bed in an Eastern European Country, 2004.

Chapter 9 From Stigma to Ignorance, Prejudice and Discrimination

Friends

They don't call me sad.
They don't call me bad.
They don't call me mad.
They don't call me.
© William McKnight

What is the basic problem? In the preceding chapters we have seen how many people with mental illness are subjected to systematic disadvantages in most areas of their lives. Why should this be so? What can we learn from other conditions whose image may have changed over time? Should we fatalistically accept that these processes of exclusion are somehow tribal, deeply rooted and resistant to change? Or it is realistic to see stigma and discrimination as cultural constructions, which we can collectively change if we understand them clearly and commit ourselves to tackle them? These issues are at the core of this chapter.

Defining terms

To begin with we should be clear about the key building blocks in thinking about stigma and all its implications, by defining key terms. We shall start with dictionary definitions as a point of reference, and then see how these relate to each other as the chapter proceeds.[1]

The starting point: stigma

The unavoidable starting point for this discussion is the idea of stigma. This term (plural stigmata) was originally used to refer to an indelible dot left on the skin after stinging with a sharp instrument, sometimes used to identify vagabonds or slaves.[2,3] The resulting mark led to the metaphorical use of 'stigma' to refer to stained or soiled individuals were who in some way morally diminished.[4,5] In modern times stigma has come to mean 'any attribute, trait or disorder that marks an individual as being unacceptably different from the 'normal' people with whom he or she routinely interacts, and that elicits some form of community sanction.'[6,7]

Box 9.1   Definitions of key terms

- *approval*: a favourable opinion
- *disadvantaged*: in socially or economically deprived circumstances.
- *dignity*: the state or quality of being worthy of honour or respect
- *discrimination*: (i) recognize a distinction: perceive or constitute the difference in or between, (ii) make an unjust distinction in the treatment of different categories of people, especially on the grounds of race, sex, or age
- *disgrace*: (i) loss of reputation as the result of a dishonourable action, (ii) a shameful and unacceptable person or thing
- *disgust*: revulsion or strong disapproval
- *esteem*: respect and admiration
- *honour*: (i) great respect or esteem, (ii) a feeling of pride and pleasure from being shown respect, (iii) a source of esteem
- *humiliation*: injure the dignity and self-respect of
- *prejudice*: preconceived opinion that is not based on reason or actual experience
- *self-respect*: pride and confidence in oneself
- *shame*: a feeling of humiliation or distress caused by the consciousness of wrong or foolish behaviour
- *stereotype*: an image or idea of a particular type of person or thing that has become fixed through being widely held
- *stigma*: a characteristic that individuals possess that (or are believed to possess) that conveys a social identity that is devalued, or a mark of disgrace associated with a particular circumstance, quality, or person[1]

The historical description of stigmatisation

However precisely we see the implications of stigma, it is clear that such processes are very long-standing. There are references to insanity, for example, from biblical times that we would now recognise at stigmatising. For example, the Babylonian king Nebuchadnezzar was punished by God for his vanity and was 'cast out from among men', ate grass and lived with wild beasts, and after returning to society declared 'my reason was restored to me'.[8, 9] He was later portrayed with 'shaggy brutishness' by William Blake.[10] In the fourth century BC Plato likened injustice to madness, and sickness of the psyche was equated with vice.[11] These historical roots to our thinking that mental disorders reflect moral failings, religious corruption, or a threat to social cohesion have been extensively described.[12–21]

Stigma and physical conditions

While this book is concerned specifically with people who have diagnoses of mental illnesses, the stigma concept has also been used extensively for some physical conditions.[22, 23] What can we learn from this work? People with HIV/AIDS have perhaps been most often described in recent years as suffering from the effects of stigmatisation.[24-26] The prominent themes in these discussions have been how far the individuals concerned are responsible (and therefore to blame) for their status,[27-29] and the balance between the need to protect public health and to respect the confidentiality and human rights of people with this diagnosis.[30-32] It is particularly important to note the during the 1990s inaccurate beliefs about the risks posed by casual social contact with people with HIV/AIDS increased, as did the belief that people with AIDS deserve their illness, but overt expression of stigma declined through this decade.[33] In other words it was not necessary for factual knowledge, or moral attitudes, to improve for behaviour to change in a postive way.

> Perhaps the reason that science struggles in the face of mental illness is that the illness is somehow bound up with their personality. This I think is dead central to the stigma issue. If the illness is in some way related to your personality, then haven't you in some way brought it on yourself? If your personality has grown to become bound up with illness, then why would anyone want to be around such an influence? Based on this, it's no wonder that people try to steer clear of the mentally ill.
>
> Robert

Epilepsy has also been extensively researched in relation to stigma.[34] A survey of over 5000 people with a diagnosis of epilepsy in 15 European countries, for example, found that half (51 per cent) reported feeling stigmatised, and that these people were more likely to also have worry, negative feelings about life, long-term health problems, injuries, and to report side effects of antiepileptic drugs.[35, 36] One of the most important findings was that the nature of the stigma experienced in these countries differed a great deal. In other words there seems to be a high level of cultural specificity in the social reactions and in the personal experiences related to epilepsy.[35]

Further, it appears that feelings of stigma are not associated with the severity of the condition in epilepsy,[37] but do have profound implications for the self-esteem[38] and the social identity of the people affected.[39] Nevertheless, as with AIDS, these social reactions are not immutable, and there is evidence from the UK that attitudes to people with epilepsy have improved in recent years, and that outmoded ideas (such as the 'epileptic personality') are now much less common.[40]

Skin conditions are also often seen to convey a sense of stigma.[41] People with vitiligo, for example (a condition in which irregular patches of skin turn white), have been found to have high rates of depression and anxiety, especially those with high levels of perceived stigma, and these individuals are more likely to react to this by avoiding social situations in which they expect to face rejection.[42]

A study of psoriasis showed that the type of visible abnormality can be important. In a UK survey stigma was higher among those people where the condition started at an early age, there was more bleeding, or they had more feelings of despair or rejection. They found another type of vicious cycle: those most in despair were less likely to accept treatment, so that their skin problems worsened and they were more likely to be rejected by others.[43] About a fifth of these people each reported over 50 episodes of 'gross rejection', most often at the gym, swimming pool, hairdresser, or at work, and among these people alcohol consumption was greater.[44]

Related work in Germany suggests that rejection by others is greater for people with abnormal 'visible parts', but that retreat from social contact is more for people affected by psoriasis in 'invisible regions',[45] such as the genital area.[46] There is some evidence from studies in Norway that adopting a more optimistic coping style can improve mental health and quality of life.[47, 48]

Research on the stigma related to skin conditions therefore suggests that the degree of visibility or concealment (in social and intimate situations), along with how the condition is construed by the person with the condition, can have very important consequences for the degree of rejection or withdrawal experienced.[49] Indeed it has been suggested that the key to understanding changing popular views of leprosy is that improved treatment methods have allowed more people with this condition to ensure that it remains invisible to onlookers.[50, 51]

Another condition in which visibility is a central feature is obesity.[52] An attempt to reduce the degree of stigmatisation (based upon ideas that obese people were lazy and lacking in self-control) was made in Kentucky by educating first year medical students about genetic predisposition and weight, and found that blaming attitudes could be reduced.[53] The attitude of the obese person may also be very influential. Researchers in New York State discovered that when obese people blamed the negative views of others upon their prejudice and discrimination, this enhanced their own mood and self-esteem.[54] Strangely enough, even some professionals who specialize in the treatment of obesity themselves have strong but implicit anti-fat attitudes.[55]

> Often I have heard comments, either said to me or about people with depression, as 'lazy'. I was constantly tired and at low periods I would take to my bed and isolate myself from the outside world.
>
> Tania

Many other physical disorders have been studied in relation to stigma.[56] They include, for example, neurological conditions,[57, 58] incontinence, the use of catheters and colostomies,[59-61] and cerebro-vascular disorders such as stroke.[62, 63] A few common themes emerge from these studies. First, the degree of social rejection is related to the visibility of the condition. Second, conditions which are perceived to be under personal control are more likely to lead to a blaming attitude and to social distancing.[64] Third, how stigma is perceived is mediated by the coping style of the person affected. Fourth, attitudes and behaviour can and do change.[11]

Degrees of rejection

What do we know about how far stigma applies to people with mental illnesses compared with other conditions? In brief, very little. As we have seen in earlier chapters, most of the literature on stigma and discrimination focuses on theories of psychological processes, attitude scales, opinion surveys, links with violence and portrayals in the media. Comparative stigma is one of the many areas about which very little has been written.[65]

There have been several studies of social distance.[66-68] These typically present a vignette or a hypothetical scenario of a person with a particular condition, and ask whether you would want to live next door to that person, let them act as a childminder to your children, or to allow your son or daughter to marry such a person.[69, 70] A series of such surveys in Germany found high levels of social distance expressed towards people with schizophrenia, and even higher levels to those with alcohol dependence.[71] A revealing US study asked employers about job offer intentions, and found that ex-convicts were seen to be more acceptable than people with mental illness, and the only group less favoured by employers were those with tuberculosis.[72] Such high levels of concern were also found in a sample of over 1500 members of the general UK population who were asked about their attitudes to people with five different conditions. Their concern levels were: stress or depression 34 per cent, epilepsy 19 per cent, heart attack 17 per cent, facial disfigurement 9 per cent, or use of a wheelchair 4 per cent.[73]

In a very detailed comparison in Kansas, over 100 undergraduate psychology students were asked to compare 66 different medical conditions along 13 dimensions, including social distance. Overall, five of these dimensions predicted rejection: severity of the condition, contagiousness, behavioural causality, availability and sexual transmission, where the last four were all closely linked to personal control. In other words, how far is the individual directly or indirectly at fault in developing the condition? In an important conclusion the authors stated, 'Severity and behavioural causality account for a significant amount of the *socially shared representation* of what makes an illness stigmatisable' (emphasis added).[64] Care is needed here. It may not necessarily follow, for example, that emphasizing the biological basis of mental illnesses will reduce stigma by reducing blame for a condition over which the person affected is assumed to have little responsibility. Indeed a German survey found the opposite.[74] *'Stigma is thus negotiable, yet it is intrinsic to the heart-felt urge to find meaning in sickness.'*[10]

Stigma can also be assessed indirectly. One particularly intriguing approach is to see whether people with a particular physical condition are treated differently if they do or not also have a diagnosis of mental illness.[75] For people with diabetes, for example (which is more common in people treated with some types of anti-psychotic medication), the quality of care was assessed by five key indicators: annual foot inspection, foot pulse examination, foot sensory examination, retina examination and a specific blood test (glycated hemoglobin). The results of the study were that people with mental illness (particularly substance misuse) were less likely to receive these recommended health checks.[76]

In terms of treatment for heart conditions, most (but not all[77]) studies also show that people with mental illness receive inferior physical healthcare. For example, careful examination of the treatment records of over 110,000 people who had acute inpatient care in the USA found that, compared to those without a mental illness, people with such conditions were less often prescribed appropriate medications,[78] and also received fewer surgical procedures.[79, 80] These care deficits were associated with higher mortality rates after heart attacks.[78] This strongly suggests that some form of direct or indirect discrimination is in operation.

Global patterns

Do we know if discrimination varies between countries and cultures? The evidence here is stronger, but still frustratingly patchy.[81] Although studies on stigma and mental illness have been carried out in many countries, few have been comparison of two or more places, or have included non-Western nations.[82]

In Africa one study described attitudes to mentally ill people in rural sites in Ethiopia. Among almost 200 relatives of people with diagnoses of schizophrenia or mood disorders, three-quarters (75 per cent) said that they had experienced stigma due to the presence of mental illness in the family, and a third (37 per cent) wanted to conceal the fact that a relative was ill. Most family members (65 per cent) said that praying was their preferred method of treating the condition.[83]

Among the general population in Ethiopia, 100 people gave their views about vignettes of people with seven types of disorder. Schizophrenia was judged to be the most severe problem, and talkativeness, aggression and strange behaviour were rated as the most common symptoms of mental illness.[84] Traditional treatment methods were preferred to treat symptoms of mental illness, and medications were favoured for physical illnesses. The authors concluded that it was important to work closely with traditional healers and to reduce 'certain harmful practices' inflicted on people with mental illness in these rural communities.

In South Africa,[85, 86] a survey of over 600 members of the public was conducted on their knowledge and attitudes towards people with mental illness.[87] Different vignettes, portraying depression, schizophrenia, panic disorder or substance misuse were presented to each person. Most thought that these conditions were either related to stress or to a lack of willpower, rather than seeing them as medical disorders. They therefore preferred to talk the problem over rather than to consult professionals. The results suggest that there is widespread misinformation about mental illness in South Africa. Among one particular group, the Xhosa, the use of traditional remedies and ancestor worship is usual, and it is common for mental distress to be explained as the influence of spirits and therefore to lie in the domain of witchdoctors.[88]

Similar findings, that a lack of willpower contributes towards mental illness, have also been observed in other non-Western countries, for example in Turkey,[89] or in Siberia and Mongolia.[74] This suggests that people in such countries may be more ready to make the individual responsible for his or her mental illness and less willing to grant the benefits of the sick role.

We have seen in previous chapters that most of the published work on stigma is by authors in the USA and Canada,[90–93] but there are also a few reports from elsewhere in the Americas and in the Caribbean.[94] In a review of studies from Argentina, Brazil, Dominica, Mexico and Nicaragua, mainly from urban sites, a number of common themes emerged. The conditions most often rated as 'mental illnesses' were the psychotic disorders, especially schizophrenia. People with higher levels of education tended to have more favourable attitudes to people with mental illness. Alcoholism was considered to be the most common type of mental disorder. Most people thought that a health professional needs to be consulted by people with mental illnesses.[95]

By comparison, a study of Inuit residents in Northern Canada (Nunavik) produced a quite different pattern. A series of vignettes were labelled as 'burdened or weighed down by thoughts', 'demon possession', or 'mental illness'. Greater social distance was shown by women, by those with higher levels of education, and by people who did not personally know someone with mental illness'. Strange behaviour was commonly described as immoral conduct, or ascribed to spirits or demons. It was particularly striking that more favourable attitudes were expressed towards people expected to have a greater chance of recovery.[96]

A great deal of work has studied the question of stigma towards mentally ill people in Asian countries and cultures.[97–99] Within China,[100] a large-scale survey was undertaken of over 600 people with a diagnosis of schizophrenia and over 900 family members.[101] Over half of the family members said that stigma had had an important effect on them and their family, and levels of stigma were higher in urban areas and for people who were more highly educated.

In relation to staff views, another study discovered far more negative views toward people with mental illness among psychiatric nurses than psychiatrists in China.[102] Even so, it seems that both Chinese doctors and nurses may differ from the general population in their views about the causes of mental illness. A survey of almost 400 people with mental illness and their relatives showed that most attributed the cause to social, interpersonal and psychological problems, whereas staff more often used a biomedical explanation for schizophrenia.[103]

As usual in the field of stigma research we find that, for some reason, schizophrenia is the primary focus of interest. It is remarkable that there are almost no studies, for example, on bipolar disorder and stigma. A comparison of attitudes to schizophrenia was undertaken in England and Hong Kong. As predicted, the Chinese respondents expressed more negative attitudes and beliefs about schizophrenia, and preferred a more social model to explain its causation. In both countries most participants, whatever their educational level, showed great ignorance about this condition.[104] This may well be one reason why most of the population in Hong Kong are very concerned about their mental health and hold rather negative views about mentally ill people.[105] Less favourable attitudes were common in those with less direct personal contact with people with mental illness (as in most Western studies), and by women (the opposite of what has been found in many Western reports).[106]

Among Chinese people with mental illness, expectations of rejection may be more common than actual experiences. Almost 200 outpatients in Hong Kong, for example, said that most people would agree that someone with a history of mental illness is likely to be untrustworthy, dangerous, looked down upon and not to be taken seriously. In terms of actual experiences of rejection, the most common was seeing offensive articles in the mass media (49 per cent), being treated as less competent (34 per cent), and being treated differently by friends after they learned about the mental illness (28 per cent). Over a half (56 per cent) concluded that their best course of action was to try to conceal the condition.[107] A similar study in Hong Kong also showed that significantly more people with schizophrenia (40 per cent) than diabetes (15 per cent) experienced stigma from family members, partners, friends and colleagues.[108]

To gain some understanding about stigma in India we also need to assemble an overall picture from a few jigsaw pieces of evidence. Among relatives of people with schizophrenia in Chennai (Madras) in Southern India, their main concerns were effects on marital prospects, fear of rejection by neighbours and the need to hide the condition from others. Higher levels of stigma were reported by women and by younger people with the condition.[109] Women who have mental illness appear to be at a particular disadvantage in India. If they are divorced, sometimes related to concerns about heredity,[110] then they often receive no financial support from their former husbands, and they and their families experience intense distress from the additional stigma of being separated or divorced.[111]

There are complex relationships in India between depression and somatic disorders. It seems that how these conditions are viewed by others plays a part in framing how psychological distress is experienced and communicated. One study in Bangalore showed higher levels of stigma among psychiatric outpatients who complained of depression than for those who described physical complaints.[112] In Kolkata (Calcutta), for example, among outpatients who met Western criteria for major depression, only five per cent complained of sadness, while half (48 per cent) described pains and other physical symptoms. This suggests that there is a congruence between the language used by individuals to describe their own suffering, and the forms of distress that are socially allowed (for example avoiding stigmatising rejection).[113–115]

These cultural influences can also shape access to treatment and care. Beliefs that mental illnesses may be caused by religious factors will encourage families to seek help from senior figures in their faith communities in many countries and cultures, and can delay seeking help from health professionals.[116] In some parts of India and Pakistan mental health service provision has been integrated into the general primary care services, and this is intended to reduce the barriers to accessing care which are related to stigma.

In fact many families may be reluctant to seek help for what they see as mental illness, wherever staff are located. Indeed research in India has found that psychiatrists are the least preferred option because of the stigma attached to such consultations, as they are elsewhere in the region.[117,118] The key barrier is the sense of shame, rather than the physical location of doctors and nurses.[119–121]

These themes also emerge from work on stigma in Japan. In particular, mental illnesses are seen to reflect a loss of control, and so are not subject to the force of willpower, both of which lead to a sense of shame.[122–124] Although it is tempting to generalize about the degree of stigma in different countries, reality may not allow such simplifications. A comparison of attitudes to mentally ill people in Japan and Bali, for example, showed that views towards people with schizophrenia were less favourable in Japan, but that people with depression and obsessive-compulsive disorder were seen to be less acceptable in Bali.[125]

What different countries do often share is a high level of ignorance and misinformation about mental illnesses. A survey of teachers' opinions in Japan and Taiwan showed that relatively few could describe the main features of schizophrenia with any accuracy. The general profile of knowledge, beliefs and attitudes was similar to that found in most Western countries, although the degree of social rejection was somewhat greater in Japan.[126]

In a unique move aimed to reduce social rejection, the name for schizophrenia has been changed in Japan. Following a decade of pressure from family member groups, including Zenkaren, the name for this condition was changed from *seishi buntetsu byo* (split-mind disorder) to *togo shiccho sho* (loss of coordination disorder).[122, 127] The previous term went against the grain of traditional, culturally valued concepts of personal autonomy, as a result of which only 20 per cent of people with this condition were told the diagnosis by their doctors.[128–130] There are indications from service users and family members that the new term is seen as less stigmatising and is more often discussed openly. This is consistent with work in Germany suggesting that giving the label 'schizophrenia' has a significant and negative effect on public perceptions.[131]

Little is written in the English language literature on stigma in Islamic communities, but despite earlier indications that the intensity of stigma may be relatively low,[99] detailed studies indicate that, on balance, it is no less than we have seen described elsewhere.[132–135] A study of 100 family members of people with schizophrenia in Morocco found that 76 per cent had no knowledge about the condition, and many considered it chronic (80 per cent), handicapping (48 per cent), incurable (39 per cent), or linked with sorcery (25 per cent). Most said that they had 'hard lives' because of the diagnosis.[136] Turning to religious authority figures is reported to be common in some Muslim countries.[137, 138] Some studies have found that direct personal contact was not associated with more favourable attitudes to people with mental illness,[139,140] especially where behaviour is seen to threaten the social fabric of the community.[141]

A large-scale survey in Istanbul in Turkey asked over 700 members of the general public about their attitudes to people with mental illness. Most

(68 per cent) thought that depression was caused by 'weak personality' and many (43 per cent) said that it caused aggression. The least favourable attitudes were found among older people.[142] Social distance was very prominent with most people (65 per cent) saying that they would not marry someone with depression, and many (40 per cent) not wanting to work with such a person.[89]

What sense can we make of all these fragments of information? Several points are clear. First there is no known country, society or culture in which people with mental illness are considered to have the same value and to be as acceptable as people who do not have mental illness. Second, the quality of information that we have is relatively poor, with very few comparative studies between countries or over time. Third, there do seem to be clear links between popular understandings of mental illness, if people in mental distress want to seek help, and whether they feel able to disclose their problems.[143] The core experiences of shame (to oneself) and blame (from others) are common everywhere stigma has been studied, but to differing extents. Where comparisons with other conditions have been made, then mental illnesses are more, or far more, stigmatised,[144,145] and have been referred to as the 'ultimate stigma'.[11] Finally, rejection and avoidance of people with mental illness appear to be universal phenomena.

Understanding stigma

There is now a voluminous literature on stigma.[6, 23, 11, 56, 90, 146–153] The stigma of mental illness is the subject of many hundreds of scientific papers.[147] The most complete model of the component processes of stigmatisation has four key components.[154] (i) Labelling, in which personal characteristics, which are signalled or noticed as conveying an important difference. (ii) Stereotyping, which is the linkage of these differences to undesirable characteristics. (iii) Separating, the categorical distinction between the mainstream/normal group and the labelled group as in some respects fundamentally different. (iv) Status loss and discrimination: devaluing, rejecting, and excluding the labelled group. Interestingly, more recently the authors of this model have added a revision to include the emotional reactions which may accompany each of these stages.[155]

Another way to look at stigma is to think of six dimensions along which it can vary: (i) concealability or visibility, (ii) its course over time, (iii) the strain on interpersonal relationships, (iv) related aesthetic qualities, (v) the cause of the disorders, and (vi) the peril or danger to others associated with the condition.[156]

Shortcomings of stigma models

A number of features have limited the usefulness of these theories.[157] First, while these processes are undoubtedly complex, the approach taken by academics has been dominated by those within social psychology or sociology,[6, 56, 23, 90] and in particular there have been relatively few connections with the fields of disability policy[158–160] or clinical practice. For example, legislation such as the Americans with Disability Act in the USA, and the Disability Discrimination Act in the UK, have been applied relatively infrequently to cases involving mental illness.[161–163]

The focus upon the core concept of stigma rather than upon prejudice and discrimination has also separated the field of mental illness from the mainstream of disability-related policy, and in particular the stigma idea has offered policy-makers and politicians few recommendations for action. Further, few lessons have been drawn with other areas of unequal treatment such as for HIV/AIDS[164,165] or sexually transmitted diseases.[49]

Overwhelmingly, most work on mental illness and stigma has been descriptive, commonly describing the results of attitude surveys or relating to the portrayal of mental illness by the media. Very little is known about effective interventions to reduce stigma.[166,167] There have been notably few contributions to this literature from service users themselves. Little has been written about the actual experiences of rejection or exclusion by people with mental illness[168–170]. There has been an underlying pessimism that stigma is deeply historically rooted and difficult to change.[10]

In stigma theories the relationship between 'perceiver' and 'target' has focused research attention upon the level of one-to-one or small-group interactions.[56] Sometimes such theories come close to seeing those who are disadvantaged as victims.[56] This tends to de-emphasize any analysis of cultural or social factors. In particular such theories rarely pay attention to questions of power in relation to people with mental illness.[92, 171] Further stigma theories have paid little attention to the structural factors which manifest the low value given to disadvantaged groups, such as relatively low levels of investment in mental health services.[172]

A further limitation of stigma-related research is that it has rarely connected to the domains of civil liberties and human rights.[173,174] For this reason there has been little use of international declarations and conventions to improve psychiatric treatment and care, especially for those undergoing compulsory treatment.[175] Further, stigma research has tended to focus upon single conditions (predominantly schizophrenia) and has shown scant regard for people who have two or more diagnoses. In particular one whole area of research that is largely absent refers to people with two forms of disadvantage, for example in relation to mental illness and ethnicity, or among mentally ill offenders. Finally, an emphasis upon individual psychological factors has meant that less attention has been given to environmental factors, for example to how reasonable adjustments at work can prevent impairments from becoming disabilities.[176]

Recently there have been early signs in the research literature of a developing focus upon discrimination. This can be seen as the behavioural consequences of stigma which act to the disadvantage of service users.[92, 157, 158, 177–79] The importance of discriminatory behaviour has been clear for many years in terms of the personal experiences of service users, in terms of devastating effects upon personal relationships, parenting and childcare, education, training, work and housing[180–184], as described in Chapters 1–5. These voices have said and that the rejecting behaviour of others may bring greater disadvantage than the primary condition itself.[185,186]

The three core problems

We shall consider later what needs to be done to allow people with mental illnesses a full opportunity for social participation (in Chapters 10 and 11). First of all we need to have a clear map to know where we are and where we want to go.

Stigma theories have not been sensitive enough to understanding of feelings and experiences of people with mental illness, nor to know what practical steps are needed to reverse social exclusion.[187] Rather stigma can be seen as an overarching term that contains three important elements:

1. problems of knowledge (ignorance)
2. problems of attitudes (prejudice)
3. and problems of behaviour (discrimination)

In terms of social psychology, these are referred to as the cognitive, affective and behavioural domains,[188,189] and each will now be discussed.

First a word is necessary here about attitudes, as much of the literature on stigma consists of attitude theories and surveys.[190,191] While on the face of it the idea of attitudes towards mental illness is clear, on closer examination it becomes less straightforward. 'Attitude' can be defined as consisting of four aspects: *cognitive* (consciously held beliefs or opinions), *affective* (emotional tone or feeling), *evaluative* (positive or negative), and *conative* (tendency towards action).[192] The concept of attitude therefore mixes, often in a rather unclear and general way (as does the stigma concept), the separate elements which are discussed in this chapter.

Ignorance: the problem of knowledge

As we have seen above, while some information is available on knowledge about mental illnesses in non-Western nations, the vast majority on stigma and discrimination information stems from the more economically developed countries. A surprisingly consistent picture emerges: wherever it has been studied it is found that general levels of knowledge about mental illness are remarkably low. One common misunderstanding, for example, is that schizophrenia means 'split mind', usually misinterpreted to mean a 'split personality' (as in the 'Dr Jekyll and Mr Hyde' story by Robert Louis Stevenson). Surveys of over 12,000 individuals in several European countries have discovered that such views are common, and are supported by many people in Austria (29 per cent), Germany (80 per cent), Greece (81 per cent), Poland (50 per cent) Slovakia 61 per cent), and Turkey (39 per cent).[148,193] Commonly older people are less knowledgable than younger.[194]

At a time when there is an unprecedented volume of information in the public domain about health problems in general, the level of general knowledge about mental illnesses is universally meagre. In a population survey in England, for example, most people (55 per cent) believed that the statement 'someone who cannot be held responsible for his or her own actions' describes a person who is mentally ill.[195] Most (63 per cent) thought that fewer that 10 per cent of the population would experience a mental illness at some time in their lives. In northern Italy it was found that people who had more information about mental illnesses were less fearful and more willing to favour working with people with a history of mental illness,[196] and exactly the same finding came from a Canadian study.[197] Most such studies agree with the findings of a Swiss survey that age matters: older people are both less well informed about mental illness and less favourable towards people with mental illnesses, although these are relatively small effects.[198] Women also tend to offer more favourable views about people with mental illness in most Western surveys,[199] such as one large study throughout Australia.[200]

There are also striking knowledge gaps about how to find help. In Scotland most children did not know what to do if they had a mental health problem or what to recommend to a friend with mental health difficulties: only 1 per cent mentioned school counselling, 1 per cent nominated helplines, 4 per cent recommended talking with friends, 10 per cent said that they would turn to a doctor, but over a third (35 per cent) were unsure where to find help.[201]

The public level of knowledge about mental illnesses and their treatments has sometimes been called 'mental health literacy'.[202, 203] In Australia over 2000 adults were asked about the features of two mental illnesses and their treatment. Most (72 per cent) could identify the key characteristics of depression, but relatively few (27 per cent) could accurately recognise schizophrenia. Many standard psychiatric treatments (such as antidepressant and antipsychotic medication, or admission to a psychiatric ward) were more often rated as harmful than helpful, and most people more readily recommended the use of vitamins.[204] Similarly, although most people in a nationwide survey in the USA agreed that psychiatric medications are effective, the majority were not willing to take such drugs themselves.[205] Also among people with depression, many have strong and often ambivalent feelings about taking antidepressant drugs, although interestingly the rate of acceptance is higher among people who have taken them for a previous episode of depression.[206, 207]

Such findings have led many, especially in Australia where much of this work has been pioneered, to conclude that it is necessary to provide far more public information on the nature of conditions such as depression, and on the treatments options which are available, so that both the general population and those people who are depressed can make decisions about getting help on a fully informed basis.[208–210] In other words, the best remedy for ignorance is information.

Is stigma getting better or worse? As we have seen elsewhere in this book, sometimes the literature is voluble (for example on risk and violence) and sometimes it whispers or even remains silent. Trends in stigma are a quiet zone. There has been active research about stigma for over half a century,[190, 191, 211–213] and over most of this time public attitude surveys have been carried out.[214, 215] Indeed most of the published work on mental health and stigma consists of attitude surveys, but very few have been repeated over time to see if attitudes are becoming more or less favourable.

The evidence we do have about trends is contradictory. In Greece, a comparison was made between public views about mental illness in 1980 and 1994.[199] Significant improvements were identified for social discrimination, restrictiveness and social integration. For example, more people said that they would accept a mentally ill person as a neighbour or work colleague. A long-term comparison of popular views about mental illness in Germany has found a hardening of opinion against people with schizophrenia,[216] but no change towards people with depression.[217] There are also some indirect indications that popular views of mental illness have changed, for example the fact that increasing numbers of people in many countries do now seek help for mental illnesses,[218] although the majority still do not.[219]

An important study in the USA compared popular views of mental illness in 1950 and 1996.[218] Over this period it found evidence that there was a broadening of what was seen as mental illness, to include non-psychotic disorders and socially deviant behaviour. The second focus of the study was on 'frightening characteristics', and the results here were less heartening. There was a significant increase (almost twofold) over the 46-year period in public expectations linking mental illness to violence in terms of extreme, unstable, excessive, unpredictable, uncontrolled or irrational behaviour. This link was especially marked for public views of psychotic disorders, whereas dangerousness was less often mentioned as typical of non-psychotic conditions in 1996. In other words depression and anxiety-related disorders had become 'less alien and less extreme', while schizophrenia and similar conditions had grown in their perceived threat.[218] The authors examined the hypothesis that closing large psychiatric hospitals had led to this greater disapproval and rejection. In fact they found the opposite: those who reported frequently seeing people in public who seemed to be mentally ill were significantly less likely to perceive them as dangerous.[220] The authors concluded that 'something has occurred in our culture that has increased the connection between psychosis and violence in the public mind'.[218]

There have also been changes in public views about mental illness in Germany. A series of surveys between 1990 and 2001 found the German public became more ready to recommend seeking help from psychiatrists or psychotherapists for people with schizophrenia or depression. In particular there was a greater willingness to accept drug treatment and psychotherapy, especially for schizophrenia. Intriguingly, respondents just as often recommended that meditation or yoga should be used.[216] The results suggested that the gap between professional and popular views on treatment was closing.[221]

There is evidence that deliberate interventions to improve public knowledge about depression can be successful. In a campaign in Australia to increase knowledge about depression and its treatment, some states and territories received this coordinated programme, while others did not.[222, 223] In areas which had received this programme people more often recognised the features of depression, were more likely to support seeking help for depression, or to accept treatment with counselling and medication.[224] The implications of these and similar findings for large-scale public education campaigns will be discussed in Chapter 11.

In Great Britain there have been conflicting findings on trends in attitudes to mental illness. A series of government surveys have been carried out from 1993 to 2003 and give a mixed picture.[225] On one hand there are some clear improvements, for example the proportion thinking that people with mental illness can be easily distinguished from 'normal people' fell from 30 to 20 per cent.[195] On the other hand views became significantly less favourable over this decade for the following items:

- it is frightening to think of people with mental problems living in residential neighbourhoods (increased from 33 per cent to 42 per cent)
- residents have nothing to fear from people coming into their neighbourhood to obtain mental health services (decreased from 70 per cent to 55 per cent)
- mental illness is far less of a danger than most people suppose (decreased from 65 per cent to 58 per cent)
- less emphasis should be placed on protecting the public from people with mental illness (decreased from 38 per cent to 31 per cent)

How is it possible that different studies show that public attitudes seem to becoming both more favourable and more rejecting at the same time? One key seems to be diagnosis. Before and after its campaign called 'Changing Minds' the UK Royal College of Psychiatrists commissioned national opinion polls of nearly 2000 adults, asking about mental illness.[226] Unusually, they asked each of the key questions separately for a series of different diagnoses. Significant changes were reported in the following percentages of people who agreed with the following items between 1998 and 2003:

- 'danger posed to others': depression (fell from 23 per cent to 19 per cent), schizophrenia (fell from 71 per cent to 66 per cent), but no change for alcoholism or drug addiction
- 'hard to talk to': depression (fell from 62 per cent to 56 per cent), schizophrenia (fell from 58 per cent to 52 per cent), alcoholism (fell from 59 per cent to 55 per cent)
- 'never fully recover': schizophrenia (decrease from 51 per cent to 42 per cent), eating disorders (increase from 11 per cent to 15 per cent), alcoholism (increase 24 per cent to 29 per cent) and drug addiction (increase from 23 per cent to 26 per cent)
- 'feel different from us': depression (decrease 43 per cent to 30 per cent), schizophrenia (decrease 57 per cent to 37 per cent), dementia (decrease 61 per cent to 42 per cent)

It is clear from these trends that a complicated picture emerges of both favourable and unfavourable change across a wide spectrum of conditions.[227] These variations suggest that public opinion surveys, which ask about 'the mentally ill' in general terms, are likely to produce a composite and possibly uninformative response which summarizes these conflicting trends. Overall it seems that popular views about depression appear to be improving in some Western countries, in terms of less social rejection, but the evidence about views about people with psychotic disorders is too confused to give a clear picture.

Common myths about disability and mental illness

It is clear that lay opinions about what mental illnesses are, and how people with these conditions should be helped, are often very different from professional views. A series of common beliefs about mental illnesses have developed, which are firmly held but not firmly based on evidence. These are often described by experts as 'myths'. Some such myths are held to apply to all disabled people,[228] including:

- disability is solely the result of biological causes
- when a disabled person faces problems, it is assumed that the impairment causes them
- it is assumed that the disabled person is a 'victim'
- it is assumed that disability if central to the disabled person's self-concept
- it is assumed that having a disability is synonymous with needing help and social support.

Other myths apply in particular to people with mental illness,[187,229,230] for example:

- schizophrenia means a split personality
- all 'schizophrenics' are violent and dangerous
- people with serious mental illness are completely disabled
- having schizophrenia means that you can never do anything with your life
- schizophrenia represents a form of creative imagination or 'inner journey'
- they're lazy and not trying
- it's all the fault of the genes
- they can't work
- they are incapable of making their own decisions
- there's no hope for people with mental illnesses
- mental illnesses cannot affect me
- mental illness is the same as mental retardation
- once people develop mental illnesses, they will never recover
- mental illnesses are brought on by a weakness of character
- psychiatric disorders are not true medical illnesses like diabetes
- mental illness is the result of bad parenting
- depression results from a personality weakness or character flaw, and people who are depressed could just snap out of it if they tried hard enough
- depression is a normal part of the ageing process

◆ if you have a mental illness, you can will it away, and being treated for a
   psychiatric disorder means you have in some way 'failed' or are weak.

That many of these ideas still have a common currency shows that the
factual understanding of mental illnesses among most members of the general
population is still very weak. In the presence of ignorance myths abound.

> I think that the reason for the stigma is firstly that the mentally ill can cause
> serious social problems including violence, threats of violence. They can be
> continually morose, talk endless streams of nonsense. They can be manipula-
> tive, attention-seeking, obsessive, arrogant. They can seem extremely lazy.
> These are all traits of people that nobody could like to be around, whether or
> not this is due to an illness. What is happening to them has no properly
> understood step by step solution, so when we see somebody in a state that is
> clearly abnormal, we are scared because we are aware that nobody really knows
> how they got this way, how to get them out of this state, or whether it will even
> be possible for them to be returned to a more normal state. I think it is much
> more scary to see a man with an amputated leg than a man with a leg in plaster,
> because we know that the leg in plaster is getting better, whereas we know that
> the amputated leg will not return as far as science allows. I think if science did
> allow the amputated leg to 'grow back' then there would be no fear of looking at
> an amputee. Similarly I don't think that the stigma and conflicting views of the
> mentally ill would exist if science allowed all the sufferers to rapidly return to
> health by a fairly unstoppable means.
>
> Robert

The advantages of stereotypes

Stereotypes are normal and are enormously useful.[211] They allow us to be
cognitive misers, and to avoid being overwhelmed by an unmanageable flood
of information from a complex world.[190] The use of stereotypes brings many
advantages.[190] It can minimize within-group differences and so reduce social
tensions among peers, colleagues or family members. Their use can elicit
stereotype-confirming behaviour, so that stereotypes may be self-fulfilling.[231]
Stereotyping may operate outside conscious awareness and so speed-up mental processing and recall, allowing split-second judgements. In particular,
stereotype-confirming information is processed more quickly than that
which is stereotype-disconfirming, and indeed blocks the latter. So using
stereotypes preserves mental resources, which are then available for other
tasks. These functional benefits mean that 'people are hardly equal opportunity perceivers; a stereotype-matching advantage dominates.'[232]

The rapid analysis of incoming information, and a clear preference to match
it to pre-existing categories, are therefore universal psychological mechanisms.
Further, stereotypes may be less damaging than has been reported. They
predict discrimination less well than do emotional prejudices.

So the use of stereotypes seems to be unavoidable. But why should they be employed with particular venom towards some categories of people? There are many theories about this. One is that a primary aim of stereotypes is to assist our social survival.[233] People's physical and psychological well-being depends upon others. To achieve survival we are therefore motivated to achieve belonging, understanding, controlling, self-enhancing and trusting. According to this approach we separate out those who threaten any of these basic resources for social survival into negatively appraised 'outgroups'.

Another view is that stigmatisation serves several further socially useful purposes.[191, 188] It may enable individuals to believe that they are good (self-enhancement), that their group is good (social identity enhancement), that they are deserving and fair (self-justification and system-justification[234]), or that their worldview is correct (anxiety-buffering or terror management). A third overall approach to the question 'Why do we stigmatise?' is that it is rooted in a basic need to live in effective groups. Stigmatisation, in this view, is a form of social control, used against those whose characteristics are seen to threaten the effective functioning of social groups.[165, 235]

Some argue that stigma has biological roots,[236] such as a tendency to herd, although this view is not strongly supported by evidence.[237] A related theory is that stigma originates in a universal human tendency to avoid danger.[238] Stigmatisation is not therefore mainly directed against individuals, but against those who are understood to pose a threat. Such understandings are socially created, and individual 'stigmatisers' are essentially only repeating (and recreating) their society's norms about what are appropriate feelings and behaviours to display to members of any threatening group.[238]

One interesting aspect of this theory is that the emotional reaction to threat may combine anxiety and fear, and that the strength of the consequent avoidant or rejecting behaviour may be increased if linked to strong negative emotions. This ties in with what we saw in Chapter 6 on the media, namely that the predominant characteristic of mental illness which is portrayed in the public domain is threat.[234, 239] In other words threat forms a conceptual bridge from ignorance to prejudice and discrimination, which are discussed next.

Prejudice: the problem of negative attitudes

If ignorance is the first great hurdle faced by people with mental illness, prejudice is the second. Although the term prejudice is used to refer to many social groups which experience disadvantage, for example minority ethnic groups, it is employed rarely in relation to people with mental illness.[68,240,241] Social psychologists have focused upon thoughts (cognition) rather than feelings (affect).[66] In particular they have long been interested in stereotypes (widely held and fixed images about a particular type of person), and degrees of social distance to such stereotypes.[190, 211, 212]

> Another thing that I was brought up with was that it was OK for women to get ill, or suffer from 'nerves', whereas a man was tough and robust enough to weather any storm life threw at him.
>
> Paul

But reactions of a host majority to act with prejudice in rejecting a minority group usually involve not just negative thoughts but also emotionally laden attitudes involving anxiety, anger, resentment, hostility, distaste, or disgust.[155] In fact prejudice may more strongly predict discrimination than do stereotypes.[189]

So-called 'gut level' prejudices[190] stem from anticipated threats, in other words how far a member of an outgroup is seen to threaten the goals or the interests of the person concerned. Anticipating harm may provoke anger (if the person seen to threaten harm does so unjustifiably), fear (if the harm is in the certain future), anxiety (if the harm is in the uncertain future), or sadness (if the harm is in the past).[190] Some writers have made a distinction between 'hot' prejudice, in which strong emotions are more prominent than negative thoughts, and 'cold' forms of rejection, for example in failing to promote a member of staff, when stereotypes are activated in the absence of negative feelings.[232]

Prejudiced emotional reactions may also be a consequence of direct contact with the 'other' group. This can be experienced as discomfort, anxiety, ambivalence, or as a rejection of intimacy.[191] Such feelings have been shown to be stronger in individuals who have a relatively authoritarian personality, and among people who believe that the world is basically just (and so people get what they deserve).[242, 243] Such emotional aspects of rejection have been studied extensively in the fields of HIV/AIDS,[33, 244] and in those conditions which produce visible marks which contravene aesthetic conventions,[245] such as the use of catheters or colostomies.[59, 61]

Interestingly, probably because research on exclusion and mental health has been almost entirely carried out using the concept of stigma rather than prejudice, there is almost nothing published about emotional reactions to people with mental illness apart from that which describes a fear of violence.[68, 198] One fascinating exception to this is work carried out in the south-eastern region of the USA, in which students were asked to imagine meeting people who either did or did not have a diagnosis of schizophrenia. All three physiological measures of stress (brow muscle tension, palm skin conductance and heart rate) showed raised during imagery with 'labelled' compared with 'non-labelled' individuals. Such tension also associated with self-reported negative attitudes of stigma towards people with schizophrenia. The authors concluded that one reason why individuals avoid those with mental illness is physiological arousal, which is experienced as unpleasant feelings.[246]

Discrimination: the problem of rejecting and avoidant behaviour

We have seen earlier in this chapter that most research on stigma and mental illness consists of attitude surveys. Much of this concerned with asking people, usually either students or members of the general public, about what they would do in imaginary situations or what they think 'most people' do, for example, when faced with a neighbour or work colleague with mental illness. Important lessons have flowed from these findings, as discussed earlier in this chapter. At the same time, this work has emphasized what 'normal' people say rather than the actual experiences of people with mental illness themselves. It also assumes that such statements (usually on knowledge, attitudes or behavioural intentions) are linked with actual behaviour, rather than assessing such behaviour directly. In short, with some clear exceptions, it has focussed on hypothetical rather than real situations,[157] shorn of emotions and feelings,[190,191] divorced from context,[178] indirectly rather than directly experienced,[247] and without clear implications for how to intervene to reduce social rejection.[248] In short, most work on stigma has been beside the point.

If we deliberately shift focus from stigma to discrimination, there are a number of distinct advantages. First attention moves from attitudes to actual behaviour, not if an employer *would* hire a person with mental illness, but if he or she *does*. Second, interventions can be tried and tested to see if they change behaviour towards people with mental illness, without *necessarily* changing knowledge or feelings. Third, people who have a diagnosis of mental illness can expect to benefit from all the relevant anti-discrimination policies and laws in their country or jurisdiction, on a basis of parity with people with physical disabilities. Fourth, a discrimination perspective requires us to focus not upon the 'stigmatised' but upon the 'stigmatiser'. In sum, this means sharpening our sights upon human rights, upon injustice and upon discrimination as actually experienced by people with mental illness.[168, 175, 249, 250]

I remember the first time a psychiatrist told me that if I had broken my leg, it would take a long time to heal and that your mind can take a long time to heal too. The day that the stigma vs. mental illness is the same as the stigma vs. a broken leg will be the time to stop talking about it, and until then I think that although the mentally ill can be a pest during the peaks of their suffering, if people are treated with respect just like you might help someone with a broken leg to walk up some stairs, that people may be able to recover quicker, and feel less isolated after.

Robert

References

1. Soanes C, Stevenson A. *Concise Oxford English Dictionary*, 11th edn. Oxford: Oxford University Press; 2003.
2. Cannan E. The stigma of pauperism. *Economic Review* 1895;380–391.
3. Thomas Hobbes of Malmesbury. *Markes of the Absurd Geometry, Rural Language, Scottish Church Politics, and Barbarisms of John Wallis Professor of Geometry and Doctor of Divinity.* London: Printed for Andrew Cooke; 1657.
4. Gilman SL. *Seeing the Insane*. Wiley: New York; 1982.
5. Gilman SL. *Difference and Pathology: Stereotypes of sexuality, race and madness*. Ithaca, New York: Cornell University Press; 1985.
6. Goffman I. *Stigma: Notes on the management of spoiled identity*. Harmondsworth, Middlesex: Penguin Books; 1963.
7. Scambler G. Stigma and disease: changing paradigms. *Lancet* 1998; 352(9133):1054–1055.
8. *The New American Bible*. Book of Daniel, Chapter 4, 1029. 1992.
9. Reaume G. Lunatic to patient to person: nomenclature in psychiatric history and the influence of patients' activism in North America. *Int J Law Psychiatry* 2002; 25(4):405–26.
10. Porter R. Can the stigma of mental illness be changed? *Lancet* 1998; 352(9133):1049–1050.
11. Falk G. *Stigma: How we treat outsiders*. New York: Prometheus Books; 2001.
12. Shorter E. *A History of Psychiatry: From the era of the asylum to the age of Prozac*. New York: John Wiley & Sons; 1997.
13. Porter R. *Mind-Forg'd Manacles*. Harmondsworth: Penguin Books; 1990.
14. Porter R. *Flesh in the Age of Reason*. London: Allen Lane; 2003.
15. Zeldin T. *An Intimate History of Humanity*. London: Vintage; 1998.
16. Sartorius N. *Fighting for Mental Health*. Cambridge: Cambridge University Press; 2002.
17. Gale C, Howard R. *Presumed Curable*. Petersfield: Wrightson Biomedical Publishing; 2003.
18. Lord JR. Lunacy law and institutional and home treatment of the insane. *Journal of Mental Science* 1923; 69,155–162.
19. Porter R. *Faber Book of Madness*. London: Faber & Faber; 1991.
20. Byrne P. Reading about psychiatric stigma. *British Journal of Psychiatry* 2001; 178:281–284.
21. Warner R. *Recovery from Schizophrenia: Psychiatry and political economy*. Hove: Brunner-Routledge; 2004.
22. Fournier E. *Stigmates Dystrophiques de L'Heredo-Syphilis*. Paris: Rueff et Cie; 1898.
23. Mason T. *Stigma and Social Exclusion in Healthcare*. London: Routledge; 2001.
24. Klitzman R, Bayer R. *Mortal Secrets: Truth and Lies in the Age of AIDS*. Baltimore, Maryland: The Johns Hopkins University Press; 2003.
25. Herek GM, Glunt EK. An epidemic of stigma. Public reactions to AIDS. *Am Psychol* 1988; 43(11):886–891.
26. Fife BL, Wright ER. The dimensionality of stigma: a comparison of its impact on the self of persons with HIV/AIDS and cancer. *J Health Soc Behav* 2000; 41(1):50–67.
27. Herek GM. Gay people and government security clearances. A social science perspective. *Am Psychol* 1990; 45(9):1035–1042.

28. Kelly JA, St Lawrence JS, Smith S Jr, Hood HV, Cook DJ. Stigmatization of AIDS patients by physicians. *Am J Public Health* 1987; 77(7):789–791.

29. Carrick R, Mitchell A, Powell RA, Lloyd K. The quest for well-being: a qualitative study of the experience of taking antipsychotic medication. *Psychol Psychother* 2004; 77(Pt 1):19–33.

30. Goldin CS. Stigmatization and AIDS: critical issues in public health. *Soc Sci Med* 1994; 39(9):1359–1366.

31. Herek GM, Capitanio JP, Widaman KF. Stigma, social risk, and health policy: public attitudes toward HIV surveillance policies and the social construction of illness. *Health Psychol* 2003; 22(5):533–540.

32. Letamo G. Prevalence of, and factors associated with, HIV/AIDS-related stigma and discriminatory attitudes in Botswana. *J Health Popul Nutr* 2003; 21(4):347–357.

33. Herek GM, Capitanio JP, Widaman KF. HIV-related stigma and knowledge in the United States: prevalence and trends, 1991–1999. *Am J Public Health* 2002; 92(3):371–377.

34. Jacoby A, Snape D, Baker GA. Epilepsy and social identity: the stigma of a chronic neurological disorder. *Lancet Neurol* 2005; 4(3):171–178.

35. Baker GA, Brooks J, Buck D, Jacoby A. The stigma of epilepsy: a European perspective. *Epilepsia* 2000; 41(1):98–104.

36. Austin JK, MacLeod J, Dunn DW, Shen J, Perkins SM. Measuring stigma in children with epilepsy and their parents: instrument development and testing. *Epilepsy Behav* 2004; 5(4):472–482.

37. Jacoby A. Felt versus enacted stigma: a concept revisited. Evidence from a study of people with epilepsy in remission. *Soc Sci Med* 1994; 38(2):269–274.

38. Westbrook LE, Bauman LJ, Shinnar S. Applying stigma theory to epilepsy: a test of a conceptual model. *J Pediatr Psychol* 1992; 17(5):633–649.

39. Jacoby A, Snape D, Baker GA. Epilepsy and social identity: the stigma of a chronic neurological disorder. *Lancet Neurol* 2005; 4(3):171–178.

40. Jacoby A. Stigma, epilepsy, and quality of life. *Epilepsy Behav* 2002; 3(6S2):10–20.

41. Vlassoff C, Weiss M, Ovuga EB, Eneanya C, Nwel PT, Babalola SS *et al.* Gender and the stigma of onchocercal skin disease in Africa. *Soc Sci Med* 2000; 50(10):1353–1368.

42. Kent G, Al'Abadie M. Psychologic effects of vitiligo: a critical incident analysis. *J Am Acad Dermatol* 1996; 35(6):895–898.

43. Ginsburg IH, Link BG. Feelings of stigmatization in patients with psoriasis. *J Am Acad Dermatol* 1989; 20(1):53–63.

44. Ginsburg IH, Link BG. Psychosocial consequences of rejection and stigma feelings in psoriasis patients. *Int J Dermatol* 1993; 32(8):587–591.

45. Schmid-Ott G, Jaeger B, Kuensebeck HW, Ott R, Lamprecht F. Dimensions of stigmatization in patients with psoriasis in a 'Questionnaire on Experience with Skin Complaints'. *Dermatology* 1996; 193(4):304–310.

46. Schmid-Ott G, Kuensebeck HW, Jaeger B, Werfel T, Frahm K, Ruitman J *et al.* Validity study for the stigmatization experience in atopic dermatitis and psoriatic patients. *Acta Derm Venereol* 1999; 79(6):443–447.

47. Wahl A, Hanestad BR, Wiklund I, Moum T. Coping and quality of life in patients with psoriasis. *Qual Life Res* 1999; 8(5):427–433.

48. Wahl A, Loge JH, Wiklund I, Hanestad BR. The burden of psoriasis: a study concerning health-related quality of life among Norwegian adult patients with psoriasis compared with general population norms. *J Am Acad Dermatol* 2000; 43(5 Pt 1):803–808.

49. Breitkopf CR. The theoretical basis of stigma as applied to genital herpes. *Herpes* 2004; 11(1):4–7.

50. Navon L. Beggars, metaphors, and stigma: a missing link in the social history of leprosy. *Soc Hist Med* 1998; 11(1):89–105.

51. Arole S, Premkumar R, Arole R, Maury M, Saunderson P. Social stigma: a comparative qualitative study of integrated and vertical care approaches to leprosy. *Lepr Rev* 2002; 73(2):186–196.

52. Lewis RJ, Cash TF, Jacobi L, Bubb-Lewis C. Prejudice toward fat people: the development and validation of the antifat attitudes test. *Obes Res* 1997; 5(4):297–307.

53. Wiese HJ, Wilson JF, Jones RA, Neises M. Obesity stigma reduction in medical students. *Int J Obes Relat Metab Disord* 1992; 16(11):859–868.

54. Crocker J, Cornwell B, Major B. The stigma of overweight: affective consequences of attributional ambiguity. *J Pers Soc Psychol* 1993; 64(1):60–70.

55. Schwartz MB, Chambliss HO, Brownell KD, Blair SN, Billington C. Weight bias among health professionals specializing in obesity. *Obesity Research* 2003; 11:1033–1039.

56. Heatherton T.F., Kleck RE, Hebl MR, Hull JG. *The Social Psychology of Stigma*. New York: Guilford Press; 2003.

57. Schrag A, Hovris A, Morley D, Quinn N, Jahanshahi M. Young- versus older-onset Parkinson's disease: impact of disease and psychosocial consequences. *Mov Disord* 2003; 18(11):1250–1256.

58. Papathanasiou I, MacDonald L, Whurr R, Jahanshahi M. Perceived stigma in spasmodic torticollis. *Mov Disord* 2001; 16(2):280–285.

59. Wilde MH. Life with an indwelling urinary catheter: the dialectic of stigma and acceptance. *Qualitative Health Research* 2003; 13:1189–1204.

60. Garcia JA, Crocker J, Wyman JF, Krissovich MMRC. Breaking the cycle of stigmatization: managing the stigma of incontinence in social interactions. *J Wound Ostomy Continence Nurs* 2005; 32(1):38–52.

61. MacDonald LD, Anderson HR. Stigma in patients with rectal cancer: a community study. *J Epidemiol Community Health* 1984; 38(4):284–290.

62. Pound P, Gompertz P, Ebrahim S. A patient-centred study of the consequences of stroke. *Clin Rehabil* 1998; 12(4):338–347.

63. Hyman MD. The stigma of stroke. Its effects on performance during and after rehabilitation. *Geriatrics* 1971; 26(5):132–141.

64. Crandall CS, Moriarty D. Physical illness stigma and social rejection. *Br J Soc Psychol* 1995; 34 (Pt 1):67–83.

65. Weiss MG. Cultural epidemiology. *Anthropology and Medicine* 2001; 8:5–29.

66. Bogardus ES. Social distance and its origins. *Journal of Applied Sociology* 1924; 9:216–226.

67. Corrigan PW, Green A, Lundin R, Kubiak MA, Penn DL. Familiarity with and social distance from people who have serious mental illness. *Psychiatr Serv* 2001; 52(7):953–958.

68. Corrigan PW, Edwards AB, Green A, Diwan SL, Penn DL. Prejudice, social distance, and familiarity with mental illness. *Schizophr Bull* 2001; 27(2):219–225.

69. Angermeyer MC, Matschinger H. [Social distance of the population toward psychiatric patients]. *Gesundheitswesen* 1996; 58(1 Suppl):18–24.

70. Angermeyer MC, Beck M, Matschinger H. Determinants of the public's preference for social distance from people with schizophrenia. *Can J Psychiatry* 2003; 48(10):663–668.

71. Angermeyer MC, Matschinger H. Social distance towards the mentally ill: results of representative surveys in the Federal Republic of Germany. *Psychol Med* 1997; 27(1):131–41.

72. Brand RC, Jr., Clairborn WL. Two studies of comparative stigma: employer attitudes and practices toward rehabilitated convicts, mental and tuberculosis patients. *Community Ment Health* J 1976; 12(2):168–175.

73. Jacoby A, Gorry J, Gamble C, Baker GA. Public knowledge, private grief: a study of public attitudes to epilepsy in the United Kingdom and implications for stigma. *Epilepsia* 2004; 45(11):1405–1415.

74. Dietrich S, Beck M, Bujantugs B, Kenzine D, Matschinger H, Angermeyer MC. The relationship between public causal beliefs and social distance toward mentally ill people. *Aust N Z J Psychiatry* 2004; 38(5):348–354.

75. Murray C, Lopez A. *The Global Burden of Disease, Volume 1. A comprehensive assessment of mortality and disability from diseases, injuries and risk factors in 1990, and projected to 2020.* Cambridge, Massachusetts: Harvard University Press; 1996.

76. Desai MM, Rosenheck RA, Druss BG, Perlin JB. Mental disorders and quality of diabetes care in the veterans health administration. *Am J Psychiatry* 2002; 159(9):1584–1590.

77. Desai MM, Rosenheck RA, Druss BG, Perlin JB. Mental disorders and quality of care among postacute myocardial infarction outpatients. *J Nerv Ment Dis* 2002; 190(1):51–53.

78. Druss BG, Bradford WD, Rosenheck RA, Radford MJ, Krumholz HM. Quality of medical care and excess mortality in older patients with mental disorders. *Arch Gen Psychiatry* 2001; 58(6):565–572.

79. Druss BG. Cardiovascular procedures in patients with mental disorders. *JAMA* 2000; 283(24):3198–3199.

80. Druss BG, Bradford DW, Rosenheck RA, Radford MJ, Krumholz HM. Mental disorders and use of cardiovascular procedures after myocardial infarction. *JAMA* 2000; 283(4):506–511.

81. Littlewood R. Cultural and national aspects of stigmatisation. In: Crisp AH, ed., *Every Family in the Land*, pp. 14–17. London: Royal Society of Medicine; 2004.

82. Fabrega H, Jr. The culture and history of psychiatric stigma in early modern and modern Western societies: a review of recent literature. *Compr Psychiatry* 1991; 32(2):97–119.

83. Shibre T, Negash A, Kullgren G, Kebede D, Alem A, Fekadu A *et al.* Perception of stigma among family members of individuals with schizophrenia and major affective disorders in rural Ethiopia. *Soc Psychiatry Psychiatr Epidemiol* 2001; 36(6):299–303.

84. Alem A, Jacobsson L, Araya M, Kebede D, Kullgren G. How are mental disorders seen and where is help sought in a rural Ethiopian community? A key informant study in Butajira, Ethiopia. *Acta Psychiatr Scand Suppl* 1999; 397:40–7.

85. Stein DJ, Wessels C, Van Kradenberg J, Emsley RA. The Mental Health Information Centre of South Africa: a report of the first 500 calls. *Cent Afr J Med* 1997; 43(9):244–246.

86. Minde M. History of mental health services in South Africa. Part XIII. The National Council for Mental Health. *S Afr Med J* 1976; 50(3F):1452–1456.

87. Hugo CJ, Boshoff DE, Traut A, Zungu-Dirwayi N, Stein DJ. Community attitudes toward and knowledge of mental illness in South Africa. *Soc Psychiatry Psychiatr Epidemiol* 2003; 38(12):715–719.

88. Cheetham WS, Cheetham RJ. Concepts of mental illness amongst the rural Xhosa people in South Africa. *Aust N Z J Psychiatry* 1976; 10(1):39–45.

89. Ozmen E, Ogel K, Aker T, Sagduyu A, Tamar D, Boratav C. Public attitudes to depression in urban Turkey - the influence of perceptions and causal attributions on social distance towards individuals suffering from depression. *Soc Psychiatry Psychiatr Epidemiol* 2004; 39(12):1010–1016.

90. Corrigan P. *On the Stigma of Mental Illness.* Washington, DC: American Psychological Association; 2005.

91. Link BG, Yang LH, Phelan JC, Collins PY. Measuring mental illness stigma. *Schizophr Bull* 2004; 30(3):511–541.

92. Estroff SE, Penn DL, Toporek JR. From stigma to discrimination: an analysis of community efforts to reduce the negative consequences of having a psychiatric disorder and label. *Schizophr Bull* 2004; 30(3):493–509.

93. Corrigan P, Thompson V, Lambert D, Sangster Y, Noel JG, Campbell J. Perceptions of discrimination among persons with serious mental illness. *Psychiatr Serv* 2003; 54(8):1105–1110.

94. Villares C, Sartorius N. Challenging the stigma of schizophrenia. *Rev Bras Psiquiatr* 2003; 25:1–2.

95. de Toledo Piza PE, Blay SL. Community perception of mental disorders – a systematic review of Latin American and Caribbean studies. *Soc Psychiatry Psychiatr Epidemiol* 2004; 39(12):955–961.

96. Kirmayer LJ, Fletcher CM, Boothroyd LJ. Inuit attitudes toward deviant behavior: a vignette study. *J Nerv Ment Dis* 1997; 185(2):78–86.

97. Ng CH. The stigma of mental illness in Asian cultures. *Aust N Z J Psychiatry* 1997; 31(3):382–390.

98. Leong FT, Lau AS. Barriers to providing effective mental health services to Asian Americans. *Ment Health Serv Res* 2001; 3(4):201–214.

99. Fabrega H, Jr. Psychiatric stigma in non-Western societies. *Compr Psychiatry* 1991; 32(6):534–551.

100. Kleinman A, Mechanic D. Some observations of mental illness and its treatment in the People's Republic of China. *J Nerv Ment Dis* 1979; 167(5):267–274.

101. Phillips MR, Pearson V, Li F, Xu M, Yang L. Stigma and expressed emotion: a study of people with schizophrenia and their family members in China. *Br J Psychiatry* 2002; 181:488–493.

102. Sevigny R, Yang W, Zhang P, Marleau JD, Yang Z, Su L *et al.* Attitudes toward the mentally ill in a sample of professionals working in a psychiatric hospital in Beijing (China). *Int J Soc Psychiatry* 1999; 45(1):41–55.

103. Phillips MR, Li Y, Stroup TS, Xin L. Causes of schizophrenia reported by patients' family members in China. *Br J Psychiatry* 2000; 177:20–25.

104. Furnham A, Chan E. Lay theories of schizophrenia. A cross-cultural comparison of British and Hong Kong Chinese attitudes, attributions and beliefs. *Soc Psychiatry Psychiatr Epidemiol* 2004; 39(7):543–552.

105. Chou KL, Mak KY, Chung PK, Ho K. Attitudes towards mental patients in Hong Kong. *Int J Soc Psychiatry* 1996; 42(3):213–9.

106. Chung KF, Chen EY, Liu CS. University students' attitudes towards mental patients and psychiatric treatment. *Int J Soc Psychiatry* 2001; 47(2):63–72.

107. Chung K, Wong M. Experiences of stigma among Chinese mental health patients in Hong Kong. *Psychiatr Bull* 2004; 28:451–454.

108. Lee S, Lee MT, Chiu MY, Kleinman A. Experience of social stigma by people with schizophrenia in Hong Kong. *Br J Psychiatry* 2005; 186:153–157.

109. Thara R, Srinivasan TN. How stigmatising is schizophrenia in India? *Int J Soc Psychiatry* 2000; 46(2):135–141.

110. Raguram R, Raghu TM, Vounatsou P, Weiss MG. Schizophrenia and the cultural epidemiology of stigma in Bangalore, India. *J Nerv Ment Dis* 2004; 192(11):734–744.

111. Thara R, Kamath S, Kumar S. Women with schizophrenia and broken marriages – doubly disadvantaged? Part II: family perspective. *Int J Soc Psychiatry* 2003; 49(3):233–240.

112. Raguram R, Weiss MG, Channabasavanna SM, Devins GM. Stigma, depression, and somatization in South India. *Am J Psychiatry* 1996; 153(8):1043–1049.

113. Chowdhury AN, Sanyal D, Dutta SK, Banerjee S, De R, Bhattacharya K *et al.* Stigma and mental illness: Pilot study of laypersons and health care providers with the EMIC in rural West Bengal, India. *International Medical Journal* 2000; 7(4):257–260.

114. Chowdhury AN, Sanyal D, Bhattacharya A, Dutta SK, De R, Banerjee S *et al.* Prominence of symptoms and level of stigma among depressed patients in Calcutta. *J Indian Med Assoc* 2001; 99(1):20–23.

115. Desjarlais R, Eisenberg L, Good B, Kleinman A. *World Mental Health. Problems and priorities in low income countries.* Oxford: Oxford University Press; 1995.

116. Conrad MM, Pacquiao DF. Manifestation, attribution, and coping with depression among Asian Indians from the perspectives of health care practitioners. *J Transcult Nurs* 2005; 16(1):32–40.

117. Chadda RK, Agarwal V, Singh MC, Raheja D. Help seeking behaviour of psychiatric patients before seeking care at a mental hospital. *Int J Soc Psychiatry* 2001; 47(4):71–78.

118. Razali SM, Najib MA. Help-seeking pathways among Malay psychiatric patients. *Int J Soc Psychiatry* 2000; 46(4):281–289.

119. James S, Chisholm D, Murthy RS, Kumar KK, Sekar K, Saeed K *et al.* Demand for, access to and use of community mental health care: lessons from a demonstration project in India and Pakistan. *Int J Soc Psychiatry* 2002; 48(3):163–176.

120. Weiss MG, Raguram R, Channabasavanna SM. Cultural dimensions of psychiatric diagnosis. A comparison of DSM-III-R and illness explanatory models in south India. *Br J Psychiatry* 1995; 166(3):353–359.

121. Weiss MG, Jadhav S, Raguram R, Vaunatsou P, Littlewood L. Psychiatric stigma across cultures: local validation in Bangalore and London. *Anthropology and Medicine* 2001; 8:71–87.

122. Desapriya EB, Nobutada I. Stigma of mental illness in Japan. *Lancet* 2002; 359(9320):1866.

123. Hasui C, Sakamoto S, Suguira B, Kitamura T. Stigmatization of mental illness in Japan: Images and frequency of encounters with diagnostic categories of mental illness among medical and non-medical university students. *Journal of Psychiatry and Law* 2000; 28(Summer):253–266.

124. Sugiura T, Sakamoto S, Kijima N, Kitamura F, Kitamura T. Stigmatizing perception of mental illness by Japanese students: comparison of different psychiatric disorders. *J Nerv Ment Dis* 2000; 188(4):239–242.

125. Kurihara T, Kato M, Sakamoto S, Reverger R, Kitamura T. Public attitudes towards the mentally ill: a cross-cultural study between Bali and Tokyo. *Psychiatry Clin Neurosci* 2000; 54(5):547–552.

126. Kurumatani T, Ukawa K, Kawaguchi Y, Miyata S, Suzuki M, Ide H *et al.* Teachers' knowledge, beliefs and attitudes concerning schizophrenia – a cross-cultural approach in Japan and Taiwan. *Soc Psychiatry Psychiatr Epidemiol* 2004; 39(5):402–409.

127. Takizawa T. Patients and their families in Japanese mental health. *New Dir Ment Health Serv* 1993;(60):25–34.

128. Goto M. [Family psychoeducation in Japan]. *Seishin Shinkeigaku Zasshi* 2003; 105(2): 243–247.

129. Kim Y, Berrios GE. Impact of the term schizophrenia on the culture of ideograph: the Japanese experience. *Schizophr Bull* 2001; 27(2):181–185.

130. Mino Y, Yasuda N, Tsuda T, Shimodera S. Effects of a one-hour educational program on medical students' attitudes to mental illness. *Psychiatry Clin Neurosci* 2001; 55(5):501–7.

131. Angermeyer MC, Matschinger H. Labeling–stereotype–discrimination. An investigation of the stigma process. *Soc Psychiatry Psychiatr Epidemiol* 2005; 40(5):391–395.

132. Karim S, Saeed K, Rana MH, Mubbashar MH, Jenkins R. Pakistan mental health country profile. *Int Rev Psychiatry* 2004; 16(1–2):83–92.

133. Al-Krenawi A, Graham JR, Kandah J. Gendered utilization differences of mental health services in Jordan. *Community Ment Health* J 2000; 36(5):501–511.

134. Al-Krenawi A, Graham JR, Ophir M, Kandah J. Ethnic and gender differences in mental health utilization: the case of Muslim Jordanian and Moroccan Jewish Israeli out-patient psychiatric patients. *Int J Soc Psychiatry* 2001; 47(3):42–54.

135. Cinnirella M, Loewenthal KM. Religious and ethnic group influences on beliefs about mental illness: a qualitative interview study. *Br J Med Psychol* 1999; 72 (Pt 4):505–524.

136. Kadri N, Manoudi F, Berrada S, Moussaoui D. Stigma impact on Moroccan families of patients with schizophrenia. *Can J Psychiatry* 2004; 49(9):625–629.

137. Al-Krenawi A, Graham JR, Dean YZ, Eltaiba N. Cross-national study of attitudes towards seeking professional help: Jordan, United Arab Emirates (UAE) and Arabs in Israel. *Int J Soc Psychiatry* 2004; 50(2):102–114.

138. Loewenthal KM, Cinnirella M, Evdoka G, Murphy P. Faith conquers all? Beliefs about the role of religious factors in coping with depression among different cultural-religious groups in the UK. *Br J Med Psychol* 2001; 74(Pt 3):293–303.

139. Arkar H, Eker D. Influence of having a hospitalized mentally ill member in the family on attitudes toward mental patients in Turkey. *Soc Psychiatry Psychiatr Epidemiol* 1992; 27(3):151–155.

140. Arkar H, Eker D. Effect of psychiatric labels on attitudes toward mental illness in a Turkish sample. *Int J Soc Psychiatry* 1994; 40(3):205–213.

141. Coker EM. Selfhood and social distance: toward a cultural understanding of psychiatric stigma in Egypt. *Soc Sci Med* 2005; 61(5):920–930.

142. Sagduyu A, Aker T, Ozmen E, Uguz S, Ogel K, Tamar D. [Relatives' beliefs and attitudes towards schizophrenia: an epidemiological investigation]. *Turk Psikiyatri Derg* 2003; 14(3):203–212.

143. Littlewood R. Cultural variation in the stigmatisation of mental illness. *Lancet* 1998; 352(9133):1056–1057.

144. Lai YM, Hong CP, Chee CY. Stigma of mental illness. *Singapore Med J* 2001; 42(3):111–114.

145. Lee S, Lee MT, Chiu MY, Kleinman A. Experience of social stigma by people with schizophrenia in Hong Kong. *Br J Psychiatry* 2005; 186:153–157.

146. Wahl OF. *Telling is a Risky Business: Mental health consumers confront stigma.* New Jersey: Rutgers University Press; 1999.

147. Pickenhagen A, Sartorius N. *The WPA Global Programme to Reduce Stigma and Discrimination because of Schizophrenia.* Geneva: World Psychiatric Association; 2002.

148. Sartorius N, Schulze H. *Reducing the Stigma of Mental Illness: A report from a global association.* Cambridge: Cambridge University Press; 2005.

149. Hayward P, Bright JA. Stigma and mental illness: A review and critique. *Journal of Mental Health* 1997; 6(4):345–354.

150. Link BG, Cullen FT, Struening EL, Shrout PE, Dohrenwend BP. A modified labeling theory approach in the area of mental disorders: An empirical assessment. *American Sociological Review* 1989; 54:100–123.

151. Link BG, Struening EL, Rahav M, Phelan JC, Nuttbrock L. On stigma and its consequences: evidence from a longitudinal study of men with dual diagnoses of mental illness and substance abuse. *J Health Soc Behav* 1997; 38(2):177–190.

152. Link BG, Phelan JC, Bresnahan M, Stueve A, Pescosolido BA. Public conceptions of mental illness: labels, causes, dangerousness, and social distance. *Am J Public Health* 1999; 89(9):1328–33.

153. Smith M. Stigma. *Advances in Psychiatric Treatment* 2002; 8:317–325.

154. Link BG, Phelan JC. Conceptualizing stigma. *Annual Review of Sociology* 2001; 27:363–385.

155. Link BG, Yang LH, Phelan JC, Collins PY. Measuring mental illness stigma. *Schizophr Bull* 2004; 30(3):511–541.

156. Jones E, Farina A, Hastorf A, Markus H, Milller D, Scott R. *Social Stigma: The psychology of marked relationships.* New York: W.H. Freeman & Co.; 1984.

157. Sayce L. Stigma, discrimination and social exclusion: what's in a word? *Journal of Mental Health* 1998; 7:331–343.

158. Sayce L. *From Psychiatric Patient to Citizen. Overcoming discrimination and social exclusion.* Basingstoke: Palgrave; 2000.

159. Corrigan PW, Penn DL. Disease and discrimination: two paradigms that describe severe mental illness. *Journal of Mental Health* 1997; 6(4):355–366.

160. Penn D, Wykes T. Stigma, discrimination and mental illness. *Journal of Mental Health* 2003; 12:203–208.

161. Glozier N. The Disability Discrimination Act 1995 and psychiatry: lessons from the first seven years. *Psychiatr Bull* 2004; 28:126–129.

162. Pardeck JT. Psychiatric disabilities and the Americans with Disabilities Act: implications for policy and practice. *J Health Soc Policy* 1998; 10(3):1–12.

163. Appelbaum PS. Discrimination in psychiatric disability coverage and the Americans With Disabilities Act. *Psychiatr Serv* 1998; 49(7):875–6, 881.

164. Aggleton P. Barcelona 2002: law, ethics, and human rights. HIV/AIDS-related stigma and discrimination: a conceptual framework. *Can HIV AIDS Policy Law Rev* 2002; 7(2–3): 115–116.

165. Perker R, Aggleton P. *HIV and AIDS-related Stigma and Discrimination: A conceptual framework and implications for action.* Rio de Janeiro: ABIA; 2002.

166. Gaebel W, Baumann AE. Interventions to reduce the stigma associated with severe mental illness: experiences from the open the doors program in Germany. *Can J Psychiatry* 2003; 48(10):657–662.

167. Pinfold V, Thornicroft G, Huxley P, Farmer P. Active ingredients in anti-stigma programmes in mental health. *International Review of Psychiatry* 2005; (in press).

168. Rose D. *Users' Voices, The perspectives of mental health service users on community and hospital care.* London: The Sainsbury Centre; 2001.

169. Crossley ML, Crossley N. 'Patient' voices, social movements and the habitus; how psychiatric survivors 'speak out'. *Soc Sci Med* 2001; 52(10):1477–1489.

170. Dinos S, Stevens S, Serfaty M, Weich S, King M. Stigma: the feelings and experiences of 46 people with mental illness. Qualitative study. *Br J Psychiatry* 2004; 184:176–181.

171. Morone JA. Enemies of the people: the moral dimension to public health. *Journal of Health Politics, Policy and Law* 1997; 22(4):993–1020.

172. Corrigan PW, Watson AC, Warpinski AC, Gracia G. Stigmatizing attitudes about mental illness and allocation of resources to mental health services. *Community Ment Health J* 2004; 40(4):297–307.

173. Amnesty International. *Ethical Codes and Declarations Relevant to the Health Professions.* London: Amnesty International; 2000.

174. Bindman J, Maingay S, Szmukler G. The Human Rights Act and mental health legislation. *Br J Psychiatry* 2003; 182:91–94.

175. Kingdon D, Jones R, Lonnqvist J. Protecting the human rights of people with mental disorder: new recommendations emerging from the Council of Europe. *Br J Psychiatry* 2004; 185:277–279.

176. Ustun TB, Cooper JE, Duuren-Kristen S, Kennedy C, Henderson G, Sartorius N. Revision of the ICIDH: mental health aspects. WHO/MNH Disability Working Group. *Disabil Rehabil* 1995; 17(3–4):202–209.

177. Sayce L. Beyond good intentions. Making anti-discrimination strategies work. *Disability & Society* 2003; 18:625–642.

178. Corrigan PW, Markowitz FE, Watson AC. Structural levels of mental illness stigma and discrimination. *Schizophr Bull* 2004; 30(3):481–491.

179. Corrigan P, Thompson V, Lambert D, Sangster Y, Noel JG, Campbell J. Perceptions of discrimination among persons with serious mental illness. *Psychiatr Serv* 2003; 54(8):1105–1110.

180. Thornicroft G, Tansella M, Becker T, Knapp M, Leese M, Schene A *et al.* The personal impact of schizophrenia in Europe. *Schizophr Res* 2004; 69(2–3): 125–132.

181. Becker DR, Drake RE. *A Working Life for People with Severe Mental Illness.* Oxford: Oxford University Press; 2003.

182. Dear M, Wolch J. *Landscapes of Despair.* Princeton, New Jersey: Princeton University Press; 1992.

183. Beeforth M, Wood H. Needs from a user perspective. In: Thornicroft G, ed., *Measuring Mental Health Needs*, 2nd edn., pp. 190–199. London: Gaskell, Royal College of Psychiatrists; 2001.

184. Dalgin RS, Gilbride D. Perspectives of people with psychiatric disabilities on employment disclosure. *Psychiatr Rehabil J* 2003; 26(3):306–10.

185. Corrigan PW, Edwards AB, Green A, Diwan SL, Penn DL. Prejudice, social distance, and familiarity with mental illness. *Schizophr Bull* 2001; 27(2):219–25.

186. Sartorius N, Schulze H. *Reducing the Stigma of Mental Illness. A Report from the global programme against stigma of the World Psychiatric Association.* Cambridge: Cambridge University Press; 2005.

187. Social Exclusion Unit. *Mental Health and Social Exclusion.* London: Office of the Deputy Prime Minister; 2004.

188. Dovidio J, Major B, Crocker J. Stigma: introduction and overview. In: Heatherton TF, Kleck RE, Hebl MR, Hull JG, eds., *The Social Psychology of Stigma*, pp. 1–28. New York: Guilford Press; 2000.

189. Dovidio J, Brigham JC, Johnson BT, Gaertner SL. Stereotyping, prejudice and discrimination: another look. In: McCrae N, Stangor C, Hewstone M, eds., *Stereotypes and Stereotyping*, pp. 276–319. New York: Guildford; 1996.

190. Fiske S.T. Stereotyping, prejudice and discrimination. In: Gilbert DT, Fiske ST, Lindzey G, eds., *The Handbook of Social Psychology*, 4th edn., pp. 357–411. Boston, Massachusetts: McGraw Hill; 1998.

191. Crocker J, Major B, Steele C. Social stigma. In: Gilbert D, Fiske ST, Lindzey G, eds., *The Handbook of Social Psychology*, 4th edn., pp. 504–533. Boston: McGraw-Hill; 1998.

192. Reber AS, Reber E.S. *Dictionary of Psychology*, 3rd edn., London: Penguin; 2001.

193. Gaebel W, Baumann A, Witte AM, Zaeske H. Public attitudes towards people with mental illness in six German cities: results of a public survey under special consideration of schizophrenia. *Eur Arch Psychiatry Clin Neurosci* 2002; 252(6):278–287.

194. Stuart H, Arboleda-Florez J. Community attitudes toward people with schizophrenia. *Canadian Journal of Psychiatry* 2001; 46:245–252.

195. Department of Health. *Attitudes to Mental Illness 2003 Report.* London: Department of Health; 2003.

196. Vezzoli R, Archiati L, Buizza C, Pasqualetti P, Rossi G, Pioli R. Attitude towards psychiatric patients: a pilot study in a northern Italian town. *Eur Psychiatry* 2001; 16(8):451–8.

197. Stuart H, Arboleda-Florez J. Community attitudes toward people with schizophrenia. *Can J Psychiatry* 2001; 46(3):245–52.

198. Lauber C, Nordt C, Sartorius N, Falcato L, Rossler W. Public acceptance of restrictions on mentally ill people. *Acta Psychiatr Scand* Suppl. 2000; 102(407):26–32.

199. Madianos MG, Economou M, Hatjiandreou M, Papageorgiou A, Rogakou E. Changes in public attitudes towards mental illness in the Athens area (1979/1980–1994). *Acta Psychiatr Scand* 1999; 99(1):73–78.

200. Jorm AF, Korten AE, Jacomb PA, Christensen H, Henderson S. Attitudes towards people with a mental disorder: a survey of the Australian public and health professionals. *Aust N Z J Psychiatry* 1999; 33(1):77–83.

201. See Me Scotland. *The Second National Public Attitudes Survey, 'Well? What do you think?'.* Edinburgh: Scottish Executive; 2004.

202. Jorm AF, Korten AE, Jacomb PA, Christensen H, Rodgers B, Pollitt P. 'Mental health literacy': a survey of the public's ability to recognise mental disorders and their beliefs about the effectiveness of treatment. *Med J Aust* 1997; 166(4):182–6.

203. Chen H, Parker G, Kua J, Jorm A, Loh J. Mental health literacy in Singapore: a comparative survey of psychiatrists and primary health professionals. *Ann Acad Med Singapore* 2000; 29(4):467–473.

204. Jorm AF, Korten AE, Jacomb PA, Christensen H, Rodgers B, Pollitt P. 'Mental health literacy': a survey of the public's ability to recognise mental disorders and their beliefs about the effectiveness of treatment. *Med J Aust* 1997; 166(4):182–186.

205. Croghan TW, Tomlin M, Pescosolido BA, Schnittker J, Martin J, Lubell K *et al.* American attitudes toward and willingness to use psychiatric medications. *J Nerv Ment Dis* 2003; 191(3):166–174.

206. Sirey JA, Meyers BS, Bruce ML, Alexopoulos GS, Perlick DA, Raue P. Predictors of antidepressant prescription and early use among depressed outpatients. *Am J Psychiatry* 1999; 156(5):690–696.

207. Sirey JA, Bruce ML, Alexopoulos GS, Perlick DA, Raue P, Friedman SJ *et al.* Perceived stigma as a predictor of treatment discontinuation in young and older outpatients with depression. *Am J Psychiatry* 2001; 158(3):479–481.

208. Jorm AF. Mental health literacy. Public knowledge and beliefs about mental disorders. *Br J Psychiatry* 2000; 177:396–401.

209. Parslow RA, Jorm AF. Improving Australians' depression literacy. *Med J Aust* 2002; 177 Suppl:S117–S121.

210. Jorm AF, Griffiths KM, Christensen H, Korten AE, Parslow RA, Rodgers B. Providing information about the effectiveness of treatment options to depressed people in the community: a randomized controlled trial of effects on mental health literacy, help-seeking and symptoms. *Psychol Med* 2003; 33(6):1071–1079.

211. Allport G. *The Nature of Prejudice*. New York: Doubleday Anchor Books; 1954.

212. Lindzey G. *The Handbook of Social Psychology*. Reading, Massachusetts: Addison-Wesley; 1954.

213. Nunnally JC. *Popular Conceptions of Mental Health*. New York: Holt, Rinehart&Winston; 1961.

214. Star SA. *What the Public Thinks about Mental Health and Mental Illness*. Indianapolis, Indiana: Paper presented at the annual meeting of the National Association of Mental Health; 1952.

215. Cumming J, Cumming E. On the stigma of mental illness. *Community Mental Health Journal* 1965; 1:135–143.

216. Angermeyer MC, Matschinger H. Have there been any changes in the public's attitudes towards psychiatric treatment? Results from representative population surveys in Germany in the years 1990 and 2001. *Acta Psychiatr Scand* 2005; 111(1):68–73.

217. Angermeyer MC, Matschinger H. Public attitudes to people with depression: have there been any changes over the last decade? *J Affect Disord* 2004; 83(2–3):177–182.

218. Phelan JC, Link BG, Stueve A, Pescosolido BA. Public conceptions of mental illness in 1950 and 1996: What is mental illness and it sit to be feared? *Journal of Health and Social Behavior* 2000; 41:188–207.

219. Kessler RC, Demler O, Frank RG, Olfson M, Pincus HA, Walters EE *et al*. Prevalence and treatment of mental disorders, 1990 to 2003. *N Engl J Med* 2005; 352(24):2515–2523.

220. Link BG, Susser E, Stueve A, Phelan J, Moore RE, Struening E. Lifetime and five-year prevalence of homelessness in the United States. *Am J Public Health* 1994; 84(12):1907–1912.

221. Angermeyer M, Matschinger H. The stigma of mental illness in Germany: a trend analysis. *International Journal of Social Psychiatry* 2005; 51; 276–284.

222. Ellis PM, Smith DA. Treating depression: the beyondblue guidelines for treating depression in primary care. 'Not so much what you do but that you keep doing it'. *Med J Aust* 2002; 176 Suppl:S77–S83.

223. Hickie I. Can we reduce the burden of depression? The Australian experience with beyond-blue: the national depression initiative. *Australas Psychiatry* 2004; 12 Suppl:S38–S46.

224. Jorm AF, Christensen H, Griffiths KM. The impact of beyondblue: the national depression initiative on the Australian public's recognition of depression and beliefs about treatments. *Aust N Z J Psychiatry* 2005; 39(4):248–254.

225. Department of Health. *Attitudes to Mental Illness Summary Report 2000*. London: Department of Health; 2000.

226. Crisp AH, Cowan L, Hart D. The College's anti-stigma campaign 1998–2003. *Psychiatr Bull* 2004; 28:133–136.

227. Crisp A, Gelder MG, Goddard E, Meltzer H. Stigmatization of people with mental illnesses: a follow-up study within the Changing Minds campaign of the Royal College of Psychiatrists. *World Psychiatry* 2005; 4:106–113.

228. Fine F, Asch A. Disability beyond stigma: social interaction, discrimination, and activism. *Journal of Social Issues* 1988; 44(1):3–23.

229. Jones S, Hayward P. *Coping with Schizophrenia: A guide for patients, families and carers*. Oxford: Oneworld Publications; 2004.

230. Hegner RE. Dispelling the myths and stigma of mental illness: the Surgeon General's report on mental health. *Issue Brief Natl Health Policy Forum* 2000;(754):1–7.

231. Sibicky M, Dovidio JF. Stigma of psychological therapy: stereotypes, interpersonal reactions, and the self-fulfilling prophecy. *Journal of Counseling Psychology* 2005; 33:148–154.

232. Fiske ST. Social cognition and social perception. *Annu Rev Psychol* 1993; 44:155–194.

233. Crandall CS. Ideology and lay theories of stigma: the justification of stigmatization. In: Heatherton TF, Kleck RE, Hebl MR, Hull JG, eds., *The Social Psychology of Stigma*, pp. 126–150. New York: Guilford; 2000.

234. Corrigan PW, Watson AC, Ottati V. From whence comes mental illness stigma? *Int J Soc Psychiatry* 2003; 49(2):142–157.

235. Neuberg SL, Smith DM, Asher T. Why people stigmatize: toward a biocultural framework. In: Heatherton TF, Kleck RE, Hebl MR, Hull JG, eds., *The Social Psychology of Stigma*, pp. 31–61. New York: Guildford; 2000.

236. Haghighat R. A unitary theory of stigmatisation: pursuit of self-interest and routes to destigmatisation. *Br J Psychiatry* 2001; 178:207–215.

237. Crisp AH. The nature of stigmatisation. In: Crisp AH, ed., *Every Family in the Land*, pp. 412–425. London: Royal Society of Medicine; 2004.

238. Stangor C, Crandall CS. Threat and the social construction of stigma. In: Heatherton TF, Kleck RE, Hebl MR, Hull JG, eds., *The Social Psychology of Stigma*, pp. 62–87. New York: Guilford; 2000.

239. Thompson AH, Stuart H, Bland RC, Arboleda-Florez J, Warner R, Dickson RA. Attitudes about schizophrenia from the pilot site of the WPA worldwide campaign against the stigma of schizophrenia. *Soc Psychiatry Psychiatr Epidemiol* 2002; 37(10):475–482.

240. Biernat M, Dovidio J. Stigma and stereotypes. In: Heatherton TF, Kleck RE, Hebl MR, Hull JG, eds., *The Social Psychology of Stigma*, pp. 88–125. New York: Guildford; 2000.

241. Veltro F, Raimondo A, Porzio C, Nugnes T, Ciampone V. [A survey on the prejudice and the stereotypes of mental illness in two communities with or without psychiatric Residential Facilities]. *Epidemiol Psichiatr Soc* 2005; 14(3):170–176.

242. Crandall CS, Eshleman A, O'Brien L. Social norms and the expression and suppression of prejudice: the struggle for internalization. *J Pers Soc Psychol* 2002; 82(3):359–378.

243. Crandall CS, Eshleman A. A justification-suppression model of the expression and experience of prejudice. *Psychol Bull* 2003; 129(3):414–446.

244. Herek GM, Capitanio JP. Public reactions to AIDS in the United States: a second decade of stigma. *Am J Public Health* 1993; 83(4):574–577.

245. Hahn H. The politics of physical differences: disability and discrimination. *Journal of Social Issues* 1988; 44:39–47.

246. Graves RE, Cassisi JE, Penn DL. Psychophysiological evaluation of stigma towards schizophrenia. *Schizophr Res* 2005; 76(2–3):317–327.

247. Repper J, Perkins R. *Social Inclusion and Recovery.* Edinburgh: Balliere Tindall; 2003.

248. Corrigan PW. Target-specific stigma change: a strategy for impacting mental illness stigma. *Psychiatr Rehabil J* 2004; 28(2):113–121.

249. Chamberlin J. User/consumer involvement in mental health service delivery. *Epidemiol Psichiatr Soc* 2005; 14; 10–14.

250. Hinshaw SP, Cicchetti D. Stigma and mental disorder: conceptions of illness, public attitudes, personal disclosure, and social policy. *Dev Psychopathol* 2000; 12(4):555–598.

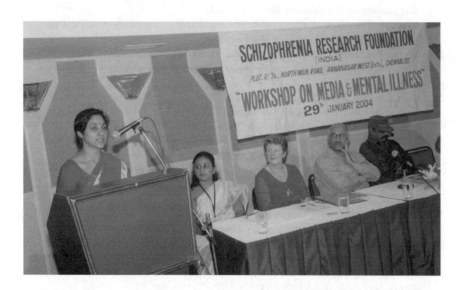

Workshop on Media and Mental Illness, Chennai, India, 2004.

Chapter 10 What works to reduce discrimination?

Challenges for service users

> I have friends from the place I hang out. I've got two healthy friends, who have invited me to their weddings, but I have never talked to them about my disease or the fact that I'm on medication. I don't want them to know, because they might not take it well and I don't want to lose them.
>
> Paraskeuas

So far we have considered three key issues in relation to mental illness: lack of knowledge (ignorance), negative attitudes (prejudice) and rejecting behaviour (discrimination). We have seen how these forces operate in relation to home life, family, personal relationships, work, neighbours, in leisure and social life and in healthcare. In the final chapter we shall turn to the question of what needs to be done by all of us to reduce these destructive influences. In this chapter we consider what can be done by people with mental illnesses themselves. It is tempting to see ignorance, prejudice and discrimination simply as what are 'done to' service users and consumers, but this is unhelpful for two reasons. First, as we saw in Chapter 8, stigmatisation is applied by people with mental illnesses to themselves as well as applied to them by others. Second, accepting the role of passive victim to stigma and discrimination is not one that assists recovery from mental illness and its consequences.[1] So this chapter will outline what can be done by consumers and service users to cope with and minimize these forces.[2]

Before deciding what to do to modify the reactions of other people, a useful starting point is to find out as much as possible about the condition itself.[3] Although in some countries it is common for clinical staff to be reluctant to inform people with mental illness about their particular diagnosis, more often staff will try to communicate something about the condition to the people they have assessed. From the point of view of medical staff, for example, although their training will usually give great emphasis to making a diagnosis, it does not attach much importance to conveying this information to the person concerned.

Most research in this area has discussed giving information about the diagnosis within a comprehensive set of interventions called psychosocial education which also includes details about what treatments are available, treatment and services, and which tries to involve family members. Psycho-social education has been found to be reasonably effective, in addition to pharmacological treatment, for schizophrenia,[4–7] and bipolar disorder,[8–12] and there is also some weaker evidence that it can improve the outcome for people with depression.[13–15]

The psycho-educational approach has been used less often for people with eating disorders,[16] anxiety-related disorders,[17] panic disorder,[18,19] and not at all for people with post-traumatic, obsessive-compulsive and personality disorders. This last group is especially important, as we saw in relation in Chapter 5 that some people with personality disorder feel unsympathetically treated by mental and physical healthcare professionals. It appears that some clinical staff have particular difficulty in giving clear diagnostic information to people they consider to have a personality disorder.[20]

> It rips me apart, let's put it that way, OK?
>
> Kim

The focus of psycho-education is to improve the understanding of their condition by the person with mental illness, and his or her family, so that this increases the likelihood of accepting treatment. While there is no doubt that this is important, as about a half of all prescribed medication is not actually taken,[21] the significance of the diagnosis goes beyond medication adherence alone. The diagnosis gives a name to what may have previously been an anonymous threat to a person's intimate sense of themself. It allows the person to meet others with the same condition and to learn how they have tried to cope. It enables the person to find out about the range of treatments for that particular condition, and how strong or weak the evidence is that they work.

Given this, it is remarkable that there has been very little research on how staff should offer diagnostic information, especially as a person who begins to experience the symptoms of mental illness will only know what most people in the general population know about mental illness – very little except for information that tends to sensationalize and brutalize the meaning of mental illness. The willingness of the people receiving diagnoses to accept the recom-mended treatment will depend to a large extent upon how far they agree with the professional assessment. How far there is agreement between, for example, the psychiatrist's diagnosis and the view of the person concerned is seldom discussed. In particular there are suggestions that clinicians may be reluctant to disclose the diagnosis,[22–24] over-confident of their therapeutic skills,[25] or pessimistic about the outlook for particular conditions.[26]

From the point of view of service users and consumers, the background knowledge they bring to a diagnostic consultation,[27] along with their own agenda,[28] attitudes to treatment,[29] hopes,[30] expectations[31] and priorities[32] will all have a bearing on what conclusions they come to after being offered a diagnosis by their physician. These issues, and wider patterns of communication,[33] have been particularly studied for general practitioners (primary care physicians).

It might be expected that in relation to mental illnesses, where there are especially controversial diagnostic practices[34] and where psychiatrists usually possess legal powers that go well beyond those available to other doctors,[35] that 'doctor-patient' communication would have been especially well researched. But this would be a mistaken assumption. Both for general aspects of communication,[36] but also in relation to specific discussions on diagnosis, little is known about what is effective or acceptable for service users, as we shall see later in this chapter. Nevertheless it is clear from service user/consumer groups that they call for a more participatory style from professionals, in which there is a greater degree of negotiation about diagnosis and treatment,[37, 38] and more joint decision-making.[39] Such groups may need to maintain active pressure for these changes to see them enter mainstream clinical practice.

Concealment and disclosure

> I have had to be careful who I tell about my illness, because a lot of the time people throw it back in your face. They say 'Well you are mad. You have to see a psychiatrist.'
>
> Louise

When a person begins to experience the features of a mental illness, then the question arises: what to tell other people? This is one of the most difficult questions of all. One way to look at this is to see the decision as a balance between the benefits and costs of disclosing information about mental illness.[40] The first possible benefit of telling someone else is to allow the other person to offer help. Help can be of four types: instrumental support (such as solving a problem), tangible support (for example donating a cooker), informational support (providing advice), or emotional support (giving reassurance).[41] Further, admitting to having a mental illness allows a person to join self-help groups, to be able to advocate for one's own treatment and care and to join groups campaigning for better mental health services. It can trigger extra welfare benefit payments if a person satisfies criteria to be in special need or be disabled. Disclosing one's diagnosis has also been described as removing the stress of having to keep it a secret.[42] It may help the person to identify others who have had similar experiences, or who can be helpful in future. Telling one's story has also been describing as a liberating and empowering experience,[41] which can reduce social isolation and loneliness.

At the same time there are a series of potential drawbacks from disclosure. It directly allows others to draw upon their own ignorance or misinformation, along with negative feelings, to react in a negatively discriminating way.[43] It means that such a declaration may be taken as a 'master status' and colour, for example, the views of doctors when investigating physical problems (see Chapter 5). Disclosure may also substantially reduce opportunities for employment, while non-disclosure prevents employers from making reasonable adjustments/accommodations. It may also lead to other forms of exclusion, for example being considered unsuitable for marriage or for child-minding. It can allow others to see your every action as related to mental illness, for example, to see a legitimate complaint or an outburst of anger as signs of the condition, and not to be taken seriously at face value. It may also mean that family members react to this information in extreme ways, for example with either avoidance or over-protection. As we have seen in previous chapters, the implications of gossip are that disclosure within smaller communities, such as villages, may mean that to tell someone will mean that everyone will know.

It is therefore clear that decisions by a person with mental illness about whom to tell, what to tell, when to tell are fraught and far from straightforward.[44,45] One practical approach is to draw up a balance sheet, for example of the short-term and long-term expected benefits and costs of concealing or disclosing, and let this framework guide such decisions.[41] Broadly speaking five different viewpoints can be adopted:[41]

1. social avoidance: avoiding people and places which might be stigmatising
2. secrecy: withholding important information but not avoiding normal settings
3. selective disclosure: giving information on diagnosis to a small group of people who are expected to understand and provide support
4. indiscriminate disclosure: telling everyone
5. broadcasting: deliberately communicating one's experiences to a large group, for example using media interviews.

But taking such decisions means making a series of guesses about how people will react if told about a mental illness. However, as we saw in Chapter 2, the reactions of others can be unexpectedly helpful or harsh, and what has been said cannot be unsaid.

> I have learnt to recognise the types of people who may be less prejudiced. Anyone humble or who knows a close friend/family member who has suffered. Anyone who has been abused, or had a stressful childhood experience e.g. coming out as a homosexual. Anyone well-travelled. Anyone with medical training. Anyone who knows many different people. I believe that the

prejudiced people are just believers in willpower and getting on with things. People who have never had a problem that they can't deal with or sidestep somehow. Their achievements in their lives rest firmly on the shoulders of their courage and determination against the odds, and frankly if others wind up mentally ill, then it's probably because they've lacked the iron will and sense to get on with things. In a cynical moment I'll say that people revel in the misfortune of others. We're built to compete and to see someone stricken with mental illness gives everyone the relief and satisfaction that it didn't happen to them.

Robert

One risk is that an anticipated tolerance for diversity may not actually happen.[46,47] A survey of over 1000 consumers of mental health services in the USA found evidence for caution here:[48]

- *'I have been treated as less competent by others when they learned I am a consumer'* (70 per cent agreed that this happened sometimes, often or very often)
- *'I have been shunned or avoided by others when it was revealed that I was a consumer'* (60 per cent agreed that this happened sometimes, often or very often)
- *'I have been advised to lower my expectations of life because I am a consumer'* (57 per cent agreed that this happened sometimes, often or very often).

This survey also found that many consumers were reluctant or very selective in disclosing information about their difficulties to others. For example regarding the statement *'I have avoided indicating on written applications that I am a consumer for fear that this information will be used against me'*, 71 per cent said that this had happened to them.

I go to interviews arranged by my personnel department, apply directly for posts that I am made aware of, but as soon as the managers are aware that I have been off work with chronic depression the interview is either cancelled or quickly terminated. The personnel department's and prospective manager's view of me has not been helped by an email sent from my previous manager which stated that following my suicide attempt I was clearly unstable and potentially a risk to others as well as myself. I only know of this email because I had asked to see my personnel file. While it was clear from the file that some pages were missing, that email had been left on, I presume inadvertently. I have now lodged an application with the Employment Tribunal on the grounds of disability discrimination in the hope that this will prompt my employer to do something.

Thomas

In some ways such decisions run parallel to those of gay people thinking about 'coming out'.[40, 49, 50] Gay and lesbian people share several characteristics with people with mental illness: their status may be concealable, it can be seen as socially abnormal, lead to problems of personal identity from early adulthood,[40] and precipitate dilemmas about disclosure that go on and on.[51, 52]

> I got a job with the Police as a 'lollipop' man (School Crossing Patrol), and everything went well until 1995, when I became ill after I had tried to study for school leaver exams, and the pressure got to me and a good friend had died after a long illness caused by cancer. I also had a lot of aggravation from a Care Worker (independent living officer), who didn't like me doing the lollipop job and kept telling me that I could be sued and even put into prison because he thought that I had not told the police that I suffered from schizophrenia. I was worried already but this made me worse, even though I had told Scotland Yard on my job application form. Within the same week, there was also an incident when I was working at a school crossing when a boy crossing the road was knocked down by a bicycle. He wasn't hurt but I got into a terrible state. I wasn't concentrating because of these problems and I felt that there could be a serious accident and I decided to leave. That night I wrote to the police and told them I suffered with schizophrenia, and they suspended me. The same day I got a medical certificate, and went on sick pay and left on health grounds six months later. During the previous three years I had had cancer twice and had developed Type 2 diabetes and immune deficiency, so I never worked again.
>
> Steven

Visibility

To a large extent the question of disclosure or concealment of having a mental illness depends upon whether it is visible or concealable. Can other people know or guess the diagnosis if the person concerned does not say so?[53] Visibility has long been seen as one of the cornerstones of many types of stigma. As we saw in Chapter 9, one influential definition put 'concealability' as the first of six key dimensions of stigma.[54] Another view is that stigmatising conditions can be divided into those which are 'discrediting' (visible) and those which are 'discreditable' (invisible).[55] Spasmodic torticollis is an example of the former,[56] while mental illnesses demonstrate the latter.[55]

Visibility has been studied in some detail for a series of physical disorders and disabilities. Skin conditions, such as scleroderma, have been a particular focus of such research.[57, 58] This work suggests that people who can minimize the visual signs of difference have more choice about whether to disclose, and will often choose not to.

Trying to maintain invisibility may itself carry hidden costs. A study in Virginia compared female students with and without eating disorders. Each group was asked to role-play having or not having an eating disorder. The groups who played a role consistent with their real life reported little distress, but those women who did have an eating disorder who were asked to play the role of not having the condition reported a continuing preoccupation with secrecy, and the need to suppress repeatedly intrusive thoughts.[59] So the price of privacy may be constant vigilance and worry about discovery.[60] This can be so severe and persistent that it has been described as a 'private hell'.[61]

But we are in deep and complex waters here. There are also psychological costs to revealing a mental illness which is concealable. One study in Connecticut examined whether the intellectual performance of college students was associated with disclosing a concealable stigma. Students with and without a history of mental illness took part. The results showed that among students who had a history of mental illness, those who revealed this did worse on the reasoning test than those who did not.[62] These fascinating results are consistent with what we saw in Chapter 8, namely the power of self-stigmatisation, and destructive vicious cycles which can start when a person expects to be devalued.

On the other side of the balance, it appears that the risk of disclosing a concealable stigma is lower for people who have high levels of social support. In a notable study in Harvard, students were asked to rate their self-esteem and mood at frequent intervals over a 11–day period. Those with concealable stigmas (students who said they were gay, that they were bulimic, or that their family earned less than $20,000 a year) reported lower self-esteem and mood than both those who had visible stigmas and those without any stigmatising characteristics. In the first group, only the presence of similar others lifted their self-esteem and mood.[63]

> Stigma still exists and probably always will when it comes to mental illness as you can't see it. Many do sympathize with say a lady who's gone through years of cosmetic surgery, her struggle to regain her self-esteem, and it's only right that we do so. Yet how many would sympathize with someone with OCD (obsessive-compulsive disorder), as you can't see it, and her struggle to regain self-esteem. Not many.
>
> Paul

Nevertheless, to think that all mental illnesses are concealable is an over-simplification. Some can lead to features that are difficult or impossible to hide, such as extreme thinness in anorexia nervosa. Others mean that considerable care is needed to maintain concealment, such as the accumulated scars of someone with borderline personality disorder who then chooses to conceal them, for example with long-sleeved clothes. Other features may be more subtle, for example some lack of facial, emotional or vocal expressiveness in people who are depressed. Small changes may be immediately noticeable to other people, such as a slightly increased delay before initiating conversation.[64–67]

Other indications of mental illness may be indirect, such as the side-effects of drugs. An example of this is tardive dyskinesia, which means repetitive or writhing movements (such as lip smacking or restless legs), which can be a consequence of taking drugs for psychotic disorders. Other visible characteristics may also reflect the condition indirectly. People whose self-esteem is low (common for many mental illnesses), or whose motivation to care for themselves is compromised, may neglect looking after their hair or personal cleanliness.[68] As we saw in Chapter 3, unemployment and material poverty are common among people with the more severe type of mental illness and this can also have visible consequences, for example in cheap clothes from second-hand shops. If a person has rapid weight gain from taking antipsychotic medication,[69] then it may be difficult to afford new clothes so what they are seen wearing is ill-fitting. People whose mental illness affects their ability to speak clearly, for example because of muddled thoughts from some psychotic disorders, can also give an immediate impression of abnormality. It is therefore misleading to think that mental illnesses are necessarily concealable sources of stigma.

Even so, as the primary difficulty is a disorder of the mind, to a large extent many people with mental illnesses may be able to conceal their condition or disability if they wish. Achieving concealability would allow choice about whether to disclose or not. Ways to conceal have not been discussed to any significant extent in relation to mental illness.[61] Such coping strategies could include intensive training on self-care, on speech patterns, on conversational ploys, on finding affordable clothing that fits, or on styles of non-verbal interaction. In short, ways of 'passing' as 'normal'. Such a strategy is controversial and some argue that people with mental illness should show pride and not deny their situation.[70] Others, nevertheless, may wish to retain or regain the ability to not stand out as different if they choose.[71]

> I think people are frightened by 'the mind illness' whereas 'physical illness' is there to be seen.
>
> Sonia

Acceptance or denial of having a mental illness

So far we have considered the options open to people with a mental illness who may not wish to reveal their condition to others. Another important option exists, namely to deny that one has a mental illness at all. Denial has been studied far more in relation to cancer[72-74] and heart disease,[75-78] than for mental illness.[79-82] Interestingly this work shows that denial can have some positive effects. There are indications that acceptance of a psychiatrist's diagnosis may vary according to the ethnic group of the patient[83,84] (for example among Puerto Ricans in Los Angeles or in black Caribbeans in London). Such views have practical implications. Not accepting that difficulties are a form of mental illness tends to lead people to stop contact with health services.[83]

> Personally I don't feel stigmatised. I'm not very different from the other people. I consider myself normal. I know nothing about stigma. People treat me good, because they don't understand that I've got something. I've got relationships with normal people. I even have a boyfriend. I would like to get a job and leave my parents' house. My problem is that I want to forget what I have, but the other people are reminding me all the time.
>
> Andriani

Rather than focus on the denial or rejection of diagnoses, more often psychiatric research has concentrated upon the concept of 'insight'.[85] Insight is a complex concept that covers awareness of the mental disorder, its symptoms, the need for treatment, its social consequences and the attribution of symptoms to mental disorder.[86,87] At present there is no clear agreement about the nature and implications of insight.[87] Put crudely, insight refers to how far a person with mental illness agrees with the diagnosis made by the psychiatrist. Research in this field has mostly concentrated upon links between insight and cognitive impairment (for example problems in concentration or memory), or with medication adherence (sometimes called compliance or concordance).[21,88–91]

Little attention has been paid to whether people with mental illness may have valid reasons to reject such diagnoses, alongside having, for example, problems with attention or concentration.[92,93] In Chapter 6 we saw that popular portrayals of mental illnesses in the media are highly selective and allow dangerousness to overshadow all other aspects of these conditions. We have also seen countless examples in Chapters 1–5 of the disadvantages experienced by people who accept a diagnosis of mental illness. It has also been found that some groups of people with higher levels of insight also show more hopelessness about the future.[94] On the face of it, therefore, there seem to be strong reasons why a person offered a diagnosis of mental illness may choose not to accept it, especially if this will mean making important sacrifices.[95,96] If we see the process of diagnosis as a type of negotiation or trade, then making a deal will depend on what exactly is being offered, with what benefits and at what price.

Surprisingly little attention has been paid by staff to giving understandable information about the diagnosis on offer, or to the types of communication (for example an exchange of views rather than a one-way flow of information) that can help or hinder the acceptance of a diagnosis.[97,98] So it is perhaps not surprising that about half of all medication prescribed for conditions such as diabetes, asthma or schizophrenia is not taken by patients.[21,99] The latter, for example, are more likely to take treatment as recommended if they have received detailed information from their doctor.[100] From a consumer perspective it may often be necessary to ask for, or even to demand, detailed information about the diagnosis and treatments being recommended before deciding whether to accept these or not.

> I was told I was ill by the psychiatrist. Manic depression was put on my prescription. I had to finally ask what manic depression was as I was not ever offered or given a leaflet with information about my illness. My doctor put bipolar on my prescription so I thought I had two things wrong with me. I had to ask about that too. When I asked for an information leaflet the psychiatrist at the resource centre could not give me a leaflet as there were none available, then, before or after. He sent me a copy from the website. Hearing someone say 'Bipolar means cruel, mean and crazy' didn't help.
>
> Justine

Coping

For people who do, at least practically, accept that they have a mental health problem then there is a need to grapple with the question: how can I cope with this? Coping has been defined as, 'a person's constantly changing cognitive and behavioural efforts to manage specific external and/or internal demands that are appraised as taxing or exceeding the person's resources'.[101] In other words, what needs to be done to survive practically and emotionally from day to day.

The challenges facing people with mental illness, including stigma and discrimination, can be seen as a series of threats. The coping strategies used by an individual (or by a group) may or not may be sufficient to outweigh the strength of the threat.[60] These threats are not only clear-cuts acts of discrimination, but also the costs of continuing vigilance against stigma, and the draining effects of uncertainty, sometimes not knowing if a bad experience was related to discrimination or not.[55] Under some circumstances denying that experiences are instances of stigma may be a postive way of coping,[60] although generally speaking the use of denial as a coping strategy is associated with poorer physical and mental health.[60] The following ways of coping with threats have been described:[102]

- ◆ avoidance
- ◆ denial
- ◆ mental disengagement
- ◆ behavioural disengagement
- ◆ acceptance

- positive reframing
- venting negative emotions
- seeking emotional support
- seeking instrumental social support
- religious coping
- suppressing activities
- active coping (problem-focused coping)
- planned problem-solving.

What does all this mean in practice? One starting point is for service users and consumers to try to eliminate the reason for discrimination, for example by trying the treatment that has been recommended to see if it works. A second option may be to compensate for the effects of the mental illness by modifying behaviour so that the problem is not visible to others, for example by changing self-care or clothing patterns. A third course of action is to deliberately decide whether to confirm or disconfirm the stereotyped expectations of others, for example by increasing effort at work to undermine employer expectations that depression is a sign of laziness, or moral weakness of will.[103]

A further means of coping with real or expected threats is avoidance.[104] As we saw in Chapter 8, anticipated discrimination can sometimes be worse than the real thing. But in everyday life both can have the same consequences: avoidance and social withdrawal. While this way of coping can minimize exposure to discrimination, it comes at the high price of losing prospects of work, marriage or intimate relationships.

One further positive method to cope with stigma is to attribute such experiences to external rather than to internal factors.[60] For example, failure in a job interview can be seen as evidence of prejudice and discrimination by an employer, rather than reflecting a personal failing (such as a lack of relevant skills for a particular post).[105,106] While this tactic has been studied in relation to discrimination against minority ethnic groups, it has not been researched for people with mental illness.

Acknowledgement is another coping option, which means acknowledging both the mental illness and also the discriminatory reactions of others. One advantage of this is to move blame from oneself onto the outside world. Using a physical disability illustration, a wheelchair user might say, 'As you can see, I use a wheelchair.' By stating the obvious, especially for a visible disability likely to trigger a stigmatising reaction, the idea is to pre-empt any reactions characterized by disdain, pity or contempt. That is, to allow others to see the person rather than the disability.

Once again we need to avoid oversimplifying complex social situations. One study of people with physical disabilities, for example, found that they received more positive reactions from others if their own initial statement was made using socially appropriate language and if they avoided giving any indications of depression.[107] A technique related to acknowledgement is to 'ask a favour' of others, which has been found with some physical disabilities to break through avoidance and to facilitate social interaction,[107] although some disabled people may see this technique as rather demeaning.

These coping strategies may be useful for people with physical disabilities, but there has been almost no research on their effectiveness in reducing prejudice or discrimination related to mental illnesses. One exception was a study in New York which investigated whether people with mental illness can reduce stigmatisation by: (i) keeping their condition a secret, (ii) educating others about their situation, or (iii) by avoiding situations in which rejection might occur. The result was that none of these coping methods was effective in diminishing stigma. In fact, the three methods produced more harm than good, in terms of increasing withdrawal and avoidance. The authors concluded that these issues are 'social problems' and not 'individual troubles'.[108]

> People view it as being mental. They don't talk about it and that makes it worse. I prefer to turn it around and make it a joke. I am not ashamed of anything. I make a joke out of it. I call it going 'nut-nut'.
>
> Emile

Self-management and recovery

Mental health services are essentially different from all other health services in that they routinely force some patients to undergo treatment. Psychiatrists are different from all other medical specialists in having such legal and professional powers to use on a regular basis. One of the consequences of having these powers is that some people with mental illness avoid mental health services for fear of having unwanted treatment forced upon them. Others who have been treated without their consent try to avoid any repetition,[109] for example, by not keeping in touch with mental health services.[110] This reluctance to lose control of treatment decisions, alongside the wish not to become stigmatised as 'insane' (the most common reason given in one Israeli study of mentally ill people who chose not to go to psychiatric services[111]), decreases the likelihood that people who need specialist help will receive it. In other words maintaining personal control over their situation is of paramount importance for many people with mental illnesses.

> My anger and rebellion against being considered a failure and invalid.[112]

One way to try to achieve such control is self-management. This involves a person with a chronic condition 'engaging in activities that protect and promote health, monitoring and managing symptoms and signs of illness, managing the impacts of illness on functioning, emotions and inter-personal relationships and adhering to treatment regimes'.[113] Self-management is often seen as one element within a partnership with treatment services who offer self-management support, defined as 'the systematic provision of education and supportive interventions by healthcare staff to increase patients' skills and confidence in managing their health problems, including regular assessment of progress and problems, goal setting, and problem-solving support'.[114]

Self-management has been developed for a wide range of chronic conditions,[115] including asthma,[116] arthritis[117] and diabetes.[118] These methods have only recently been used by people with mental illnesses,[119,120] including those with diagnoses of depression,[121,122] panic disorder, phobias and obsessive-compulsive disorder,[123] and psychotic disorders.[124,125]

Self-management covers the range from approaches which are a type of do-it-yourself for consumers,[126] through to programmes which are 'professional-based interventions designed to help consumers and professionals collaborate in the treatment of mental illness, reduce susceptibility to relapses, and develop effective coping strategies for the management of symptoms'.[120] For example, consumers' views can shape their care through the use of crisis plans and advance directives.[127,128] Four particular elements appear to be most beneficial:[119,120]

- psycho-education
- strategies addressing medication non-adherence
- relapse prevention training
- coping skills training.

The self-management viewpoint starts with evidence of what works for long-term conditions and then seeks to empower people with those conditions to get the best treatment possible. It assumes that the full range of evidence-based treatments should be available to each individual. For many types of mental illness this will mean a combination of pharmacological, psychological and social interventions.[129–132]

Self-management may be able to contribute indirectly towards reducing discrimination towards individuals with mental illnesses if they fully or partially recover. This may reduce stigma to some extent, although we have seen that even people who fully recover from a period of mental illness can still be discriminated against because they have such a history. Interestingly, self-management has not yet been applied directly to reducing stigma or discrimination.

The idea of recovery has become increasingly important in recent years.[133] Although there is no consensus on what this term means,[134] it is usually used in a wider sense than to mean a complete cure.[135] More often the term is now used by consumers to mean, for example, 'enjoying the pleasures life has to offer, pursuing personal dreams and goals, developing rewarding relationships, and learning to cope with or grow past one's mental illness despite symptoms or setbacks',[120] or 'reducing relapses, becoming free of symptoms, staying out of the hospital or getting a job'.[120] The term is an indication that service users and consumers are taking the initiative in defining their own goals and the language which best supports this.[136–139]

Another type of initiative which consumers can take on their own behalf consists of empowerment and self-advocacy.[140,141] An empowerment orientation by consumers is positively associated with quality of life, self-esteem, social support and psychiatric symptoms.[142] Indeed empowerment has been described as the opposite of self-stigmatisation.[143,144] Specific ways in which people with mental illness can gain empowerment include the following:[145]

- participating in formulating care and crisis plans[146]
- using cognitive-behavioural therapy to reverse negative self-stigma[147,148]
- running regular assessments of consumer satisfaction with services[149]
- creating user-led and user-run services[37,150,151]
- developing peer support worker roles in mainstream mental healthcare[152]
- asking employers to give positive value for experience of mental illness[153,154]
- being actively involved in evaluation and research.[155,156]

Collective approaches to reducing discrimination

Apart from what individual people can do to reduce discrimination, what can groups do in terms of collective action?[110,157–159] First, consumer groups can protest against misrepresentations of mental illnesses and campaign for more accurate and fair portrayals.[160–164] Already at the local, national, and international levels consumer groups have started anti-stigma organisations which include, from many different perspectives, the following:

- Mad Pride
- MindFreedom
- StigmaBusters
- National Anti-Stigma Clearing House
- National Mental Health Awareness Campaign
- National Mental Health Association Stigma Watch
- Mental Health Self-Help Network
- Campaign to Complain.[165]

Yet it is not clear if such collective protest is effective. A part of the motivation for such protests consists of a moral appeal for fairness, which can have a paradoxical effect. Recipients of such admonishments can respond with negative feelings about being told what to think.[166,167] Although there are some examples of television programmes or newspaper stories being reconsidered because of coordinated protests by consumer groups,[167] these are few and the impact of anti-stigma activities is not well understood.[160,163]

A study in Chicago, for example, compared education, direct contact and protest upon views about schizophrenia.[162] Education had no effect on college students' views about physical disabilities but did produce more favourable views about depression, psychosis, cocaine addiction and learning disability (mental retardation). Direct contact between the students and consumers produced even more favourable changes in views about depression and psychosis, but protest alone produced no change in views about any of these conditions. These results support a great deal of other research suggesting that direct contact between people with mental illness and others can improve stigmatising views and discriminatory behaviour, and this will be discussed in more detail in Chapter 11.

Media involvement

A further way in which people with a diagnosis of mental illness can take action to reduce prejudice and discrimination is to contribute to the coverage of mental health issues in the print, broadcast and electronic media.[107,168] As we saw in Chapter 6, although mental illness-related stories and features are covered relatively often, it is rare for people with mental illness to be quoted in their own words.[169] More often journalists will 'editorialize', usually in ways that are consistent with pre-existing popular views of mental illness. In particular, it is rare to feature stories about people who have recovered from a mental illness.[170] One way to redress this deficit is to create 'speakers' bureaux', which are groups of service users able to give positive accounts about mental illness to the media. Such bureaux have been established for several types of physical disability.[171–174] There is no published research about their effectiveness, and indeed consumer-led attempts to reduce stigmatisation have so far hardly been researched at all.[175] Nevertheless, speakers' bureaux can be seen as promising candidate interventions, because, as we shall see now in Chapter 11, there is strong evidence for the positive effects of direct personal contact with mentally ill people in reducing discrimination.

> I'm a human being, with all the feelings that brings, but stigma makes my life harder to bear.
>
> Maria

References

1. Noh S, Kaspar V. Perceived discrimination and depression: moderating effects of coping, acculturation, and ethnic support. *Am J Public Health* 2003; 93(2):232–238.

2. Corrigan PW, Calabrese JD, Diwan SE, Keogh CB, Keck L, Mussey C. Some recovery processes in mutual-help groups for persons with mental illness; I: qualitative analysis of program materials and testimonies. *Community Ment Health J* 2002; 38(4):287–301.

3. Kilian R, Holzinger A, Angermeyer MC. ['It may be somewhat more demanding sometimes, but also more interesting'. Psychiatrists evaluate the impact of psychoeducation on outpatient treatment of schizophrenia]. *Psychiatr Prax* 2001; 28(5):209–213.

4. Hogarty GE, Anderson CM, Reiss DJ, Kornblith SJ, Greenwald DP, Ulrich RF *et al.* Family psychoeducation, social skills training, and maintenance chemotherapy in the aftercare treatment of schizophrenia. II. Two-year effects of a controlled study on relapse and adjustment. Environmental-Personal Indicators in the Course of Schizophrenia (EPICS) Research Group. *Arch Gen Psychiatry* 1991; 48(4):340–347.

5. Dixon L, Adams C, Lucksted A. Update on family psychoeducation for schizophrenia. *Schizophr Bull* 2000; 26(1):5–20.

6. McFarlane WR, Dixon L, Lukens E, Lucksted A. Family psychoeducation and schizophrenia: a review of the literature. *J Marital Fam Ther* 2003; 29(2):223–245.

7. Pekkala E, Merinder L. *Psychoeducation for schizophrenia*. Cochrane Database Syst Rev 2002;(2):CD002831.

8. Colom F, Lam D. Psychoeducation: improving outcomes in bipolar disorder. *Eur Psychiatry* 2005; 20; 359–364.

9. Gonzalez-Pinto A, Gonzalez C, Enjuto S, Fernandez de CB, Lopez P, Palomo J *et al.* Psychoeducation and cognitive-behavioral therapy in bipolar disorder: an update. *Acta Psychiatr Scand* 2004; 109(2):83–90.

10. Michalak EE, Yatham LN, Wan DD, Lam RW. Perceived quality of life in patients with bipolar disorder. Does group psychoeducation have an impact? *Can J Psychiatry* 2005; 50(2):95–100.

11. Miklowitz DJ, George EL, Richards JA, Simoneau TL, Suddath RL. A randomized study of family-focused psychoeducation and pharmacotherapy in the outpatient management of bipolar disorder. *Arch Gen Psychiatry* 2003; 60(9):904–912.

12. Vieta E. Improving treatment adherence in bipolar disorder through psychoeducation. *J Clin Psychiatry* 2005; 66 Suppl 1:24–29.

13. Glick ID, Burti L, Okonogi K, Sacks M. Effectiveness in psychiatric care. III: Psychoeducation and outcome for patients with major affective disorder and their families. *Br J Psychiatry* 1994; 164(1):104–106.

14. Srinivasan J, Cohen NL, Parikh SV. Patient attitudes regarding causes of depression: implications for psychoeducation. *Can J Psychiatry* 2003; 48(7):493–495.

15. Dowrick C, Dunn G, yuso-Mateos JL, Dalgard OS, Page H, Lehtinen V *et al.* Problem solving treatment and group psychoeducation for depression: multicentre randomised controlled trial. Outcomes of Depression International Network (ODIN) Group. *BMJ* 2000; 321(7274):1450–1454.

16. Andrewes DG, O'Connor P, Mulder C, McLennan J, Derham H, Weigall S *et al.* Computerised psychoeducation for patients with eating disorders. *Aust N Z J Psychiatry* 1996; 30(4):492–497.

17. Chavira DA, Stein MB. Combined psychoeducation and treatment with selective serotonin reuptake inhibitors for youth with generalized social anxiety disorder. *J Child Adolesc Psychopharmacol* 2002; 12(1):47–54.

18. Baillie AJ, Rapee RM. Predicting who benefits from psychoeducation and self help for panic attacks. *Behav Res Ther* 2004; 42(5):513–527.

19. Dannon PN, Iancu I, Grunhaus L. Psychoeducation in panic disorder patients: effect of a self-information booklet in a randomized, masked-rater study. *Depress Anxiety* 2002; 16(2):71–76.

20. Lequesne ER, Hersh RG. Disclosure of a diagnosis of borderline personality disorder. *J Psychiatr Pract* 2004; 10(3):170–176.

21. McDonald HP, Garg AX, Haynes RB. Interventions to enhance patient adherence to medication prescriptions: scientific review. *JAMA* 2002; 288(22):2868–2879.

22. Fisher M. Telling patients with schizophrenia their diagnosis. Patients expect a diagnosis. *BMJ* 2000; 321(7257):385.

23. Clafferty RA, McCabe E, Brown KW. Telling patients with schizophrenia their diagnosis. Patients should be informed about their illness. *BMJ* 2000; 321(7257):384–385.

24. Green RS, Gantt AB. Telling patients and families the psychiatric diagnosis: a survey of psychiatrists. *Hosp Community Psychiatry* 1987; 38(6):666–668.

25. Harman JS, Brown EL, Have TT, Mulsant BH, Brown G, Bruce ML. Primary care physicians attitude toward diagnosis and treatment of late-life depression. *CNS Spectr* 2002; 7(11):784–790.

26. Laukkanen E, Korhonen V, Peiponen S, Nuutinen M, Viinamaki H. A pessimistic attitude towards the future and low psychosocial functioning predict psychiatric diagnosis among treatment-seeking adolescents. *Aust N Z J Psychiatry* 2001; 35(2):160–165.

27. Elwyn G, Edwards A, Britten N. What information do patients need about medicines? 'Doing prescribing': how doctors can be more effective. *BMJ* 2003; 327(7419):864–867.

28. Barry CA, Bradley CP, Britten N, Stevenson FA, Barber N. Patients' unvoiced agendas in general practice consultations: qualitative study. *BMJ* 2000; 320(7244):1246–1250.

29. Britten N, Ukoumunne OC, Boulton MG. Patients' attitudes to medicines and expectations for prescriptions. *Health Expect* 2002; 5(3):256–269.

30. Britten N, Ukoumunne O. The influence of patients' hopes of receiving a prescription on doctors' perceptions and the decision to prescribe: a questionnaire survey. *BMJ* 1997; 315(7121):1506–1510.

31. Britten N. Patients' expectations of consultations. *BMJ* 2004; 328(7437):416–417.

32. Britten N. Does a prescribed treatment match a patient's priorities? *BMJ* 2003; 327(7419):840.

33. Stevenson FA, Cox K, Britten N, Dundar Y. A systematic review of the research on communication between patients and health care professionals about medicines: the consequences for concordance. *Health Expect* 2004; 7(3):235–245.

34. Szasz T. Psychiatric diagnosis, psychiatric power and psychiatric abuse. *J Med Ethics* 1994; 20(3):135–138.

35. Rogers A, Day JC, Williams B, Randall F, Wood P, Healy D *et al.* The meaning and management of neuroleptic medication: a study of patients with a diagnosis of schizophrenia. *Soc Sci Med* 1998; 47(9):1313–1323.

36. Britten N. Psychiatry, stigma, and resistance. Psychiatrists need to concentrate on understanding, not simply compliance. *BMJ* 1998; 317(7164):963–964.

37. Chamberlin J. User/consumer involvement in mental health service delivery. *Epidemiol Psichiatr Soc* 2005; 14; 10–14.

38. Thornicroft G, Tansella M. Growing recognition of the importance of service user involvement in mental health service planning and evaluation. *Epidemiol Psichiatr Soc* 2005; 14(1):1–3.

39. Entwistle V. Trust and shared decision-making: an emerging research agenda. *Health Expect* 2004; 7(4):271–273.

40. Corrigan P.W. Dealing with stigma through personal disclosure. In: Corrigan PW, ed., *On the Stigma of Mental Illness. Practical strategies* for research and social change, pp. 257–280. Washington DC: American Psychological Press; 2005.

41. Corrigan PW, Lundin R. *Don't Call Me Nuts: Coping with the Stigma of Mental Illness.* Chicago Illinois: Recovery Press; 2001.

42. Breitkopf CR. The theoretical basis of stigma as applied to genital herpes. *Herpes* 2004; 11(1):4–7.

43. Eisenberg L. Violence and the mentally ill: victims, not perpetrators. *Arch Gen Psychiatry* 2005; 62(8):825–826.

44. Dalgin RS, Gilbride D. Perspectives of people with psychiatric disabilities on employment disclosure. *Psychiatr Rehabil J* 2003; 26(3):306–10.

45. Dickerson FB, Sommerville J, Origoni AE, Ringel NB, Parente F. Experiences of stigma among outpatients with schizophrenia. *Schizophr Bull* 2002; 28(1):143–155.

46. Hinshaw SP, Cicchetti D. Stigma and mental disorder: conceptions of illness, public attitudes, personal disclosure, and social policy. *Dev Psychopathol* 2000; 12(4):555–598.

47. Jones AH. Mental illness made public: ending the stigma? *Lancet* 1998; 352(9133):1060.

48. Wahl OF. *Telling is a Risky Business: Mental health consumers confront stigma.* New Jersey: Rutgers University Press; 1999.

49. Corrigan P. Beat the stigma: come out of the closet. *Psychiatr Serv* 2003; 54(10):1313.

50. Corrigan PW, Matthews A. Stigma and disclosure: implications for coming out of the closet. *Journal of Mental Health* 2003; 12(3):235–248.

51. Derlega VJ, Chaikin AL. Norms affecting self-disclosure in men and women. *J Consult Clin Psychol* 1976; 44(3):376–380.

52. Klitzman R, Bayer R. *Mortal Secrets: Truth and lies in the age of AIDS.* Baltimore, Maryland: The Johns Hopkins University Press; 2003.

53. Joachim G, Acorn S. Stigma of visible and invisible chronic conditions. *J Adv Nurs* 2000; 32(1):243–248.

54. Jones E, Farina A, Hastorf A, Markus H, Milller D, Scott R. *Social Stigma: the psychology of marked relationships.* New York: W.H. Freeman & Co.; 1984.

55. Goffman I. *Stigma: Notes on the management of spoiled identity.* Harmondsworth, Middlesex: Penguin Books; 1963.

56. Papathanasiou I, MacDonald L, Whurr R, Jahanshahi M. Perceived stigma in spasmodic torticollis. *Mov Disord* 2001; 16(2):280–285.

57. Joachim G, Acorn S. Life with a rare chronic disease: the scleroderma experience. *J Adv Nurs* 2003; 42(6):598–606.

58. Acorn S, Joachim G, Wachs JE. Scleroderma: living with unpredictability. *AAOHN J* 2003; 51(8):353–357.

59. Smart L, Wegner DM. Covering up what can't be seen: concealable stigma and mental control. *J Pers Soc Psychol* 1999; 77(3):474–486.

60. Miller CT, Major B. Coping with stigma and prejudice. In: Heatherton TF, Kleck RE, Hebl MR, Hull JG, eds., *The Social Psychology of Stigma*, pp. 243–272. New York: Guilford; 2000.

61. Smart L, Wegner D. The hidden costs of hidden stigma. In: Heatherton TF, Kleck RE, Hebl MR, Hull JG, eds., *The Social Psychology of Stigma*, pp. 220–242. New York: Guilford; 2000.

62. Quinn DM, Kahng SK, Crocker J. Discreditable: stigma effects of revealing a mental illness history on test performance. *Pers Soc Psychol Bull* 2004; 30(7):803–815.

63. Frable DE, Platt L, Hoey S. Concealable stigmas and positive self-perceptions: feeling better around similar others. *J Pers Soc Psychol* 1998; 74(4):909–922.

64. Brebion G, Amador X, Smith M, Malaspina D, Sharif Z, Gorman JM. Depression, psycho-motor retardation, negative symptoms, and memory in schizophrenia. *Neuropsychiatry Neuropsychol Behav Neurol* 2000; 13(3):177–183.

65. Brebion G, Smith MJ, Widlocher D. Discrimination and response bias in memory: effects of depression severity and psychomotor retardation. *Psychiatry Res* 1997; 70(2):95–103.

66. Lemke MR, Puhl P, Koethe N, Winkler T. Psychomotor retardation and anhedonia in depression. *Acta Psychiatr Scand* 1999; 99(4):252–256.

67. Iverson GL. Objective assessment of psychomotor retardation in primary care patients with depression. *J Behav Med* 2004; 27(1):31–37.

68. Getty C, Perese E, Knab S. Capacity for self-care of persons with mental illnesses living in community residences and the ability of their surrogate families to perform health care functions. *Issues Ment Health Nurs* 1998; 19(1):53–70.

69. Newcomer JW. Second-generation (atypical) antipsychotics and metabolic effects: a com-prehensive literature review. *CNS Drugs* 2005; 19 Suppl. 1:1–93.

70. Pinfold V. 'Building up safe havens... around the world': users' experiences of living in the community with mental health problems. *Health Place* 2000; 6(3):201–212.

71. Penn DL, Kohlmaier JR, Corrigan PW. Interpersonal factors contributing to the stigma of schizophrenia: social skills, perceived attractiveness, and symptoms. *Schizophr Res* 2000; 45(1–2):37–45.

72. Kreitler S. Denial in cancer patients. *Cancer Invest* 1999; 17(7):514–534.

73. Charavel M, Bremond A. Problem of perception and denial of illness by women who have had breast cancer. *Eur J Cancer Prev* 1995; 4(3):259–260.

74. Maguire P, Faulkner A. Communicate with cancer patients: 2. Handling uncertainty, collu-sion, and denial. *BMJ* 1988; 297(6654):972–974.

75. Prince PN, Prince CR. Perceived stigma and community integration among clients of assertive community treatment. *Psychiatr Rehabil J* 2002; 25(4):323–331.

76. Levenson JL, Mishra A, Hamer RM, Hastillo A. Denial and medical outcome in unstable angina. *Psychosom Med* 1989; 51(1):27–35.

77. Levenson JL, Kay R, Monteferrante J, Herman MV. Denial predicts favorable outcome in unstable angina pectoris. *Psychosom Med* 1984; 46(1):25–32.

78. Folks DG, Freeman AM, III, Sokol RS, Thurstin AH. Denial: predictor of outcome following coronary bypass surgery. *Int J Psychiatry Med* 1988; 18(1):57–66.

79. Frankel FH. What's in a name? The 'mental health' euphemism and the consequences of denial. *Hosp Community Psychiatry* 1975; 26(2):104–106.

80. Lamb HR. The denial of severe mental illness. *Psychiatr Serv* 1997; 48(11):1367.

81. Munetz MR. Denial of mental illness. *Psychiatr Serv* 1998; 49(4):536.

82. Sussman S. Denial of mental illness. *Psychiatr Serv* 1998; 49(4):536–537.

83. Ortega AN, Alegria M. Denial and its association with mental health care use: a study of island Puerto Ricans. *J Behav Health Serv Res* 2005; 32(3):320–331.

84. Perkins RE, Moodley P. Perception of problems in psychiatric inpatients: denial, race and service usage. *Soc Psychiatry Psychiatr Epidemiol* 1993; 28(4):189–193.

85. Amador XF, David A. *Insight and Psychosis: Awareness of illness in schizophrenia and related disorders.* Oxford: Oxford University Press; 2004.

86. Cooke MA, Peters ER, Kuipers E, Kumari V. Disease, deficit or denial? Models of poor insight in psychosis. *Acta Psychiatr Scand* 2005; 112(1):4–17.

87. Mintz AR, Dobson KS, Romney DM. Insight in schizophrenia: a meta-analysis. *Schizophr Res* 2003; 61(1):75–88.

88. Gray R, Wykes T, Gournay K. From compliance to concordance: a review of the literature on interventions to enhance compliance with antipsychotic medication. *J Psychiatr Ment Health Nurs* 2002; 9(3):277–284.

89. Sanz M, Constable G, Lopez-Ibor I, Kemp R, David AS. A comparative study of insight scales and their relationship to psychopathological and clinical variables. *Psychol Med* 1998; 28(2):437–446.

90. David A, van OJ, Jones P, Harvey I, Foerster A, Fahy T. Insight and psychotic illness. Cross-sectional and longitudinal associations. *Br J Psychiatry* 1995; 167(5):621–628.

91. Schwartz RC. The relationship between insight, illness and treatment outcome in schizophrenia. *Psychiatr Q* 1998; 69(1):1–22.

92. Morgan K. Perception of psychosis in patients. *Epidemiol Psichiatr Soc* 2004; 13:222–226.

93. Benkert O, Graf-Morgenstern M, Hillert A, Sandmann J, Ehmig SC, Weissbecker H *et al.* Public opinion on psychotropic drugs: an analysis of the factors influencing acceptance or rejection. *J Nerv Ment Dis* 1997; 185(3):151–8.

94. Carroll A, Pantelis C, Harvey C. Insight and hopelessness in forensic patients with schizophrenia. *Aust N Z J Psychiatry* 2004; 38(3):169–173.

95. Schwenk TL. The stigmatisation and denial of mental illness in athletes. *Br J Sports Med* 2000; 34(1):4–5.

96. Borges Z. It is within ourselves that we start to overcome prejudice. *Lancet* 2004; 363(9416):1220.

97. Stevenson FA, Cox K, Britten N, Dundar Y. A systematic review of the research on communication between patients and health care professionals about medicines: the consequences for concordance. *Health Expect* 2004; 7(3):235–245.

98. Goldberg RW, Green-Paden LD, Lehman AF, Gold JM. Correlates of insight in serious mental illness. *J Nerv Ment Dis* 2001; 189(3):137–145.

99. Sayre J. The patient's diagnosis: explanatory models of mental illness. *Qual Health Res* 2000; 10(1):71–83.

100. MacPherson R, Jerrom B, Hughes A. A controlled study of education about drug treatment in schizophrenia. *British Journal of Psychiatry* 1996; 168:709–717.

101. Lazarus.R.S., Folkman S. *Stress, Appraisal and Coping.* New York: Springer; 1984.

102. Carver CS, Scheier MF, Weintraub JK. Assessing coping strategies: a theoretically based approach. *J Pers Soc Psychol* 1989; 56(2):267–283.

103. Karasz A. Cultural differences in conceptual models of depression. *Soc Sci Med* 2005; 60(7):1625–1635.

104. Swim JK, Cohen LL, Hyers LL. Experiencing everyday prejudice and discrimination. In: Swim JK, Stangor C, eds., *Prejudice: the Target's Perspective*, pp. 37–60. San Diego, California: Academic Press; 1998.

105. Crocker J, Cornwell B, Major B. The stigma of overweight: affective consequences of attributional ambiguity. *J Pers Soc Psychol* 1993; 64(1):60–70.

106. Crocker J, Quinn DM. Social stigma and the self: meanings, situations, and self-esteem. In: Heatherton TF, Kleck RE, Hebl MR, Hull JG, eds., *The Social Psychology of Stigma*, pp. 153–183. New York: Guilford; 2000.

107. Hebl MR, Kleck RE. The social consequences of physical disability. In: Heatherton TF, Kleck RE, Hebl MR, Hull JG, eds., *The Social Psychology of Stigma*, pp. 419–439. New York: Guilford; 2000.

108. Link BG, Mirotznik J, Cullen FT. The effectiveness of stigma coping orientations: can negative consequences of mental illness labeling be avoided? *J Health Soc Behav* 1991; 32(3):302–320.

109. Fennell P. *Treatment Without Consent: Law, psychiatry and the treatment of mentally disordered people since 1845.* London: Routledge; 1995.

110. Chamberlin J. *On Our Own: Patient-controlled alternatives to the mental health system.* New York: McGraw-Hill; 1979.

111. Ben-Noun L. Characterization of patients refusing professional psychiatric treatment in a primary care clinic. *Isr J Psychiatry Relat Sci* 1996; 33(3):167–174.

112. Martyn D. *The Experiences and Views of Self-management of People with a Schizophrenia Diagnosis.* London: Rethink; 2005.

113. Gruman J, Von Korff M. *Indexed Bibliography on Self-Management for People with Chronic Disease.* Washington DC: Center for Advancement in Health; 1996.

114. Adams K, Greiner AC, Corrigan JM. *Report of a Summit.* The 1st Annual Crossing the Quality Chasm Summit – A Focus on Communities. Washington DC: Institute of Medicine of the National Academies. The National Academic Press; 2004.

115. Newman S, Steed L, Mulligan K. Self-management interventions for chronic illness. *Lancet* 2004; 364(9444):1523–1537.

116. Guevara JP, Wolf FM, Grum CM, Clark NM. Effects of educational interventions for self management of asthma in children and adolescents: systematic review and meta-analysis. *BMJ* 2003; 326(7402):1308–1309.

117. Keysor JJ, DeVellis BM, DeFriese GH, DeVellis RF, Jordan JM, Konrad TR *et al.* Critical review of arthritis self-management strategy use. *Arthritis Rheum* 2003; 49(5):724–731.

118. Steed L, Cooke D, Newman S. A systematic review of psychosocial outcomes following education, self-management and psychological interventions in diabetes mellitus. *Patient Educ Couns* 2003; 51(1):5–15.

119. Mueser KT, Corrigan PW, Hilton DW, Tanzman B, Schaub A, Gingerich S *et al.* Illness management and recovery: a review of the research. *Psychiatr Serv* 2002; 53(10):1272–1284.

120. Gingerich S, Mueser KT. Illness management and recovery. In: Drake RE, Merrens MR, Lynde DW, eds., *Evidence-Based Mental Health Practice: A textbook.* New York: Norton; 2006 (in press).

121. Williams C, Whitfield G. Written and computer-based self-help treatments for depression. *Br Med Bull* 2001; 57:133–144.

122. Griffiths KM, Christensen H, Jorm AF, Evans K, Groves C. Effect of web-based depression literacy and cognitive-behavioural therapy interventions on stigmatising attitudes to depression: randomised controlled trial. *Br J Psychiatry* 2004; 185:342–349.

123. Barlow JH, Ellard DR, Hainsworth JM, Jones FR, Fisher A. A review of self-management interventions for panic disorders, phobias and obsessive-compulsive disorders. *Acta Psychiatr Scand* 2005; 111(4):272–285.

124. Stevens S, Sin J. Implementing a self-management model of relapse prevention for psychosis into routine clinical practice. *J Psychiatr Ment Health Nurs* 2005; 12(4):495–501.

125. Naoki K, Nobuo A, Emi I. [Randomized controlled trial on effectiveness of the community re-entry program to inpatients with schizophrenia spectrum disorder, centering around acquisition of illness self-management knowledge]. *Seishin Shinkeigaku Zasshi* 2003; 105(12):1514–1531.

126. Charlton BG. Self-management of psychiatric symptoms using over-the-counter (OTC) psychopharmacology: The S-DTM therapeutic model – Self-diagnosis, self-treatment, self-monitoring. *Med Hypotheses* 2005; 65(5):823–828.

127. Henderson C, Flood C, Leese M, Thornicroft G, Sutherby K, Szmukler G. Effect of joint crisis plans on use of compulsory treatment in psychiatry: single blind randomised controlled trial. *BMJ* 2004; 329(7458):136–138.

128. Swanson J, Swartz M, Ferron J, Elbogen EB, Van Dom R. Psychiatric advance directives among public mental health consumers in five U.S. cities: prevalence, demand, and correlates. Journal of the American Academy of Psychiatry and the Law 2005; 34;43–57.

129. Whitty P, Gilbody S. NICE, but will they help people with depression? The new National Institute for Clinical Excellence depression guidelines. *Br J Psychiatry* 2005; 186:177–178.

130. Hargreaves S. NICE guidelines address social aspect of schizophrenia. *BMJ* 2003; 326(7391):679.

131. Drake RE, Mueser KT, Torrey WC, Miller AL, Lehman AF, Bond GR *et al.* Evidence-based treatment of schizophrenia. *Curr Psychiatry Rep* 2000; 2(5):393–397.

132. Neumeyer-Gromen A, Lampert T, Stark K, Kallischnigg G. Disease management programs for depression: a systematic review and meta-analysis of randomized controlled trials. *Med Care* 2004; 42(12):1211–1221.

133. Turner-Crowson J, Wallcraft J. The recovery vision for mental health services and research: a British perspective. *Psychiatr Rehabil J* 2002; 25(3):245–254.

134. Anthony W. Recovery from mental illness: The guiding vision of the mental health service system in the 1990s. *Psychosocial Rehabilitation Journal* 1993; 16:11–23.

135. Deegan PE. Recovery and empowerment for people with psychiatric disabilities. *Soc Work Health Care* 1997; 25(3):11–24.

136. Perkins RE, Repper JM. Exclusive language? In: Mason JM, Carlisle C, Waternaux C, Whitehead E, eds., *Stigma and Social Exclusion in Healthcare*, pp. 147–157. London: Routledge; 2001.

137. Markowitz FE. Modeling processes in recovery from mental illness: relationships between symptoms, life satisfaction, and self-concept. *J Health Soc Behav* 2001; 42(1):64–79.

138. Wallcraft J. Mental health. Pay attention. *Health Serv J* 2003; 113(5858):28–29.

139. Read J, Baker S. *Not Just Sticks and Stones. A survey of the stigma, taboos, and discrimination experienced by people with mental health problems.* London: MIND; 1996.

140. Corrigan PW. Empowerment and serious mental illness: treatment partnerships and community opportunities. *Psychiatr Q* 2002; 73(3):217–228.

141. Corrigan PW, Garman AN. Considerations for research on consumer empowerment and psychosocial interventions. *Psychiatr Serv* 1997; 48(3):347–352.

142. Corrigan PW, Faber D, Rashid F, Leary M. The construct validity of empowerment among consumers of mental health services. *Schizophr Res* 1999; 38(1):77–84.

143. Corrigan P.W., Calabrese JD. Strategies for assessing and diminishing self-stigma. In: Corrigan PW, ed., *On the Stigma of Mental Illness. Practical strategies for research and social change*, pp. 239–256. Washington DC: American Psychological Association; 2005.

144. Ritsher JB, Otilingam PG, Grajales M. Internalized stigma of mental illness: psychometric properties of a new measure. *Psychiatry Res* 2003; 121(1):31–49.

145. Corrigan PW. Don't call me nuts: an international perspective on the stigma of mental illness. *Acta Psychiatr Scand* 2004; 109(6):403–404.

146. Sutherby K, Szmukler GI, Halpern A, Alexander M, Thornicroft G, Johnson C *et al.* A study of 'crisis cards' in a community psychiatric service. *Acta Psychiatr Scand* 1999; 100(1): 56–61.

147. Kuipers E, Garety P, Dunn G, Bebbington P, Fowler D, Freeman D. CBT for psychosis. *Br J Psychiatry* 2002; 181:534.

148. Pilling S, Bebbington P, Kuipers E, Garety P, Geddes J, Orbach G *et al.* Psychological treatments in schizophrenia: I. Meta-analysis of family intervention and cognitive behaviour therapy. *Psychol Med* 2002; 32(5):763–782.

149. Ruggeri M, Lasalvia A, Bisoffi G, Thornicroft G, Vazquez-Barquero JL, Becker T *et al.* Satisfaction with mental health services among people with schizophrenia in five European sites: results from the EPSILON Study. *Schizophr Bull* 2003; 29(2):229–245.

150. Warner R, Huxley P, Berg T. An evaluation of the impact of clubhouse membership on quality of life and treatment utilization. *Int J Soc Psychiatry* 1999; 45(4):310–320.

151. Dixon L, Krauss N, Lehman A. Consumers as service providers: the promise and challenge. *Community Ment Health J* 1994; 30(6):615–625.

152. Allen MH, Carpenter D, Sheets JL, Miccio S, Ross R. What do consumers say they want and need during a psychiatric emergency? *J Psychiatr Pract* 2003; 9(1):39–58.

153. Becker DR, Drake RE. *A Working Life for People with Severe Mental Illness.* Oxford: Oxford University Press; 2003.

154. Henry AD, Nicholson J, Clayfield J, Phillips S, Stier L. Creating job opportunities for people with psychiatric disabilities at a university-based research center. *Psychiatr Rehabil J* 2002; 26(2):181–190.

155. Trivedi P, Wykes T. From passive subjects to equal partners: qualitative review of user involvement in research. *British Journal of Psychiatry* 2002; 181:468–472.

156. Thornicroft G, Rose D, Huxley P, Dale G, Wykes T. What are the research priorities of mental health service users? *Journal of Mental Health* 2002; 11:1–5.

157. Anspach RR. From stigma to identity politics: political activism among the physically disabled and former mental patients. *Soc Sci Med [Med Psychol Med Sociol]* 1979; 13A(6):765–773.

158. Fine F, Asch A. Disability beyond stigma: social interaction, discrimination, and activism. *Journal of Social Issues* 1988; 44(1):3–23.

159. Rose D, Lucas J. The user and survivor movement in Europe. In: Knapp M, McDaid D, Mossialos E, Thornicroft G, eds., *Mental Health Policy and Practice Across Europe. The Future Direction of Mental Health Care.* Milton Keynes: Open University Press; 2006 (in press).

160. Raymond CA. Political campaign pinpoints 'stigma hurdle' facing nation's mental health community. *JAMA* 1988; 260(10):1338–1339.

161. Shaughnessy P. Not in my back yard. Stigma from a personal perspective. In: Mason T, Carlisle C, Watkins C, Whitehead E, eds., *Stigma and Social Exclusion in Healthcare*, pp. 181–189. London: Routledge; 2001.

162. Corrigan PW, River LP, Lundin RK, Penn DL, Uphoff-Wasowski K, Campion J *et al.* Three strategies for changing attributions about severe mental illness. *Schizophr Bull* 2001; 27(2):187–195.

163. Corrigan PW, River LP, Lundin RK, Wasowski KU, Campion J, Mathisen J *et al.* Predictors of participation in campaigns against mental illness stigma. *J Nerv Ment Dis* 1999; 187(6):378–380.

164. Sayce L. *From Psychiatric Patient to Citizen. Overcoming discrimination and social exclusion.* Basingstoke: Palgrave; 2000.

165. Wilson M. MIND's Respect Campaign – an overview. In: Crisp A, ed., *Every Family in the Land*, pp. 376–379. London: Royal Society of Medicine; 2004.

166. Corrigan PW, Penn DL. Lessons from social psychology on discrediting psychiatric stigma. *Am Psychol* 1999; 54(9):765–776.

167. Watson AC, Corrigan P.W. Challenging public stigma: a targeted approach. In: Corrigan PW, ed., *On the Stigma of Mental Illness. Practical strategies for research and social change*, pp. 281–295. Washington DC: American Psychological Association; 2005.

168. Philo G. Users of services, carers and families. In: Philo G, ed., *Media and Mental Distress*, pp. 105–114. London: Longman; 1996.

169. Crossley ML, Crossley N. 'Patient' voices, social movements and the habitus; how psychiatric survivors 'speak out'. *Soc Sci Med* 2001; 52(10):1477–1489.

170. Nairn RG, Coverdale JH. People never see us living well: an appraisal of the personal stories about mental illness in a prospective print media sample. *Aust N Z J Psychiatry* 2005; 39(4):281–287.

171. Goldman KD, Schmalz KJ. Speak-Easy: setting up a speakers bureau. *Health Promot Pract* 2003; 4(4):357–361.

172. Seely T. Speakers Bureau continues to get more requests. *Mich Med* 1996; 95(11):34.

173. Chester SD. St. Mary's Hospital. A speakers bureau helps a hospital share its mission. *Health Prog* 1992; 73(9):66–67.

174. Strother L. AIDS Speakers Bureau – activities update. *Mich Med* 1988; 87(12):761–762.

175. Hess RE, Clapper CR, Hoekstra K, Gibison FP, Jr. Empowerment effects of teaching leadership skills to adults with a severe mental illness and their families. *Psychiatr Rehabil J* 2001; 24(3):257–265.

1.

2.

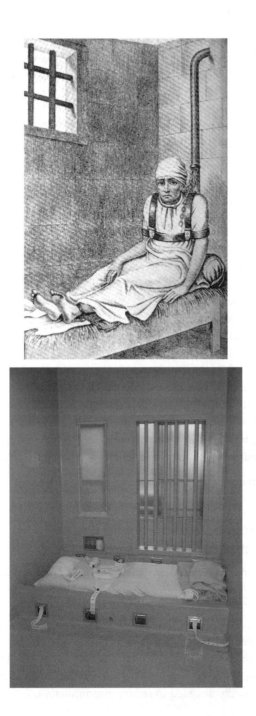

1. Eighteenth century female patient chained to a post.
2. Bed with straps for restraint, Japan, 2005

Chapter 11 What works to reduce discrimination?

Challenges for everyone

I think when there is stigma, there is often ignorance around the corner.

Robert

What needs to be done? The previous chapter argued that people with mental illness can actively challenge the ignorance, prejudice and discrimination they routinely face. Yet these attacks on their identity, their integrity and their reputation are in large part made by people who do not have a mental illness. In other words, everyone has particular responsibilities to work to stop such exclusion. The action described here can therefore be seen as a manifesto against stigma and discrimination.

This chapter gives details about what can and should be done at the following levels:[1] (i) with individuals who have a mental illness and with their families, (ii) at the local level, for example in neighbourhood initiatives, (iii) at the national level, for instance in using disability discrimination laws,[2] or monitoring how far they observe in practice the national and international laws and standards which they have signed, and (iv) internationally.

The overall thing is that I'm no longer the person I used to be.

Diana

Action with people with mental illness and their families

Well I suffer from some sort of mental illness. I wish I could get more reading about it. I'm not sure if it's schizophrenia, but I obviously do suffer from a mental illness.

Jean, who has a diagnosis of schizophrenia

First, staff in general health and mental health services can support action taken by consumers directly on their own behalf, as described in the previous chapter. Second, staff can supplement their current range of treatments with measures specifically designed to reduce discrimination.

The worst thing about my illness was in the high, manic phase, which is the part that the public seemed to understand much less. What I found most difficult was that people can't distinguish what to count as part of you and what to count as part of the illness.

Robert

As we have seen in every chapter of this book, popular knowledge about mental illnesses is a potent cocktail of profound ignorance[3] and pernicious misinformation.[4] Professionals working in mental health services are mistaken if they think that their initial task is simply to provide neutral, factual information to a person newly diagnosed a having a mental illness.

(On having been given a diagnosis of schizophrenia) 'Certainly to my self-esteem, to the people I go to church with, the people that I've worked with, to my family, to former friends, it's been a big disadvantage.

Jean

Predominant views of mental illnesses are so negative that mental health staff need to understand that the diagnoses that they offer may be seen as most unwelcome. One challenge facing staff is to develop ways of providing diagnostic information that are more acceptable to people with these conditions. It is likely that these new methods will start by having to undo misunderstandings about, for example, what schizophrenia means. Staff also need to appreciate better what psychiatric diagnoses mean from the perspective of the people on the receiving end.

They tried to make me take Prozac in the evening, without explaining why. So I refused and put them in the drawer. I refuse to be treated like that. So now I don't like hospitals, and I won't go to one unless I'm on my last legs. I'm scared of what they would do to me. And never again will I try to get help for my phobia ... because I don't like the way I'm treated by people because of being under psychiatric care. I'd rather suffer. If this is what happens to me, and I can speak for myself, what happens to people who have severe mental health problems?.

Eva

By extension, building on the evidence from psycho-educational interventions described in Chapter 10, mental health professionals need to give more clear and accurate information to consumers and to family members about diagnoses, both about what they do and what they do not mean, and to explicitly undermine popular misconceptions. One issue that is likely to be central to such programmes is to stress that mental illnesses tend not to arise because of something that the affected person has done or not done.[5] In other words, the person affected is not responsible for becoming unwell, and should not additionally suffer by being blamed for causing the condition.

> I've got family and relatives in America who see me as a sort of like, a weak person or an Uncle Tom. They don't particularly like the fact that I'm mentally ill. They just see me as stupid and inadequate, feeble.
>
> Jean

The evidence is clear that attitudes towards mentally ill people are more favourable where the public believe that the condition has arisen 'through no fault of their own'.[6-12] It is therefore important, for consumers and for family members, to be given information clearly describing what is known about the causes of mental illnesses, given in a rounded way that does not over-rely on any one particular causative model as the 'answer', and which does not suggest that responsibility for the onset lies with the person affected or with the family.[13,14]

> Well, he's looking down on me. I've told people that I suffer from depression and people they just change their opinion towards me.
>
> Kim

Such information about causes is important not just for consumers directly, but also to provide family members with knowledge that they can use against the 'stigma by association' that they suffer in turn.[15,16] In other words to arm relatives with the information they need so that they can tell their friends, neighbours and colleagues that the condition affecting their relation is no-one's 'fault'.[17,18] Some particular myths may need be to be openly under-mined, for example that people with psychotic disorders are usually danger-ous, that depression indicates laziness or a lack of willpower, or that anxiety disorders are a sign of person weakness.[19-21]

> I always get this remark that I should take it easy, I shouldn't stress myself as if I'm a weakling, or maybe because of what has happened to me I can no longer do things that I used to do and I don't like that. I want to feel like everybody else.
>
> Diana

One way to do this is to develop information packs, for routine use with consumers and their families, not only on what mental illnesses are, but also on what they are not.[22] This would mean spelling out common myths and undermining their existence through providing clear counter-information. As such approaches are not routinely used now, they need to developed, tested and refined with consumers and family members.[23] Such information packs will need to be tested as part of integrated information and treatment pro-grammes, specifically developed for people with different conditions.[24-26] This will include balanced information about violence and mental illness, to correct misinformation or exaggerated concerns.[27]

Such approaches may be explicitly based upon stereotype suppression so that popular stereotypes and misperceptions are acknowledged and then rebutted.[28,29] Additional modules are likely to be necessary so that people with a history of mental illness can develop and rehearse a 'storyline' about their condition, which allows them to tell their story in a largely positive way that does not alienate other people. This is based on the assumption that people with mental illness are usually capable of acting in their own best interests – not an assumption widely held by professional groups in some countries. Table 11.1 summarizes some of the actions which are necessary at the individual level.

> Well there was this guy I was involved with when I was about 25, and he said that one of his friends had blurted out that he had ended up with a mental cripple.
>
> Teresa

Action at the local level

Work

For adults with mental illness, perhaps the single most important step to support a process of recovery is to work.[30–32] Employment offers social networks, a route out of poverty, and a source of social status in market economies As we saw in Chapter 3, rates of unemployment for people with psychotic disorders, for example, are in often in excess of 75 per cent. Over time, unemployment often leads to a loss of confidence, and a sense of being without any social value. Interestingly, less economically developed countries appear to be more successful than industrialized nations in providing opportunities for meaningful employment.[33,34] Sheltered employment does not usually lead to

Table 11.1 Action for individuals with mental illness and their families

Action	By
◆ Develop new ways to offer diagnoses	◆ Mental health staff
◆ Have information packages for service users/consumers and family members that explain causes, nature, treatments and prognoses of different types of mental illness	◆ Mental health staff, consumer and families
◆ Actively provide factual information against popular myths	◆ Mental health staff
◆ Develop and rehearse accounts of mental illness experiences which do not alienate other people	◆ Mental health staff and consumer groups

real jobs. While there is a wide range of types of vocational rehabilitation, sheltered work and day care, few have been shown to be effective in achieving open market employment.[35–41]

> I lost my job. I was unwell. I was having a lot of difficulties. I couldn't tolerate being sacked again. I've given up. Once bitten once twice shy.
>
> Kim

One positive option is supported work schemes, in which people with a history of mental illness are supported by job coaches (employment advisers) to find a paid job and to continue in work.[38,42–44] Problems with concentration and memory can harm a person's chance of getting or keeping a job,[45] and it is likely that some people will need both occupational support to find jobs, and psychological treatment to help them with their cognitive problems.[46–48]

The evidence for such supported work schemes is now increasingly strong and studies typically find that about 50 per cent of people receiving such support gain paid jobs, compared with about 20 per cent of people in more traditional sheltered occupation (segregated facilities for disabled people).[36] The key principles of the supported work approach are: (i) competitive employment as the goal, (ii) rapid job search and placement, (iii) integration of vocational rehabilitation and mental health services, (iv) attention to the mentally ill person's preferences, (v) continuous assessment, and (vi) time unlimited support.[31,49] Implementing such schemes on a routine basis presents great challenges to mental health and employment services.

There is one way to jump-start this process: to encourage health and social care agencies to see the experience of mental illness as a positive attribute when hiring staff. In many countries the health and social services are substantial forces in the labour market, for example the National Health Service in the UK is the largest employer in Europe. Paradoxically, as we saw in Chapter 5, such organisations have been particularly poor both in keeping staff who become mentally ill, and in taking on new staff who have a history of mental illness.[50–52] They can do this by making it clear that a personal knowledge of mental illness, for example as a consumer or a carer, is seen as a positive advantage for qualified applicants.

A study in Connecticut, for example, found that former consumers had the same ability to work as case managers as anyone else.[53] Another approach is to develop new roles, such as peer support worker,[54] in which a former consumer is employed within a mental health team. His or her experience is seen as a particular asset, for example in engaging consumers in treatment, as long as this does not contravene international standards, such as those monitored by the

Committee for the Prevention of Torture and Inhuman or Degrading Treatment or Punishment.[55,56] However this is done, it means reversing the common tendency in human service organisations to see workers as either healthy and strong and the donors of care, or as weak and vulnerable recipients. They need to stop shunning 'wounded healers'.[57,58]

> Well when I was first having my first breakdown I used to work for a super-market and I kept on breaking down and they kept on taking me back. Because I think they valued the amount of work that I did. I was told by managers that I was a good worker ... they wouldn't sack me ... and every time I fell ill and went into hospital they always took me back ... on about four occasions.
>
> Teresa

For some people with mental illness, allowances needs to be made at work for their personal requirements. In parallel with the modifications made for people in wheelchairs, people with mental health-related disabilities may need (but this should not be assumed) what are called 'reasonable adjustments', or 'reasonable accommodations',[59,60] in line with the relevant disability laws.[61–67]

What does this mean in practice?[68] One of the challenges here is that while employers can understand the need for an entrance ramp for people in wheelchairs, often they do not know how to apply this concept to people with mental illnesses. It can be argued that these provisions should be made available to everyone, not only those people who have already developed a disability.[30] Such support may assume different forms such as:

- for people with concentration problems, having a quieter work place with fewer distractions rather than a noisy open plan office, with a rest area for breaks
- more or more frequent supervision than usual to give feedback and guidance on job performance
- allow a person to use headphones to block out distracting noise
- flexibility in work hours so that they can attend their healthcare appointments, or work when not impaired by medication
- buddy/mentor scheme to provide on-site orientation, and assistance
- clear person specifications, job descriptions and task assignments to assist people who find ambiguity or uncertainty hard to cope with
- for people likely to become unwell for prolonged periods it may be necessary to make contract modifications to specifically allow whatever sickness leave they need
- a more gradual induction phase, for example with more time to complete tasks, for those who return to work after a prolonged absence, or who may have some cognitive impairment

- improved disability awareness in the workplace to reduce stigma and to underpin all other accommodations
- reallocation of marginal job functions which are disturbing to an individual
- allow use of accrued paid and unpaid leave for periods of illness.

At the same time such accommodations may be resented by regular staff, who see these as preferential conditions which they cannot themselves enjoy. For this reason it is vital for trades unions to be fully involved in such negotiations, and to ensure that people without mental illness do not suffer duress as a result of these policies. Also work adjustments can only apply to people who disclose their mental illness (or history) and we have seen in previous chapters that this is a sharp and unforgiving double-edged sword.[69]

The accommodations needed by an individual may well change over time and need to be reviewed regularly. Clear arrangements on confidentiality are necessary, in other words, if a job applicant does disclose having a mental illness and receives accommodations, who needs to know this? In particular, for people working in the same organisation in which they are treated for their mental illness, specific safeguards are needed to see that the confidentiality of clinical information is safeguarded.[70]

Where employers, especially small organisations and those without a human resources department, are unaware of the relevant disability laws, it is important to inform them of their statutory obligations.[71] Employers' concerns may be exaggerated. For example a survey in England found that among employers with physically disabled employees more than half did not need to make any adjustments to the physical environment. Where changes were needed, they were usually not costly or difficult to make.[72]

> I haven't applied for any jobs since I've become ill. To stop me applying is a part of the anxieties and the things that I have as part of the syndrome of mine and is just lack of confidence you know. Thought processes and memories are kind of damaged. I mean I can't think as fast as before I was ill. And I have trouble with the memory. I don't really have that much ambitious goals, just get a decent job and you know a decent reasonable living. That's what I wanted to do. But I haven't been able to do that yet because of my illness so far. But I feel much better now I'm getting ready to get back to employment.
>
> Leroy

As we saw in Chapter 7, many people with mental illness experience demoralization, reduced self-esteem, loss of confidence and sometimes depression.[73–77] It is therefore likely that support programmes assisting people with mental illness to gain employment will need to assess whether structured psychological treatment is also needed.[78–80]

I would have gone back to university back in the early 90s but there's no way I could get in with my mental health, ... because I had such low self-esteem and because I didn't think I could get those jobs or university places because of my mental health problems.

Jean

Anti-discrimination interventions for targeted groups

It has long been known that direct personal contact with people with mental illness is one of the most potent ways to improve attitudes towards people with mental illness.[81–87] It appears that to be effective this requires direct face-to-face contact, the opportunity to meet someone who can relate their experiences clearly and without attacking the audience, and the chance to see this as a condition affecting a real person (rather than thinking of 'the mentally ill' in the abstract). Such day-to-day and face-to-face contacts are one important element in normalizing the experience of mental illness.

I have three best friends that take me as I am, phobias and all. My main friend, David, has a better understanding of my phobias because he has gone through it with me, as we have been friends since I was 12 years old.

Eva

For this reason there has been a trend in recent years to move away from large-scale mental health awareness campaigns towards local programmes which are targeted to specific groups.[88–90] In the anti-stigma network of the World Psychiatric Association (called 'Open the Doors'), for example, such interventions have most often been applied to medical staff, journalists, school children, police, employers and church leaders.[91–95]

Children

Within schools, for example, there have been a series of studies which have educated students about mental illnesses to reduce ignorance, prejudice and discrimination.[96] In Germany these took place against a background where many young people were very poorly informed about these issues.[97] The intervention programme led to a substantial reduction in the use of negative stereotypes by 14–18 year olds.[98,99] In Chicago and Texas mental health awareness programmes had a similar impact.[100,101] In England 14-year-old school students received both factual information about mental illnesses and detailed discussions with a mental health service consumer and showed improvements in several aspects of their knowledge and attitudes,[102,103] and the same findings came from a Canadian intervention study.[104] This is all the more remarkable since attitudes to mental illness otherwise seem to remain stable from the kindergarten stage throughout childhood.[105]

Such changes may have very important implications because many young people have low levels of information and negative feelings about mental illness, leading them to be reluctant to seek help.[106,107]

Educational interventions alone have tended to produce little change. It is the direct contribution of service users/consumers that seems to be the key active ingredient to these programmes.[103] The nature and the context of the contact are important. The most effective contact is with a person who moderately disconfirms a pre-existing stereotype. Indeed, behaviour consistent with a stereotype can reinforce it or make it worse, while individuals who appear to strongly disconfirm stereotypes can be dismissed as 'special exceptions'.[108] To decrease stigma, social contact with people with mental illness also needs to have:[109] (i) the same status for the different groups involved, (ii) shared goals for the session or programme, (iii) a tone of collaboration rather than competition, and (iv) senior managerial support for the initiative.

> The only practical way to stop stigma and discrimination is by better education of schoolchildren at an early age and to reinforce this message through lifelong learning. Each course or class should not only start with 'household' messages about fire escapes, etc., but that bullying or discrimination will not be tolerated whilst on the course
>
> Paul

Police

A second example of successful targeted interventions concerns the police.[110] The content of the intervention will necessarily vary here. Many police officers have frequent contact with people with mental illness, usually at times of crisis. On the other hand, they may have little or no experience of meeting people with psychotic disorders who are well at the time. Studies in Israel, for example, have found levels of knowledge among the police to be the same as in the general population.[111]

Police attitudes may even be less favourable than popular opinions. An intervention programme in Chicago found that the police tended to discount information from victims or eyewitnesses who had a mental illness, in the belief that they were not credible informants.[112,113] Such misunderstandings can have very serious consequences. A series of fatal shootings of suspects (some of whom were mentally ill) by police officers in Victoria, Australia, led to Project Beacon in which all police officers in the state received mandatory training about mental illnesses. The number of fatalities among people with mental illness stopped until the programme was discontinued.[114]

Healthcare staff

Another key target group is healthcare professionals. As we saw in Chapter 5, consumers surprisingly often describe that their experiences of general health-care and mental healthcare staff reveal levels of ignorance, prejudice and discrimination that they find deeply distressing. This has been confirmed in studies in Australia, Brazil, Canada, Croatia, England, Malaysia, Spain and Turkey,[115–123] Based on the principle 'catch them young', several programmes have given anti-stigma interventions to medical students.[120,124–127] As is usual in the field of stigma and discrimination, there is more research describing stigma than assessing which interventions are effective. In Japan one study found that the traditional medical curriculum led to mixed results: students became more accepting of mentally ill people and mental health services, and more optimistic about the outlook with treatment, but there was no impact on their views about how far people with mental illness should have their human rights fully observed.[128] Positive changes in all of these domains were achieved with a one-hour supplementary educational programme.[129]

Interestingly, it seems that psychiatrists may not be in the best position to lead such educational programmes. Studies in Switzerland found no overall differences between the general public and psychiatrists in terms of social distance to mentally ill people.[130] Psychiatry itself tries to walk the narrow tightrope between the physical/pharmacological and psychological/social poles.[131] Clinicians who keep contact with people who are unwell, and who selectively stop seeing people who have recovered, may therefore develop a pessimistic view of the outlook for people with mental illnesses.[132] On balance there is mixed evidence about whether psychiatrists can be seen as stigmatisers or destigmatisers.[133] Mental health nurses have also been found to have more and less favourable views about people with mental illness than the general public.[117] Interestingly, nurses, like the general population, tend to be more favourable if they have a friend who is mentally ill, in other words if there is a perceived similarity and equality with the person affected.[134]

In this case what should mental health staff do? Later in this chapter we shall see that direct involvement in the media is a vital route that professionals can use more often, with proper preparation and training. They also need to set their own house in order by promoting information within their training curricula, continuing professional development (continuing medical educa-tion) and relicensing/revalidation procedures which ensures that they have accurate information, for example, on recovery.[135]

Further, in future practitioners need to pay greater attention to what con-sumers and family members say about their experiences of discrimination, for example in relation to work or housing. Staff can also work directly with consumers to combat social exclusion, such as against repressive or regressive mental health laws.[136] Third, it is clear that consumer groups increasingly seek to change to the terms of engagement between mental health professionals and consumers, and to move from paternalism to negotiation.[137] Vehicles to support shared decision-making include: crisis plans,[138] (which seem able to reduce the frequency of compulsory treatment[139]), advance directives,[140] shared care agreements[141] and consumer-held records.[142] The key issue is that many consumers want direct participation in their own care plans.[143]

> I also have trouble with the small of my back. It gives out every now and then, but it's been getting worse. So I tried to get help for that, but the doctor asked me how long had I been under a psychiatrist? I asked him what that had to do with a bad back, but he dismissed it as a part of my mental health problem. When I told him the only problem I have is a phobia, he didn't want to know, and gave me painkillers, which they know I can't take because they make my stomach bleed. So now I don't go to the doctor anymore. I still have bad irritable bowel syndrome and back problems, but I'm not going to keep being fobbed off and treated like I'm stupid every time I go there.
>
> Eva

Further target groups for reducing discrimination

At the local level other targeted interventions are important. Landlords may need information on the facts about dangerousness to counteract their reluctance to lease/let apartments. Judges and lawyers can benefit from education about how far people with mental illness are responsible for their conditions, both in relation to sentencing, and to their options for referral of individuals to mental health services. Local policy-makers need to be informed if their financial allocations for mental health care show unintended systemic/structural discrimination against people with mental rather than physical disorders. Researchers need to establish whether claims that smaller, community-based mental health centres are less stigmatising are true or not.[144–146]

Action at the national level

Agreeing useful concepts

What needs to be done at the national level, or at the regional level in federated governments? The starting point is to appreciate that the forms of stigmatisation described in this book are widespread, severe and incompatible with a humane society. It is fair to say, in every country where this has been examined, that people with mental illness are one of the most discriminated-against groups.[147] For example, a survey in 15 European countries showed that 87 per cent thought that people with mental health problems or learning disabilities would have less chance of finding a job than anyone else.[148,149]

It is also necessary to stress that this is a changeable situation. We know that the nature and degree of discrimination seems to have improved for particular disorders (e.g. AIDS/HIV),[150] for people identified by their social characteristics (e.g. single parents), and for ethnic and cultural groups (at least in terms of overt racism). These changes have followed social and political recognition that these issues are problems which have been confronted by concerted educational, cultural and legal action.[151]

One necessary step to tackle stigmatisation in relation to mental illness is to frame the problems in ways that lead to action. As we saw in Chapter 9, the framework proposed in this book is to see stigma as made up of three distinct problems:

The problem of knowledge:	*Ignorance*
The problem of attitudes:	*Prejudice*
The problem of behaviour:	*Discrimination*

Seen in this way working with school children, for example, becomes more manageable, namely to develop effective interventions in at least one of these three problem areas. While this is easy to say, these steps are formidable to achieve in practice.

What concepts are useful? Three views are most common: the biomedical model (essentially locating the key problems within the individual), the individual growth model (suggesting a continuum between emotional well-being and ill health), and the disability-inclusion model (which identifies the main problems as how society reacts to disabled individuals).[152,153] Each has strengths for particular purposes, for example the brain disease approach is yielding rapid progress in relation to understanding Alzheimer's disease. For the purposes of reducing discrimination, however, the disability-inclusion model is the strongest conceptual approach.

The disability-inclusion model

One advantage of framing the social problems faced by people with mental illness as disabilities is that such individuals have legal rights to particular benefits, rather than be assessed as 'worthy poor' to receive discretionary charity.[154] One barrier is that there is no internationally agreed legal definition of disability.[155] Within the European Union (EU), for example, there has been a paradigm shift from a charity-based to a rights-based disability policy. On this basis disabled individuals are able to benefit from exercising their legal entitlements using disability discrimination laws. Such laws offer direct recourse for disabled people, but also send a powerful message that discrimination is wrongful and erects unfair barriers to prevent disabled people taking a full part in society.

These laws should go further. Within the EU at present the only area in which it is unlawful to discriminate on grounds of disability is employment. There is no disability discrimination directive (as there is for race) which outlaws discrimination in education, social security, healthcare, or in the supply of goods and services. Mental health professionals and consumer's groups can find common cause by actively lobbying for such legal changes.

Nevertheless even when a disability-inclusion approach is used, the details of its application may be counterproductive. For example, the Americans with Disability Act applies to people who are substantially limited in a range of daily activities. The stereotypical image shaping this definition is again a person with severe physical impairments, the person who is 'truly disabled' (most often embodied in the image of a person in a wheelchair).[64,65,155] The UK Disability Discrimination Act, for example, uses the following definition:

> A person has a disability for the purposes of this Act if he has a physical or mental impairment which has a substantial and long-term adverse affect on his ability to carry out normal day-to-day activities.
>
> Disability Discrimination Act UK, 1995

A wider approach is that which is sometimes called social adaptation. This sees the problem lying in the interaction of how people with impairments cope within particular environments. To use a physical analogy, the user of a wheelchair is not disabled if moving around a workplace is possible with lifts, ramps and elevators, whereas only having stairs in a building will profoundly disable that person. In other words, it is a question of the match between particular impairments and the adaptation of the environment to minimize disabling consequences.

This approach has not so far been systematically applied in the field of mental health.[156] It would mean, for example, assessing the needs of person when returning to work after a period of depression, but who has not yet fully recovered, and then making particular changes to his or her work setting. This might mean, for example, reducing the ambient noise level if noise sensitivity is a problem. This social model of disability sees social attitudes and their consequences as imposing disabling limitations upon people with impairments. This approach has been influential among groups advocating for people with physical disabilities for over 30 years.[154,157]

A related view, which also sees individual people with disabilities directly within their environment, refers to social exclusion and social inclusion.[32,149] This perspective stresses the importance of reduced participation in:

'consumption, production, social participation and political participation'.[158,159] In particular this view often advocates measures to support people with mental illness in the workplace.[160]

Going further, a counter-reaction to the 'worthy poor' view, is to see people with disabilities as having just the same rights to active citizenship as everyone else.[161,162] The idea of citizenship can have several advantages. It allows service users and consumers to challenge narrow disease-based definitions of disability. It supports the assumption that the human rights of mentally ill people should be respected. It offers a benchmark to assess the success of measures for self-determination. It acts as a point of reference in calls for social change. It fixes a responsibility with governments to respond to legitimate demands for parity of treatment, and to respond by committing resources. It provides a basis for routine consultation with mentally ill people on all measures that affect them, and legitimates their voice.[163] It offers a point of shared aspiration for people across many disability groups, around which they can organise. It moves away from a social response based upon pity, or the 'stigma of benevolence'.[86,164] Finally, this approach assumes the innate dignity of all concerned.[149,152,153]

Public knowledge and information

The evidence shows that members of the general public paradoxically have remarkably little accurate factual knowledge about mental illnesses, although most do know someone affected.[165] The extent of ignorance is hard to underestimate with some surveys showing that many people cannot distinguish between epilepsy, mental illness and learning disability (mental retardation). It is therefore perhaps less surprising to find that public attitudes on how to treat people with mental illness are sharply different from those of professionals. For example, one study in Switzerland found that the general public were very restrictive about how to treat people with mental illness. Compared with psychiatrists, the public were more likely to support withdrawing driving licences (7 per cent vs. 54 per cent), suggesting abortions to mentally ill women who are pregnant (6 per cent vs. 19 per cent), or withdrawing the right to vote (1 per cent vs. 17 per cent).[166]

We cannot resist several conclusions. Despite the profusion of news and feature stories on health topics in the mass media, the level of accurate knowledge about mental illnesses in the general population is low. The information that is mostly present in the public domain emphasizes the danger of violence from mentally ill people almost to the exclusion of all other aspects. Such a body of public knowledge presents a solid rock of ignorance, which is a serious barrier to seeking help. Such popular views promote social exclusion not social inclusion.

What remedies are available? In North America public opinion surveys have been conducted for over half a century,[167–174] usually limiting themselves to describing popular opinion. An exception was an intervention programme in Saskatchewan in Canada, which found that most people were reluctant to have close contact with mentally ill people and that attempts to reduce social distance were unsuccessful, indeed producing hostility to research staff.[170,175] Relatively early, therefore, it became common to think that public education campaigns rarely produced meaningful and sustained change.

More recent evidence has begun to challenge this received wisdom, and suggests that campaigns to raise the level of 'literacy' about mental illness can have a positive effect, as they have had for HIV/AIDS.[176,177] In Australia 'beyondblue' is a concerted programme to convey accurate information about depression. Its initial evaluation showed a series of benefits including better community recognition of people with depression, reforms in life insurance and income protection and the initiation of awareness and intervention programmes in schools.[178,179] An important aspect of this programme is that some of the Australian States and Territories have a high level of exposure to the beyondblue intervention, and others a low level of exposure, to allow a comparison of the impact. Compared with the low-exposure States, the high-exposure States had greater change in beliefs about some treatments for depression, particularly counselling and medication, and a higher recognition of the benefits of help-seeking in general. Between 1995 and 2003 the recognition of depression improved greatly throughout all of Australia, but slightly more so in the high-exposure states.[180]

In Germany, public attitudes surveys have been conducted since 1990 and show that over the following decade the German public became more ready to recommend help from psychiatrists or psychotherapists for schizophrenia or major depression. There was also an increase in the willingness to recommend treatment, especially drug treatment or psychotherapy for people with schizophrenia. Since there are no controlled comparisons of interventions over that period for the whole country, it is possible that these favourable changes are more linked to improvements in treatment services than to any public information campaigns.[181,182] At the same time contradictory evidence has emerged in Germany that attitudes to people with this condition have worsened in recent years, despite a greater appreciation of the biological causes of schizophrenia which was expected to engender greater public sympathy.[183]

There have been several national initiatives in England. The Defeat Depression campaign targeted primary care practitioners as well as members of the general public with information about depression.[184-186] The results showed modest but positive changes in attitudes to depression, particularly favouring counselling, but antidepressants were seen as addictive and less effective.[187] Among family doctors 40 per cent reported that they had improved their recognition and treatment of depression, and this was especially so for younger doctors and those who had undertaken previous psychiatric training.[188] At the same time it needs to be appreciated that because there was no clear-cut comparison between regions which did or did not receive the interventions, it is possible that these changes were not related to the campaign.

In Scotland there has been a series of coordinated anti-stigma activities since 2002, called 'See Me'. Initial assessments of a nationwide publicity campaign indicate that over half of the public sampled could recall seeing some of the campaign material and that by far the most effective channel to reach the public is television.[189] A series of annual public opinion surveys will provide information on whether popular attitudes change over the period that the campaign takes place.[190] We need to interpret such findings with some caution. For example public attitudes to people with mental illness improved during the 1990s in the absence of a national intervention programme. So such secular trends can take place alongside specific measures, and only the use of a comparison group, such as in Australia, can reveal if such changes are caused by a campaign or by other factors.

Successful initiatives in providing effective public educational materials are hampered by a lack of strong evidence about what works. Without such evidence a series of beliefs are commonly held by those active in the health education field,[152] namely that:

◆ *mental illness and mental health should be described as a continuum*
◆ *it is helpful to stress how common mental illness are*
◆ *governments should act to promote more positive popular attitudes*
◆ *groups with less favourable attitudes to people with mental illness should be particularly targeted*
◆ *a stress on positive mental health will also bring favourable attitude changes to people with severely disabling mental illnesses*
◆ *measures designed to encourage people to talk about mental illness will have positive consequences*
◆ *interventions should stress that the public should show greater tolerance or acceptance of diversity.*

In fact there is evidence that each of these assumptions is wrong.[152] So it is fair to say that at present little is known about which methods of conveying information to mass audiences are likely to be more effective. A series of techniques are possible contenders, including personal testimonies by people with mental illness, incorporating mental illness related story lines into popular drama, such as 'soap operas', using commercial brand awareness public relations methods, adapting such techniques for 'social marketing',[191] or deliberately associating mental illness themes with positive attributes (such as creativity by producing exhibitions of excellent art by people with mental illness).[192] Each of these deserves to be implemented and assessed to see whether they work or not.

> As far as people like me are concerned, I guess that if the Disability Discrimination Act had been in force when I had my last job, then I guess that I wouldn't have been sacked. I was sacked for taking time off work due to mental health problems, and what they should have done was given me a less stressful job within the organisation, but I was medically retired. I think that my psychiatric history has been a disadvantage right from the beginning really. My father wanted to have me exorcised when it first cropped up. Even when I went to study for a higher degree, I had been a teacher, and none of the rest of my cohort had been teachers, but they were all given teaching duties, which I thought was really, really unfair, because there was nothing to prevent me taking a seminar, but they thought that I was going to take an axe to the class or something like that.
>
> Veronica.

Legal changes

Legal measures need to be used more often in the future to protect people with mental illness from unfair discrimination. Laws such as the Americans with Disability Act in the USA,[68] and the Disability Discrimination Acts in the UK and Australia, have been framed primarily in relation to physical disability, and their achievements for people with mental illnesses have been few and disappointing.[66,152,193,194]

It is clear that such laws need to be either amended or interpreted in ways that provide legal parity for people with physical and mental disabilities in terms of their entitlements to work. The creation, amendment and implementation of such policies and laws are likely to be better done if people with mental illness are directly involved at each stage.[137,195–201] This is directly in line with the relevant United Nations 'Standard Rule' which states that '*States should invite persons with disabilities and their families and organizations to participate in public education programmes concerning disability matters*'.[202] Similar sentiments are the subject of official statements within Europe:

> Significant advances will not be made, however, without the necessary political will and commitment of legislators to realistic policies. The constructive involvement of all actors, including persons with mental disabilities them-

selves, their families, politicians, the legal and medical professions and NGOs is vital. These actors are partners, not antagonists, and they all have a contribution to make.[203]

The first step is therefore the introduction, where they do not exist, of laws to counteract discrimination against disabled people. Countries doing this can draw upon the experience of those who have already enacted such legislation.[149,151] Where these laws are already on the statute books, it is likely that they may need to be amended or interpreted to allow them to be applied fairly both to people whose disabilities are from physical and from mental conditions.

Experience of such laws is now accumulating and indeed almost a quarter (23 per cent) of all cases pursued under the UK Disability Discrimination Act (DDA) in the last ten years were by people with mental illness. But the limitations of the initial implementation of these laws are now becoming clear, and can lie in the detail of their drafting.[204] For example, a review of the DDA in practice by the Disability Rights Commission in England has proposed that it should be unlawful for employers to ask job applicants questions about disability except in highly specified circumstances. Further they suggest that to qualify as disabled there should be impairments of 'normal day to day activities' that include both physical and mental impairments.[205] Where impairments are disclosed then it is still a common experience for people with mental illness to be treated as a member of a category, for example as unsuitable to be a teacher because of a diagnosis of bipolar disorder, rather than to be assessed on their individual merits.[149]

> The very first case the British Disability Rights Commission took up under the Disability Discrimination Act 1995 was for a man with a diagnosis of depression who had lost his job as accountant working in local government. He won the case and was awarded £120,000 in compensation for estimated lost income.[149]

In the European Union anti-discrimination laws are now mandatory under the Article 13 Directive. Such laws must make illegal all discrimination in the workplace on grounds that include disability. They must also set up institutions to enforce these laws. The time is therefore right to share experience between different countries on how successful such laws have been in reducing discrimination against people with mental illness, and to understand more clearly what is required both for new legislation elsewhere, and for amendments to existing laws that fall short of their original intentions.[60, 149, 193, 206, 207]

Even when countries do have laws designed to protect individuals with disabilities from discrimination, they may apply them narrowly only to people with very severe problems, or they may be interpreted in the courts to apply particularly to physically disabilities. In words, where these provisions are applied to people with mental illnesses, they may be used without parity. The Australian DDA, for example, applies to people with physical disability with more than five per cent impairment, but to claim for psychiatric injury it is necessary to have about twice this level of impairment.[208] The principle of parity needs to be applied across all the ministries of government that have an impact on the daily life of people with mental illness, so that it will no longer be possible to visit social care homes in eastern Europe for example, and be confronted by many toothless residents, who clearly do not have parity in terms of dental care.

Insurance and welfare benefits

A series of further policy areas require special attention.[209] Insurance is a distinct problem for many people with mental illnesses.[62, 210] One survey in Britain found that a quarter of the people with mental illness questioned said that they had been refused insurance or other financial services.[211] This may well be unlawful. In the UK the Disability Discrimination Act (DDA) 1995 makes it illegal to provide goods, facilities and services to a disabled person (including people with mental illness) on terms which are unjustifiably different from those given to other people. Since 1996, this Act has made it illegal to refuse insurance, or charge higher premiums, unless the company can demonstrate statistically higher risks as a direct result of a specific mental health condition for that particular individual. However, people are reluctant to take out cases against big institutions and only a small handful of cases under the DDA have been successful.

Because of widespread concerns that discrimination makes access to insurance difficult for disabled people, the Association of British Insurers has produced a Code of Practice for its members whose practices should:

- *be fair and reasonable in its dealings with disabled people (including people with mental health problems)*
- *account for any difference in treatment between disabled and non-disabled people*
- *show that insurers' decisions must be based on information relevant to the assessment of the risk to be insured and from a reliable source, which may include: actuarial or statistical data, medical research information, a medical report, or an opinion on an individual from a reliable source*
- *make sure that their information is accurate and that their use of it is reasonable*

◆ *show the disabled person has a higher risk; if not, there should be no differentiation in their treatment.*[212]

But in fact many insurance application forms ask for details of pre-existing conditions, and refuse cover if such conditions are present.[213] As many mental illnesses are either long-lasting or have cycles of relapse and remission, this disqualifies many people with mental illness from being insured.[67]

Welfare benefit rules also erect formidable and complex barriers to employment for many people with mental illnesses. These appear to be worse in the UK than in the USA, where disincentives from health insurance have a greater impact.[151,214] What is needed are more imaginative and flexible arrangements (such as the provision of wage subsidies, higher levels of 'earnings disregard', raising the minimum wage, or guaranteeing jobs at non-poverty wages for all but the most disabled people)[31] so that people who have been unemployed, often for long periods, can take paid work without reckoning that this will mean an unacceptable risk to a secure income by losing welfare benefits. Specific legal provisions which discriminate against people with mental illness, such as their prohibition to serve on juries, also need to be reappraised and amended or repealed where necessary.[215]

The media

The media play a critical and formative role in contributing to the pool of public knowledge about mental illnesses, as we have seen in Chapter 6.[216] The evidence is overwhelming that the mass media, as a whole, portray mental illnesses in negative ways that evoke fear and anxiety. They offer strong indications of what emotional reactions are appropriate towards people with mental illnesses. In general, film, television and newspapers are united in their emphasis upon threat and risk. In short the factual information contained in most mass media coverage of mental health issues is grossly unbalanced, and the emotional tone that it adopts is one that directly supports the view that mentally ill people deserve to be shunned.

The effect of these media contributions is profound. These core repeated themes overwhelmingly reinforce only the most negative interpretations of what mental illnesses mean, and how to react to those affected. If we consider their role in terms of the three key problems of stigma (ignorance, prejudice and discrimination) then it is fair to conclude that they do more to distribute inaccurate than accurate information, more to foster negative than positive attitudes, and that their combined effect increases rather than decreases discrimination against people with mental illness.[217]

What can realistically be expected from these media? Their practitioners are quick to say that their role is more to entertain than to inform, more to cover the newsworthy than the worthy, and more to command audiences and markets by connecting with popular concerns, rather than to perform health education.

As has happened in relation to coverage of ethnical and racial issues, it is necessary to bring social and cultural pressure upon those producing content for the film, newspaper and television industries to give greater coverage to what people with mental illnesses say, in their *own* words. As we saw earlier, most news or feature items either include professional 'expert' contributions, or use editorialized journalistic content in which service users' views are reinterpreted to fit the overall storyline. To allow this to take place on a routine basis it may be necessary to fund, establish and maintain speakers' bureaux for groups of service users and consumers who wish to work with the media (see Chapter 10). Such personal disclosure can be particularly stressful, and service user and consumer groups will need to make careful arrangements for preparation, debriefing and other ongoing support. Here a disability rights approach may offer useful parallels, as in recent years there have been gradual improvements in how some physical disabilities are portrayed.[218]

An additional response is to provide media response units which monitor coverage of mental health themes and which issue rapid rebuttals, objections or complaints where necessary.[219] For example in Australia, the StigmaWatch programme run by SANE Australia, has pressed journalists to provide balanced mental health coverage, as does Stigma Stopwatch in Scotland.[220, 221] These groups protest against misrepresentations of mental illness and campaign for more accurate and fair portrayals.[174, 222–224] At present there is no formal evidence about the impact of such media watch intervention, which usually grow from the actions of local self-help organisations, and then go on to build larger national and international coalitions,[152] examples of which are given in Chapter 10.

Also unevaluated are more subtle approaches which are referred to as 'cultural seeding'.[225] This is somewhat similar to 'product placement' in films in that a signal is conveyed to the audience without it being explicit. The key message is integrated into a 'media vehicle', not as direct advertising, but embedded in an information source in which the audience invests legitimacy. The aim is to create a contagious idea.[225] For example at a prominent awards ceremony, a new award could be added for an outstanding programme, film or newspaper report produced by someone known to have a mental illness. A related approach is to see the negative associations of mental illnesses as a problem of branding, and to adopt standard public relations and marketing techniques to the 'rebranding' of their reputations. Such a coordinated and market-orientated approach has not so far been applied in any concerted way in the mental health field.[225]

Cultural barriers can be erected by policy-makers, as they have been in relation to discrimination on the basis of ethnicity, when reporting mental illness. Just as it has recently become more unacceptable to use terms which are regarded, for example by African-Americans, as abusive or disrespectful, this process has begun to be applied to some groups of disabled people.[226] Although terms such as 'cripple', or 'spastic' now have less currency in some parts of the English speaking world, no such cultural pressures have so far been meaningfully applied to the mass media or to the legal profession, so that the terms they use avoid causing offence. In England for example the term 'Not guilty by reason of insanity' is in continued use.

The development of 'good reporting guidelines' needs to be done with care, and the mental health field can learn from how this has been successful done in other areas of discrimination.[227–230] The key is to see the use of derogatory terminology as a form of real discrimination, rather than as a vague form of stigma, and to put political and social pressure upon governmental bodies and media organisations to apply the same restraints as they often do to words that may be seen as racist. In the UK, for example, the Code of Practice of the National Union of Journalists of 1998 states:[231]

> A journalist shall only mention a person's age, race, colour, creed, illegitimacy, disability, marital status, gender or sexual orientation if this information is strictly relevant. A journalist shall neither originate nor process material which encourages discrimination, ridicule, prejudice or hatred on any of the above-mentioned grounds.

Voluntary codes of practice, such as this, have so far failed to make any substantial impact on the reporting of mental illness. On the other hand there is some evidence that the introduction of guidelines on the reporting of suicides[232, 233] can produce real benefits.[234]

> It was definitely a disadvantage ... what I was trying to do was to compare the stigma attached to me with the stigma attached to being black. OK I was lost for words and I didn't quite explain myself properly because I was trying to say that it's wrong to be discriminated against blacks, but it's wrong to be discriminated against mental people.
>
> Kim

The plain fact is that at present there are no effective constraints upon the print, broadcast, electronic and film media from using grossly discriminatory portrayals of people with mental illness as a matter of routine.[88, 226, 235–242] Despite this there is some evidence that accurate, let alone sympathetic, portrayals of people with mental illnesses, in documentary films for example, can produce favourable changes in viewers' attitudes.[243, 244] As voluntary guidelines have not reduced media misrepresentation, another approach is to apply directly the full force of law so that offensive references to mentally ill people are treated as no more acceptable than racist references or comments that incite religious hatred.

Another channel for counter-balancing information to enter the public domain is for mental health professionals to contribute directly, as outlined in Chapter 6. There are stringent professional limitations in most countries to prevent psychiatrists from commenting upon individual cases, to safeguard confidential clinical information.[245] At the same time, most journalists covering mental health stories will want to report the stories of individuals and families. One way to address this double bind is for mental health staff to join forces with service user/consumers speakers' bureaux, so that professionals can comment upon the particular cases of those people with mental illness who give their consent for this, especially if they also contribute directly to the content of the story.[246, 247]

Research

With the exception of social contact as discussed above, we have little evidence for other effective interventions against stigma at present. Therefore we need to assess each new anti-stigma intervention to see if it actually works or not. The candidate interventions shown in Tables 11.1–11.3, for example, need to be assessed to see if they produce positive changes for: (i) knowledge about mental illnesses, (ii) attitudes towards mentally ill people, and (iii) negative discriminatory behaviour. Without evaluation, the effects of anti-stigma initiatives remain unknown, and so knowledge cannot be shared on what works to reduce stigma and discrimination.[103, 248–50]

Much of the research which has been done in this field rests on the largely untested assumption that knowledge change leads to attitude change, and that these produce behaviour change to reduce discrimination. Unfortunately a large body of work in health psychology suggests that the interrelationships between knowledge, attitudes and behaviour are far from simple.[251–255] If the main issue is to reduce discriminatory behaviour, then the challenge for researchers is to measure which interventions (whether aimed at knowledge, attitude or behaviour change) do in fact diminish discrimination.[248, 249]

Evidence in one particular area of research is notably absent: multiple discrimination. Although is it commonly accepted in the mental health field that some people are subjected to several different types of stigma at the same

Table 11.2 Action at the local level

Action	By
◆ Introduction-supported work schemes	◆ Mental health services with specialist independent sector providers
◆ Psychological treatments to improve cognition, self-esteem and confidence	◆ Mental health and general health services
◆ Health and social care explicitly give credit to applicants with a history of mental illness when hiring staff	◆ Health and social care agencies
◆ Provision of reasonable adjustments/accommodations at work	◆ Mental health providers engaging with employers and business confederations
◆ Inform employers and service providers and educators of their legal obligations under disability laws – and wider equalities laws for people facing multiple discrimination, e.g. on grounds of race, gender etc.	◆ Employers' confederations
◆ Deliver and evaluate the widespread implementation of targeted interventions with targeted groups including school children, police and healthcare staff	◆ Education, Police and Health commissioning and providing authorities
◆ Provide accurate data on mental illness recovery rates to mental health and primary care practitioners	◆ Professional training and accreditation organisations
◆ Implementation of measures to support care plans negotiated between staff and consumers	◆ Mental health provider organisations and consumer groups

time, research about this is very scarce.[256, 257] These claims have been made, for instance, for people who both have a mental illness and who:

- ◆ are non-white (in white host population countries)[258–261]
- ◆ have a forensic history or criminal justice record[262]
- ◆ have learning disability/mental retardation[263]
- ◆ have drug or alcohol misuse or dependence[264, 265]
- ◆ are older adults[266]

Table 11.3 Policy action needed at the national level

Action	By
◆ Use a social model of disability that refers to human rights, social inclusion and citizenship	◆ Governments and non-governmental organisations (NGOs) to change core concepts
◆ Enact and enforce disability discrimination law that give parity to people with physical and mental disabilities	◆ Parliament and government
◆ Inform employers, service providers, and educators of their legal obligations under these laws	◆ Ministry of Employment or equivalent
◆ Interpret anti-discrimination laws in relation to mental illness	◆ Judiciary and legal profession
◆ Establish service user speakers' bureaux to offer content to news stories and features on mental illness	◆ NGOs and other national level service user groups
◆ Provide and evaluate media watch response units to press for balanced coverage	◆ Statutory funding for NGOs to provide media watch teams
◆ Share between countries the experience of disability discrimination acts	◆ Legislators, lawyers, advocates and consumer groups
◆ Understand and implement international legal obligations under binding declarations and covenants	◆ NGOs to communicate legal obligations of all stakeholders, and health and social care inspection agencies to audit how far these obligations are respected in practice
◆ Audit compliance with codes of good practice in providing insurance	◆ Associations of insurers with service user organisations and mental health NGOs
◆ Providing economic incentives rather than disincentives to disabled people ready to return to work	◆ work and Pensions ministry to introduce new and flexible arrangements for disabled people to work with no risk to their income
◆ Change law to allow people with a history of mental illness to serve on juries with a presumption of competence	◆ Ministry of Justice to ensure fair access to jury service[215]

Without such research, we do not know the answers to many important questions including:

◆ are members of ethnic minorities who are mentally ill more discriminated against than members of the host population who have a mental illness?

- do self-stigma and self-discrimination in relation to mental illness vary according to experience of, for example, prior racial discrimination?
- if multiple discrimination does exist, does it have an effect on willingness to seek treatment, accept treatment recommendations and remain in contact with mental health services on a voluntary basis?
- which interventions are effective to reduce discrimination against those with multiply stigmatised characteristics?

Coordinating anti-discrimination action

To ensure that anti-stigma measures are implemented, governments need to make a clear commitment to redress such injustices. This is often best begun with a national anti-stigma plan. There are examples in the USA (within the Surgeon General's Report),[267–269] and in the Presidents' New Freedom Commission on Mental Health,[270] in Australia in the series of National Plans,[271] and in England with specific plans related to stigma and to social exclusion.[32, 272, 273] Such policies are necessary but not sufficient. There is a dishonourable tradition of these plans being naively or cynically published by governments with no intention to act upon them. There needs to be an accompanying action plan with all the mechanisms necessary for implementation: lists of specified tasks allocated to named organisations, budgetary allocations for this extra work, timescales attached to each task, reporting lines to assess progress to the stated targets, and a performance management system which will give rewards to organisations meeting their targets and sanctions to those which do not. Without such levers to force action, then anti-stigma plans will be as disreputable as the people they claim to assist.[274, 151]

Action at the international level

What action is necessary which is best done at the international level? Such contributions, so far removed from the everyday lives of people, may be hardly noticeable unless they are very sharply focused and coherent. Setting international standards for national polices can be one useful intervention. For example the World Health Organisation (WHO) has published standards to guide countries in producing or revising mental health laws.[275] This covers advice on:

- access to care
- confidentiality

- if an individual has characteristics which are stigmatised, e.g. mental illness and a criminal justice system record, is the total amount of discrimination the sum of these two or more or less?

- ◆ assessments of competence and capacity
- ◆ involuntary treatment
- ◆ consent
- ◆ physical treatments
- ◆ seclusion
- ◆ restraint
- ◆ privacy of communications
- ◆ appeals against detention
- ◆ review procedures for compulsory detention.[275]

Such guidelines are needed. At present 25 per cent of countries worldwide do not have legislation related to mental health treatment, and for those that do, half of these enacted its law over 15 years ago. Generally lower income countries are more likely to have older legislation.[276]

International organisation, such as the WHO can also contribute towards better care and less discrimination by indicating the need for national mental health policies, and by giving guidance on their content. In 2005, for example, only 62 per cent of countries in the world had a mental health policy.[276] In Europe Health Ministers have signed a Mental Health Declaration and Action Plan which set the following priorities:

- ◆ foster awareness of mental illness
- ◆ tackle stigma, discrimination and inequality
- ◆ provide comprehensive, integrated care systems,
- ◆ support a competent, effective workforce,
- ◆ recognise the experience and knowledge of services users and carers.[277–279]

Human rights

As shown throughout this book people with mental illnesses in many countries are treated in ways which prevent them from exercising many of their basic human rights. It is hardly an exaggeration to say that we can estimate the value attached to people in this category quite precisely from seeing how much or how little attention is paid to ensuring that they are treated in fully humane ways.[280–282]

> All persons have the right to the best available mental heath care, which shall be part of the health and social care system.[283]

Nations have responsibilities towards everyone in their jurisdiction under international law. Where there is any conflict with domestic law, law at the international level is superior. Even if international treaties are not expressly reflected in domestic laws, they are binding on states once they are ratified. All of the general international human rights treaties protect the rights of people with mental illness through the principles of equality and non-discrimination, while more specific standards exist in relation to people with mental illness.

The primary source of international human rights within the United Nations (UN) is the Universal Declaration of Human Rights (UDHR), which refers to civil, political, economic, social and cultural rights. Civil and political rights, such as the right to liberty, to a fair trial, and to vote, are set out in an internationally binding treaty, the International Covenant on Civil and Political Rights (ICCPR), which has not been ratified by only seven nations including China.[284] Economic, social and cultural rights, such as the rights to an adequate standard of living, the highest attainable standard of physical and mental health, and to education, are described in a second binding treaty, the International Covenant on Economic, Social and Cultural Rights (ICESCR), which has not been ratified by the USA.

The UN High Commissioner for Human Rights (OHCHR) reports to the UN General Assembly on the implementation of the rights protected by these human rights treaties. Countries which have ratified these binding treaties are then obliged under international law to guarantee to every person on their territory, without discrimination, all the rights enshrined in both pieces of legislation.[284-287]

The body which monitors implementation of the ICESCR is the Committee on Economic, Social and Cultural Rights (CESCR). In a special report explaining how the ICESCR relates specifically to the rights of people with disabilities, the Committee stated:

> The obligation of States party to the Covenant to promote progressive realisation of the relevant rights to the maximum of their available resources clearly requires Governments to do much more than merely abstain from taking measures which might have a negative impact on persons with disabilities. The obligation in the case of such a vulnerable and disadvantaged group is to take positive action to reduce structural disadvantages and to give appropriate preferential treatment to people with disabilities in order to achieve the objectives of full participation and equality within society for all persons with disabilities. This almost invariably means that additional resources will need to be made available for this purpose and that a wide range of specially tailored measures will be required.[288]

More specifically in relation to mental illness, the UN Principles for the Protection of Persons with Mental Illness and for the Improvement of Mental Health Care were adopted in 1991, and elaborate the basic rights and freedoms of people with mental illness that must be secured if states are to be in full compliance with the ICESCR. The 'The Right to Mental Health' is stated in Article 12 of the ICESCR, which provides the right of everyone to the 'enjoyment of the highest attainable standard of physical and mental health', and identifies some of the measures states should take 'to achieve the full realisation of this right'.

These 'Mental Illness Principles' apply to all people with mental illness, and to all people admitted to psychiatric facilities, whether or not they are diagnosed as having a mental illness. They provide criteria for the determination of mental illness, protection of confidentiality, standards of care, the rights of people in mental health facilities, and the provision of resources. Mental Illness Principle 1 lays down the basic foundation upon which nations' obligations towards people with mental illness are built: that 'all persons with a mental illness, or who are being treated as such persons, shall be treated with humanity and respect for the inherent dignity of the human person', and 'shall have the right to exercise all civil, political, economic, social and cultural rights as recognised in the Universal Declaration of Human Rights, the International Covenant on Economic, Social and Cultural Rights, the International Covenant on Civil and Political Rights and in other relevant instruments'. It also provides that 'all persons have the right to the best available mental health care'. As the United Nations' health agency, the World Health Organisation (WHO) gives substance to the UN's understanding of what is meant by 'the best available mental health care'.[275]

In addition to these agreements, 46 member states of the Council of Europe are bound or guided by a series of arrangements.[289, 290] These include the 1950 European Convention on Human Rights and Fundamental Freedoms (ECHR), and the European Committee for the Prevention of Torture and Inhuman or Degrading Treatment or Punishment (CPT).

There is no international consensus on which principles are of overriding importance in their application to mental health. Rather we have a series of treaties, conventions, covenants, declarations and consensus statements at the national or international level. Despite this, it is possible to synthesize the most common themes and to apply them to any particular country. Table 11.4 shows one example of this approach, as applied to countries within the UK, using 12 core principles.[291]

The overarching theme that lies behind these declarations is the pursuit of justice: that people with mental illness should be treated fairly, and should receive assistance in relation to their needs, and be free from unfair discrimination. This also means that people with disabilities from mental illnesses should be treated with parity in comparison to people with disabilities from physical conditions.[292, 293]

> They also forced me to eat. They divided up the servings with the strictest sense of justice, each according to her need.
>
> Isabelle Allende[294]

Table 11.4 Fundamental principles relevant to the mental health policies and mental health laws

Principle	England		Scotland 2003	United Nations (UN) 1991	WHO 2001	World Psychiatric Association 1996 (WPA)
	National Service Framework for Mental Health (NSFMH) 1999	Social Exclusion Unit (SEU) 2003				
1. Participation in care	Involve service users		Regard to past and present wishes of person, … full participation		Consumer involvement … right to information and participation	Person should be accepted as a partner by right in therapeutic process
2. Therapeutic benefit to the individual person	Effective care	Effective care to prevent crises	Importance of providing maximum benefit to person	Right to the best available mental health care. Every person shall have the right to receive such health and social care as is appropriate to his or her health needs … in the best interest of the person	Efficient treatment	Providing the best therapy available consistent with accepted scientific knowledge. Treatment must always be in the best interest of the person
3. Choice of acceptable treatments	Acceptable care & choice	Genuine choices	Importance of providing appropriate services to person		Wide range of services	Allow the person to make free and informed decisions

Table 11.4 (Continued)

Principle	England		Scotland 2003	United Nations (UN) 1991	WHO 2001	World Psychiatric Association 1996 (WPA)
	National Service Framework for Mental Health (NSFMH) 1999	Social Exclusion Unit (SEU) 2003				
4. Non-discrimination	Non-discriminatory	Fair access regardless of ethnicity, gender, age or sexuality	Have regard to encouragement of equal opportunities	These principles shall be applied without discrimination of any kind	Equality and non-discrimination	Fair and equal treatment of the mentally ill. Discrimination by psychiatrists on the basis of ethnicity or culture, whether directly or by aiding others, is unethical
5. Access	Accessible			Every person shall have the right to be treated and cared for, as far as possible, in the community in which he or she lives	Local services	
6. Safety	Promote safety			To protect the health or safety of the person concerned or of others, or otherwise to protect public	Physical integrity of service user	

7. Autonomy and empowerment	Independence	Maintain employment	safety, order, health or morals or the fundamental rights and freedoms of others Treatment … directed towards preserving and enhancing personal autonomy	Person empowerment, autonomy	Provide the person with relevant information so as to empower
8. Appropriate family involvement in care		Social and family participation	Have regard to needs and circumstances of person's carer	Partnership with families, involvement of local community	Psychiatrist should consult with the family
9. Dignity			Treated with humanity and respect for the inherent dignity of the human person	Preserve dignity	Psychiatrists to be guided primarily by the respect for persons and concern for their welfare and integrity, … to safeguard the human dignity
10. Least restrictive form of care		Have regard to minimum restriction of the freedom of the person necessary	Every person shall have the right to be treated in the least restrictive environment		Therapeutic interventions that are least restrictive to the freedom of the person

(Continued)

Table 11.4 (*Continued*)

| Principle | England | | United Nations (UN) 1991 | WHO 2001 | World Psychiatric Association 1996 (WPA) |
	National Service Framework for Mental Health (NSFMH) 1999	Social Exclusion Unit (SEU) 2003	Scotland 2003		
11. Advocacy			Have regard to views of person's named person, carer, guardian, welfare attorney			
12. Capacity				The person whose capacity is at issue shall be entitled to be represented by a counsel		

What actions stem from these lofty declarations? First, they are little known. Despite the status of many of these documents as legally binding agreements, it is rare to see them mentioned at all in mental health policies or in practice guidelines, so the first step is to ensure that those setting national polices are fully aware of their legal and ethical obligation. International and national advocacy groups are in the strongest position to remind governments and professional groups of these duties.

It is also vital that there are bodies which monitor how far the specified human rights are respected or violated, and groups such as Amnesty International, Global Initiative on Psychiatry, Mental Disability Advocacy Center and Mental Disability Rights International play a leading role in this regard. At present no comprehensive data are collected internationally on human rights violations and such a baseline is necessary to track whether the situation improves or deteriorates in future. To achieve this it is necessary for specific governmental organisations, or relevant NGOs, to initiate ongoing audits, with full legal access to the relevant institutions.

There is also a need to understand international trends in stigmatisation and discrimination. No regular information is gathered to know whether stigmatising attitudes and discriminatory behaviour are getting worse or better in different countries. So it is necessary to create an international knowledge base of effective interventions against discrimination, and to do this research commissioners need to support research to examine the cost-effectiveness of candidate interventions to reduce discrimination in cross-cultural settings.

The way that mental illnesses are portrayed to the public does affect popular views. What is far less clear is whether describing particular mental illnesses as substantially biochemical or genetic 'brain diseases' in origin reduces stigma. There is conflicting evidence that such medicalized explanations either decrease social rejection by locating the cause of the condition outside the control and responsibility of the individual,[295] or increase social exclusion if the condition is seen as genetically based and so also potentially affecting other family members.[85,152,296–302]

In addition, concerted international efforts are needed to initiate and sustain programmes to reduce stigmatisation. The World Psychiatric Association has made a major contribution in this way with its Campaign to Fight Stigma because of Schizophrenia.[303] Such initiatives would be strengthened by active participation from groups such as the International Council of Nurses, International Federation of Social Workers and the International Psychological Association. The European Employment Framework Directive is a further example of a positive international initiative.[149]

How far do particular diagnostic labels assist or hinder people with these conditions? The term schizophrenia, for example, is usually connected by the public with ideas of unpredictability, threat and violence. So is there any value in changing the name of the condition? This is unknown. In other domains of medicine there are numerous example of name changes which were intended to make a condition more speakable, for example, Hansen's disease (leprosy), or Down syndrome ('mongolism'). There is also active debate on whether the term 'chronic fatigue syndrome' should be replaced by an eponym. Indeed conditions allied to Down syndrome have changed name repeatedly over the last century without clear evidence that this has been beneficial.[304]

In Japan the phrase used for schizophrenia was changed after a long-running campaign by the family organisation Zenkaren. Professionals now consider that this new term ('integration disorder syndrome') is more often used, and less stigmatising that the previous word ('mind-split-disease').[305] While there have been proposals to rename this condition as, for example, Kraepelin–Bleuler Disease, so far there is no evidence that this would contribute to decreasing discrimination.[305–309]

> After my breakdown in 1999 I found that hospitals and psychiatry had changed in the sense that I was not only told my diagnosis but participated in drawing up my care plan; the secrecy I had known had gone along with those large hospitals.
>
> Paul

Yet words and images do matter.[310–312] Terminology has become the arena for a power struggle in recent years. At one extreme are those who describe 'research subjects', and 'schizophrenics' as being categorically different from people who are well. On the other hand are advocates of terms such as 'service user', 'consumer', 'survivor', 'client' or who have use the 'person with ...' formula (e.g. person with a diagnosis of depression[313]) to indicate variations in human diversity.[314]

Similarly visual language plays an important role in encapsulate the meaning of mental illness. Many films, for example, combine stereotyped cinematographic imagery, combined with emotionally expressive music and editorial techniques,[315,316] to convey the cognitive and emotional content about what mental illnesses mean.[317–319] Just as it has become more difficult to distribute films which are explicitly racist or anti-Semitic, so the international media, especially television, internet and cinema, have a potentially vital role to play in a seismic culture change – recasting the terms in which mental illnesses are heard and seen and understood and accepted.[320]

Conclusion: demolishing structural discrimination

Despite the realization, for almost a century now,[81] that discrimination against people with mental illness is both common and severe, little real progress has been made in most countries to ensure social inclusion. While there is some evidence that attitudes, especially towards people with depression, are improving,[321,180] attitudes in England toward people with mental illnesses as a whole have substantially deteriorated in recent years.[322] The idea of parity with people with other forms of disability, let alone with non-disabled people, is very far from the everyday experience of most people with mental illnesses.

> All the time … you're treated like an idiot or a child.
>
> Rachel

As the rejection of people with mental illness is both widespread (affecting every aspect of personal, social and work life),[323,324] and often appears not to be intentional, the totality of such exclusion has been described as *structural discrimination*.[325–327] This is similar to the idea of institutional racism,[328] which Lord MacPherson described in these terms:

> Taking all that we have heard and read into account we grapple with the problem. For the purposes of our Inquiry the concept of institutional racism, which we apply, consists of: the collective failure of an organisation to provide an appropriate and professional service to people because of their colour, culture, or ethnic origin. It can be seen or detected in processes, attitudes and behaviour which amount to discrimination through unwitting prejudice, ignorance, thoughtlessness and racist stereotyping which disadvantage minority ethnic people … It persists because of the failure of the organisation openly and adequately to recognise and address its existence and causes by policy, example and leadership. Without recognition and action to eliminate such racism it can prevail as part of the ethos or culture of the organisation. It is a corrosive disease.[328]

Just as concerted social and cultural and legal measures have been necessary to begin to reverse discrimination against black and minority ethnic communities in the UK or the USA, so the same determination is now necessary to promote the social inclusion of people with mental illness within society.

The steps outlined above in Tables 11.1–11.3 are an agenda for change. To inform the pursuit of these goals it is essential to understand the real experiences of discrimination by people with mental illness,[137,227,329–332] and their priorities for change. What this amounts to is no less than the need to demolish both direct and structural discrimination against people with mental illness.

Such a coordinated attack on discrimination depends upon recognition that mental illnesses can produce very serious impairments, for example, in concentration or memory. While these can be minimized by a favourable environment, the severity of the primary problems should not be denied or minimized. This will mean that for some people with mental illness, at least for periods when the symptoms and features of the condition are more prominent, it is difficult to advocate on their own behalf, and even harder to join with others to campaign for their common interests.

> You can't separate you from the illness and lack of self-esteem.
>
> Rachel

In broader political terms, it is clear from every chapter of this book that the social and lobbying power of people with mental illness and their advocates is weak. Indeed one of the central paradoxes of this book is that while up to three-quarters of adults know someone directly who has been affected by a mental illness, we act as if nobody knows anything.[165] This is both ignorance and denial on an astonishing scale. Perhaps Rachel (see Chapter 3) comes close to the truth when she asks if many of us are frightened of how close we are to mental illness:

> Everybody knows very little about it. Because most of the publicity is negative, about violence and so on. There's no information for people, is there? And also they don't like talking about it, and half of them are worried they got a little bit of something themselves.

If it is fair to conclude that people with mental illness are politically weak (it is often said in political circles that there are no votes in mental illness), then what are the implications?[333] One consequence is that those in the mental health field who do have resources at their disposal should selectively provide financial and human support to service user and consumer groups, at a respectful distance, so that these groups can develop, flourish and identify their own priorities and decide how they can exert pressure to achieve their goals. This can be as simple as making direct financial grants to self-help groups, or providing office and meeting rooms. This means providing these resources for consumers locally, nationally and internationally, to match the levels at which action is needed.

When it comes to campaigning for fundamental issues, a practical approach is for local and national agencies to set aside their differences and to find common cause. In some areas such coordinating groups are called forums, peak bodies, alliances or consortia. What they have in common is a recognition that what they can achieve together, in political terms, is greater that their individual impact. Core issues able to unite such coalitions are likely to be parity in funding, the use of disability discrimination laws for people with mental illness-related disabilities, and the recognition of international human rights conventions in practice.[334–337]

> There is a lot of unhelpful rivalry and an antagonism between different non-governmental organisations.
>
> Rachel

Going further, there is a basic problem in every country in the world: that the supply of treatment and care is less or far less than the actual need. Even in the best-resourced countries fully half of all people with mental illnesses receive no effective help.[338] This fraction is at the root of the problem. Many people do not reveal their distress, even to their closest family members for fear of rejection, in anticipation of being shunned. Where they do mention their difficulties, then family members may well react without understanding or sympathy, and discourage them from embarrassing the family by telling others. And even when people do go to a primary care practitioner, most of the time their mental illness is not recognised, and even less often is it treated properly.[339] The clear need is to provide acceptable care and assistance to people with mental illness on a far greater scale than has ever been done before.

If taboo means 'a social or religious custom placing prohibition or restriction on a particular thing or person',[340] then is mental illness its strongest remaining taboo? Certainly the ways in which many people with mental illness are left in social,[324] material[323] and cultural poverty[341–343] suggest that our societies allow, if not to deliberately orchestrate,[344] a form of 'structural violence' against this category of people.[345]

Yet many people with mental illness do cope. Earlier we have seen examples of such resilience. Jasmine has begun a part-time computing course, and still hopes to train as a nursery nurse (Chapter 1). Narayan did get the help he needed when he was homeless and is now preparing to work again (Chapter 2). Rachel has found ways to compensate or even over-compensate for her difficulties, to choose whether or not to disclose her condition when applying for work, and to rely upon her sheer ability to stay in work, '*Usually once I get there, they realise I'm competent*' (Chapter 3). Despite many serious setbacks Veronica continues in full-time work and is winning promotion to the higher levels of her organisation (Chapter 4). Diana found that her family suddenly rallied around her when she really needed their support, and now she has the dilemma of knowing how to ask them not to stifle her as she regains confidence, and to know when she is 'ready' to increase from part-time to full-time work (Chapter 5). Leroy thinks that having a clear-cut diagnosis has been useful for him as he tries to rebuild his life: *'It has helped with myself to get to grips with my illness. To have a better understanding of my illness you know ... I've been given some material ... it's helpful yes, very much so'* (Chapter 8).

In historical terms, the recognition of both individual and systemic discrimination against people with mental illness is a very recent phenomenon.[149,195,249,275,325,346–349] In the future we may well see that from this recognition grows a civil rights movement dedicated to the liberation of people with mental illness from being marginalized, from being excluded, and from being shunned.

> At the end of the day, I am still a person. I hold down a good job. I go out. I have a family. It's just an illness.
>
> Emile

References

1. Thornicroft G, Tansella M. *The Mental Health Matrix: A manual to improve services.* Cambridge: Cambridge University Press; 1999.
2. Cox RA. Avoiding discrimination against disabled people. *BMJ* 1996; 313(7069):1346–1347.
3. Caruso DR, Hodapp RM. Perceptions of mental retardation and mental illness. *Am J Ment Retard* 1988; 93(2):118–124.
4. Hugo CJ, Boshoff DE, Traut A, Zungu-Dirwayi N, Stein DJ. Community attitudes toward and knowledge of mental illness in South Africa. *Soc Psychiatry Psychiatr Epidemiol* 2003; 38(12):715–719.
5. Corrigan PW, Rowan D, Green A, Lundin R, River P, Uphoff-Wasowski K *et al.* Challenging two mental illness stigmas: personal responsibility and dangerousness. *Schizophr Bull* 2002; 28(2):293–309.
6. Trute B, Tefft B, Segall A. Social rejection of the mentally ill: a replication study of public attitude. *Soc Psychiatry Psychiatr Epidemiol* 1989; 24(2):69–76.
7. Steins G, Weiner B. The influence of perceived responsibility and personality characteristics on the emotional and behavioral reactions to people with AIDS. *J Soc Psychol* 1999; 139(4):487–495.
8. Corrigan P, Markowitz FE, Watson A, Rowan D, Kubiak MA. An attribution model of public discrimination towards persons with mental illness. *J Health Soc Behav* 2003; 44(2):162–179.
9. Corrigan PW. Mental health stigma as social attribution: implications for research methods and attitude change. *Clinical Psychology: Science and Practice* 2000; 7(1):48–67.
10. Furnham A, Chan E. Lay theories of schizophrenia. A cross-cultural comparison of British and Hong Kong Chinese attitudes, attributions and beliefs. *Soc Psychiatry Psychiatr Epidemiol* 2004; 39(7):543–552.
11. Jason LA, Taylor RR, Plioplys S, Stepanek Z, Shlaes J. Evaluating attributions for an illness based upon the name: chronic fatigue syndrome, myalgic encephalopathy and Florence Nightingale disease. *Am J Community Psychol* 2002; 30(1):133–148.

12. Ozmen E, Ogel K, Aker T, Sagduyu A, Tamar D, Boratav C. Public attitudes to depression in urban Turkey - the influence of perceptions and causal attributions on social distance towards individuals suffering from depression. *Soc Psychiatry Psychiatr Epidemiol* 2004; 39(12):1010–1016.

13. Wahl OF, Harman CR. Family views of stigma. *Schizophr Bull* 1989; 15(1):131–139.

14. Berkowitz R, Shavit N, Leff JP. Educating relatives of schizophrenic patients. *Soc Psychiatry Psychiatr Epidemiol* 1990; 25(4):216–220.

15. Angermeyer MC, Schulze B, Dietrich S. Courtesy stigma – a focus group study of relatives of schizophrenia patients. *Soc Psychiatry Psychiatr Epidemiol* 2003; 38(10):593–602.

16. Norvilitis JM, Scime M, Lee JS. Courtesy stigma in mothers of children with attention-deficit/hyperactivity disorder: a preliminary investigation. *J Atten Disord* 2002; 6(2):61–68.

17. Kommana S, Mansfield M, Penn DL. Dispelling the stigma of schizophrenia. *Psychiatr Serv* 1997; 48(11):1393–1395.

18. Szmukler G, Kuipers E, Joyce J, Harris T, Leese M, Maphosa W *et al.* An exploratory randomised controlled trial of a support programme for carers of patients with a psychosis. *Soc Psychiatry Psychiatr Epidemiol* 2003; 38(8):411–418.

19. Penn DL, Kommana S, Mansfield M, Link BG. Dispelling the stigma of schizophrenia: II. The impact of information on dangerousness. *Schizophr Bull* 1999; 25(3):437–446.

20. Pilling S, Bebbington P, Kuipers E, Garety P, Geddes J, Orbach G *et al.* Psychological treatments in schizophrenia: I. Meta-analysis of family intervention and cognitive behaviour therapy. *Psychol Med* 2002; 32(5):763–782.

21. Davidson J. Contesting stigma and contested emotions: Personal experience and public perception of specific phobias. *Soc Sci Med* 2005; 61; 2155–2164.

22. Penn DL, Guynan K, Daily T, Spaulding WD, Garbin CP, Sullivan M. Dispelling the stigma of schizophrenia: what sort of information is best? *Schizophr Bull* 1994; 20(3):567–578.

23. Solomon P, Draine J, Mannion E, Meisel M. Impact of brief family psychoeducation on self-efficacy. *Schizophr Bull* 1996; 22(1):41–50.

24. Gonzalez-Pinto A, Gonzalez C, Enjuto S, Fernandez de CB, Lopez P, Palomo J *et al.* Psychoeducation and cognitive-behavioral therapy in bipolar disorder: an update. *Acta Psychiatr Scand* 2004; 109(2):83–90.

25. Gingerich S, Mueser KT. Illness management and recovery. In: Drake RE, Merrens MR, Lynde DW, eds., *Evidence-based Mental Health Practice: a textbook.* New York: Norton; 2005.

26. Mueser KT, Gingerich S. *Coping with Schizophrenia: A guide for families.* New York: Guilford Press; 2005.

27. Penn DL, Martin J. The stigma of severe mental illness: some potential solutions for a recalcitrant problem. *Psychiatr Q* 1998; 69(3):235–247.

28. Penn DL, Corrigan PW. The effects of stereotype suppression on psychiatric stigma. *Schizophr Res* 2002; 55(3):269–276.

29. Crandall CS, Eshleman A. A justification-suppression model of the expression and experience of prejudice. *Psychol Bull* 2003; 129(3):414–446.

30. Warr P. *Work, Unemployment and Mental Health.* Oxford: Oxford University Press; 1987.

31. Warner R. *Recovery from Schizophrenia: Psychiatry and political economy.* Hove: Brunner-Routledge; 2004.

32. Social Exclusion Unit. *Mental Health and Social Exclusion.* London: Office of the Deputy Prime Minister; 2004.

33. Jablensky A, Sartorius N, Ernberg G, Anker M, Korten A, Cooper JE *et al*. Schizophrenia: manifestations, incidence and course in different cultures. A World Health Organization ten-country study. *Psychol Med Monogr Suppl.* 1992; 20:1–97.

34. Cooper J, Sartorius N. Cultural and temporal variations in schizophrenia: a speculation on the importance of industrialization. *Br J Psychiatry* 1977; 130:50–55.

35. Marshall M, Crowther R, Almaraz-Serrano A, Creed F, Sledge W, Kluiter H *et al*. Systematic reviews of the effectiveness of day care for people with severe mental disorders: (1) acute day hospital versus admission; (2) vocational rehabilitation; (3) day hospital versus outpatient care. *Health Technol Assess* 2001; 5(21):1–75.

36. Twamley EW, Jeste DV, Lehman AF. Vocational rehabilitation in schizophrenia and other psychotic disorders: a literature review and meta-analysis of randomized controlled trials. *J Nerv Ment Dis* 2003; 191(8):515–523.

37. Boardman J, Grove B, Perkins R, Shepherd G. Work and employment for people with psychiatric disabilities. *Br J Psychiatry* 2003; 182:467–468.

38. Lehman AF, Goldberg R, Dixon LB, McNary S, Postrado L, Hackman A *et al*. Improving employment outcomes for persons with severe mental illnesses. *Arch Gen Psychiatry* 2002; 59(2):165–172.

39. Drake RE, Goldman HH, Leff HS, Lehman AF, Dixon L, Mueser KT *et al*. Implementing evidence-based practices in routine mental health service settings. *Psychiatr Serv* 2001; 52(2):179–182.

40. Bond GR, Resnick SG, Drake RE, Xie H, McHugo GJ, Bebout RR. Does competitive employment improve nonvocational outcomes for people with severe mental illness? *J Consult Clin Psychol* 2001; 69(3):489–501.

41. Warner R. Environmental interventions in schizophrenia. 2: The community level. *New Dir Ment Health Serv* 1999;(83):71–84.

42. Becker DR, Drake RE. *A Working Life for People with Severe Mental Illness*. Oxford: Oxford University Press; 2003.

43. Marwaha S, Johnson S. Schizophrenia and employment - a review. *Soc Psychiatry Psychiatr Epidemiol* 2004; 39(5):337–349.

44. Dixon L, Goldberg R, Lehman A, McNary S. The impact of health status on work, symptoms, and functional outcomes in severe mental illness. *J Nerv Ment Dis* 2001; 189(1):17–23.

45. Gold JM, Goldberg RW, McNary SW, Dixon LB, Lehman AF. Cognitive correlates of job tenure among patients with severe mental illness. *Am J Psychiatry* 2002; 159(8):1395–1402.

46. McGurk SR, Mueser KT, Pascaris A. Cognitive training and supported employment for persons with severe mental illness: one-year results from a randomized controlled trial. *Schizophr Bull* 2005; 31; 898–909.

47. Wexler BE, Bell MD. Cognitive remediation and vocational rehabilitation for schizophrenia. *Schizophr Bull* 2005; 31; 931–941.

48. Vauth R, Corrigan PW, Clauss M, Dietl M, Dreher-Rudolph M, Stieglitz RD *et al*. Cognitive strategies versus self-management skills as adjunct to vocational rehabilitation. *Schizophr Bull* 2005; 31(1):55–66.

49. Bond GR. Principles of individual placement and support. *Psychiatric Rehabilitation Journal* 1998; 22(11):23.

50. Repper J, Perkins R. *Social Inclusion and Recovery*. Edinburgh: Balliere Tindall; 2003.

51. Perkins R, Evenson E, Davidson B. *The Pathfinder User Employment Programme*. London: South West London and St. George's Mental Health NHS Trust; 2000.

52. Perkins R, Selbie D. Decreasing employment discrimination against people who have experienced mental health problems in a mental health trust. In: Crisp A, ed., *Every Family in the Land*, pp. 350–355. London: Royal Society of Medicine; 2004.

53. Chinman MJ, Rosenheck R, Lam JA, Davidson L. Comparing consumer and nonconsumer provided case management services for homeless persons with serious mental illness. *J Nerv Ment Dis* 2000; 188(7):446–453.

54. Meehan T, Bergen H, Coveney C, Thornton R. Development and evaluation of a training program in peer support for former consumers. *International Journal of Mental Health Nursing* 2002; 11:34–39.

55. Lewis O. Mental disability law in central and Eastern Europe: paper, practice, promise. *Journal of Mental Health Law* 2002; 8:293–303.

56. Lewis O. Protecting the rights of people with mental disabilities: the European Convention on Human Rights. *European Journal of Health Law* 2002; 9:293–320.

57. Frank H, Paris J. Psychological factors in the choice of psychiatry as a career. *Can J Psychiatry* 1987; 32(2):118–122.

58. Jackson SW. The wounded healer. *Bull Hist Med* 2001; 75(1):1–36.

59. Mancuso L. Reasonable accommodation for workers with psychiatric disabilities. *Psychosocial Rehabilitation Journal* 1990; 14:3–19.

60. Zuckerman D. Reasonable accommodations for people with mental illness under the ADA. *Mental and Physical Disability Law Reporter* 1993; 17:311–319.

61. Americans With Disabilities Act 42 U.S.C. [S][S]12101–12213 (1990). Washington DC: 1990.

62. Appelbaum PS. Discrimination in psychiatric disability coverage and the Americans With Disabilities Act. *Psychiatr Serv* 1998; 49(7):875–6, 881.

63. Pardeck JT. Psychiatric disabilities and the Americans with Disabilities Act: implications for policy and practice. *J Health Soc Policy* 1998; 10(3):1–12.

64. Petrila J. The U.S Supreme Court narrows the definition of disability under the Americans With Disabilities Act. *Psychiatr Serv* 2002; 53(7):797–798, 801.

65. Petrila J, Brink T. Mental illness and changing definitions of disability under the Americans With Disabilities Act. *Psychiatr Serv* 2001; 52(5):626–630.

66. Glozier N. The Disability Discrimination Act 1995 and psychiatry: lessons from the first seven years. *Psychiatr Bull* 2004; 28:126–129.

67. Association of British Insurers. *An Insurer's Guide to the Disability Discrimination Act 1995*. London: Association of British Insurers; 2003.

68. Corrigan PW, Lundin R. *Don't Call Me Nuts: Coping with the Stigma of Mental Illness*. Chicago Illinois: Recovery Press; 2001.

69. Davidson B, McCallion H. Is it ok to lie about your mental health when applying for a job? *Nurs Times* 2001; 97(13):17.

70. Connelly K. *Consumer Involvement in the Workplace Report*. Vancouver, British Colombia: Greater Vancouver Mental Health Service Society; 1998.

71. Britt TW. The stigma of psychological problems in a work environment: Evidence from the screening of service members returning from Bosnia. *Journal of Applied Social Psychology* 2000; 30(8):1599–1618.

72. Institute of Employment Studies and MORI. *Impact on Small Business of Lowering the Disability Discrimination Act Part II Threshold*. Stratford on Avon: Disability Rights Commission; 2001.

73. Camp DL, Finlay WM, Lyons E. Is low self-esteem an inevitable consequence of stigma? An example from women with chronic mental health problems. *Soc Sci Med* 2002; 55(5):823–834.

74. Hayward P, Wong G, Bright JA, Lam D. Stigma and self-esteem in manic depression: an exploratory study. *J Affect Disord* 2002; 69(1–3):61–67.

75. Link BG, Struening EL, Neese-Todd S, Asmussen S, Phelan JC. Stigma as a barrier to recovery: the consequences of stigma for the self-esteem of people with mental illnesses. *Psychiatr Serv* 2001; 52(12):1621–1626.

76. Wright ER, Gronfein WP, Owens TJ. Deinstitutionalization, social rejection, and the self-esteem of former mental patients. *J Health Soc Behav* 2000; 41(1):68–90.

77. Crocker J, Quinn DM. Social stigma and the self: meanings, situations, and self-esteem. In: Heatherton TF, Kleck RE, Hebl MR, Hull JG, eds., *The Social Psychology of Stigma*, pp. 153–183 New York: Guilford; 2000.

78. Proudfoot J, Gray J, Carson J, Guest D, Dunn G. Psychological training improves mental health and job-finding among unemployed people. *Int Arch Occup Environ Health* 1999; 72 Suppl.:S40–S42.

79. Brown JS, Elliott SA, Boardman J, Ferns J, Morrison J. Meeting the unmet need for depression services with psycho-educational self-confidence workshops: preliminary report. *Br J Psychiatry* 2004; 185:511–515.

80. Hall PL, Tarrier N. The cognitive-behavioural treatment of low self-esteem in psychotic patients: a pilot study. *Behav Res Ther* 2003; 41(3):317–332.

81. Bogardus ES. Social distance and its origins. *Journal of Applied Sociology* 1924; 9:216–226.

82. Alexander LA, Link BG. The impact of contact on stigmatizing attitudes toward people with mental illness. *Journal of Mental Health* 2003; 12(3):271–289.

83. Couture SM, Penn DL. Interpersonal contact and the stigma of mental illness: a review of the literature. *Journal of Mental Health* 2003;(15):291–305.

84. Read J, Law A. The relationship of causal beliefs and contact with users of mental health services to attitudes to the 'mentally ill'. *Int J Soc Psychiatry* 1999; 45(3):216–229.

85. Dietrich S, Beck M, Bujantugs B, Kenzine D, Matschinger H, Angermeyer MC. The relationship between public causal beliefs and social distance toward mentally ill people. *Aust N Z J Psychiatry* 2004; 38(5):348–354.

86. Corrigan PW, Edwards AB, Green A, Diwan SL, Penn DL. Prejudice, social distance, and familiarity with mental illness. *Schizophr Bull* 2001; 27(2):219–225.

87. Angermeyer MC, Matschinger H. [Social distance of the population toward psychiatric patients]. *Gesundheitswesen* 1996; 58(1 Suppl):18–24.

88. Corrigan PW. Target-specific stigma change: a strategy for impacting mental illness stigma. *Psychiatr Rehabil J* 2004; 28(2):113–121.

89. Estroff SE, Penn DL, Toporek JR. From stigma to discrimination: an analysis of community efforts to reduce the negative consequences of having a psychiatric disorder and label. *Schizophr Bull* 2004; 30(3):493–509.

90. Holmes EP, Corrigan PW, Williams P, Canar J, Kubiak MA. Changing attitudes about schizophrenia. *Schizophr Bull* 1999; 25(3):447–456.

91. Gaebel W, Baumann AE. ['Open the doors' – the antistigma program of the World Psychiatric Association]. *MMW Fortschr Med* 2003; 145(12):34–37.

92. Pickenhagen A, Sartorius N. *The WPA Global Programme to Reduce Stigma and Discrimination Because of Schizophrenia.* Geneva: World Psychiatric Association; 2002.

93. Thompson AH, Stuart H, Bland RC, Arboleda-Florez J, Warner R, Dickson RA. Attitudes about schizophrenia from the pilot site of the WPA worldwide campaign against the stigma of schizophrenia. *Soc Psychiatry Psychiatr Epidemiol* 2002; 37(10):475–482.

94. Sartorius N, Schulze H. *Reducing the Stigma of Mental Illness: A Report from a Global Association.* Cambridge: Cambridge University Press; 2005.

95. Warner R. Local projects of the world psychiatric association programme to reduce stigma and discrimination. *Psychiatr Serv* 2005; 56(5):570–575.

96. Secker J, Armstrong C, Hill M. Young people's understanding of mental illness. *Health Educ Res* 1999; 14(6):729–739.

97. Schulze B, Angermeyer MC. What is schizophrenia? Secondary school students' associations with the word and sources of information about the illness. *Am J Orthopsychiatry* 2005; 75(2):316–323.

98. Schulze B, Richter-Werling M, Matschinger H, Angermeyer MC. Crazy? So what! Effects of a school project on students' attitudes towards people with schizophrenia. *Acta Psychiatr Scand* 2003; 107(2):142–150.

99. Angermeyer MC, Schulze B. Reducing the stigma of schizophrenia: understanding the process and options for interventions. *Epidemiol Psichiatr Soc* 2001; 10(1):1–5.

100. Watson AC, Otey E, Westbrook AL, Gardner AL, Lamb TA, Corrigan PW *et al.* Changing middle schoolers' attitudes about mental illness through education. *Schizophr Bull* 2004; 30(3):563–572.

101. Battaglia J, Coverdale JH, Bushong CP. Evaluation of a Mental Illness Awareness Week program in public schools. *Am J Psychiatry* 1990; 147(3):324–329.

102. Pinfold V, Toulmin H, Thornicroft G, Huxley P, Farmer P, Graham T. Reducing psychiatric stigma and discrimination: evaluation of educational interventions in UK secondary schools. *Br J Psychiatry* 2003; 182:342–6.

103. Pinfold V, Thornicroft G, Huxley P, Farmer P. Active ingredients in anti-stigma programmes in mental health. *International Review of Psychiatry* 2005; (in press).

104. Pinfold V, Stuart G, Thornicroft G, Arboleda-Florez J. The impact of mental health awareness programmes in schools in the UK and Canada. *World Psychiatry* 2005; 4,S1: 50–54.

105. Weiss MF. Children's attitudes toward the mentally ill: an eight-year longitudinal follow-up. *Psychol Rep* 1994; 74(1):51–56.

106. Parslow R, Jorm A, Christensen H, Jacomb P. Factors associated with young adults' obtaining general practitioner services. *Aust Health Rev* 2002; 25(6):109–118.

107. Wright A, Harris MG, Wiggers JH, Jorm AF, Cotton SM, Harrigan SM *et al.* Recognition of depression and psychosis by young Australians and their beliefs about treatment. *Med J Aust* 2005; 183(1):18–23.

108. Watson AC, Corrigan PW. Challenging public stigma: a targeted approach. In: Corrigan PW, ed., *On the Stigma of Mental Illness. Practical strategies for research and social change,* pp. 281–295. Washington DC: American Psychological Association; 2005.

109. PettigrewT.F, Tropp LR. Does intergroup contact reduce prejudice: recent meta-analytic findings. In: Oskamp S, ed., *Reducing Prejudice and Discrimination,* pp. 93–114. M. Kahwah New Jersey: Erlbaum; 2000.

110. Watson AC, Ottati V, Lurigio A, Corrigan PW. Stigma and the police. In: Corrigan PW, ed., *On the Stigma of Mental Illness,* pp. 197–217. Washington, DC: American Psychological Association; 2005.

111. Kimhi R, Barak Y, Gutman J, Melamed Y, Zohar M, Barak I. Police attitudes toward mental illness and psychiatric patients in Israel. *J Am Acad Psychiatry Law* 1998; 26(4):625–630.

112. Watson AC, Corrigan PW, Ottati V. Police responses to persons with mental illness: does the label matter? *J Am Acad Psychiatry Law* 2004; 32(4):378–385.

113. Watson AC, Corrigan PW, Ottati V. Police officers' attitudes toward and decisions about persons with mental illness. *Psychiatr Serv* 2004; 55(1):49–53.

114. Wallace C, Mullen PE, Burgess P. Criminal offending in schizophrenia over a 25-year period marked by deinstitutionalization and increasing prevalence of comorbid substance use disorders. *Am J Psychiatry* 2004; 161(4):716–727.

115. Lawrie SM, Martin K, McNeill G, Drife J, Chrystie P, Reid A *et al.* General practitioners' attitudes to psychiatric and medical illness. *Psychol Med* 1998; 28(6):1463–1467.

116. Caldwell TM, Jorm AF. Mental health nurses' beliefs about interventions for schizophrenia and depression: a comparison with psychiatrists and the public. *Aust N Z J Psychiatry* 2000; 34(4):602–611.

117. Caldwell TM, Jorm AF. Mental health nurses' beliefs about likely outcomes for people with schizophrenia or depression: a comparison with the public and other healthcare professionals. *Aust N Z J Ment Health Nurs* 2001; 10(1):42–54.

118. Filipcic I, Pavicic D, Filipcic A, Hotujac L, Begic D, Grubisin J *et al.* Attitudes of medical staff towards the psychiatric label 'schizophrenic patient' tested by an anti-stigma questionnaire. *Coll Antropol* 2003; 27(1):301–307.

119. Mas A, Hatim A. Stigma in mental illness: attitudes of medical students towards mental illness. *Med J Malaysia* 2002; 57(4):433–444.

120. Mukherjee R, Fialho A, Wijetunge A, Checinski K, Surgenor T. The stigmatisation of psychiatric illness: the attitudes of medical students and doctors in a London teaching hospital. *Psychiatr Bull* 2002; 26:178–181.

121. Rodrigues CR. [Comparison of the attitudes of Brazilian and Spanish medical students towards mental disease]. *Actas Luso Esp Neurol Psiquiatr Cienc Afines* 1992; 20(1):30–41.

122. Roth D, Antony MM, Kerr KL, Downie F. Attitudes toward mental illness in medical students: does personal and professional experience with mental illness make a difference? *Med Educ* 2000; 34(3):234–236.

123. White R. Stigmatisation of mentally ill medical students. In: Crisp A, ed., *Every Family in the Land*, pp. 365–366. London: Royal Society of Medicine; 2004.

124. Hasui C, Sakamoto S, Suguira B, Kitamura T. Stigmatization of mental illness in Japan: Images and frequency of encounters with diagnostic categories of mental illness among medical and non-medical university students. *Journal of Psychiatry and Law* 2000; 28(Summer):253–266.

125. Arkar H, Eker D. Influence of a three-week psychiatric training programme on attitudes toward mental illness in medical students. *Soc Psychiatry Psychiatr Epidemiol* 1997; 32(3):171–176.

126. Chew-Graham CA, Rogers A, Yassin N. 'I wouldn't want it on my CV or their records': medical students' experiences of help-seeking for mental health problems. *Med Educ* 2003; 37(10):873–880.

127. Lethem R. Mental illness in medical students and doctors: fitness to practice. In: Crisp A, ed., *Every Family in the Land*, pp. 356–364. London: Royal Society of Medicine; 2004.

128. Mino Y, Yasuda N, Kanazawa S, Inoue S. Effects of medical education on attitudes towards mental illness among medical students: a five-year follow-up study. *Acta Med Okayama* 2000; 54(3):127–132.

129. Mino Y, Yasuda N, Tsuda T, Shimodera S. Effects of a one-hour educational program on medical students' attitudes to mental illness. *Psychiatry Clin Neurosci* 2001; 55(5):501–7.

130. Lauber C, Anthony M, jdacic-Gross V, Rossler W. What about psychiatrists' attitude to mentally ill people? *Eur Psychiatry* 2004; 19(7):423–427.

131. Luhrmann TM. *Of Two Minds.* New York: Vintage Books; 2000.

132. Burti L, Mosher LR. Attitudes, values and beliefs of mental health workers. *Epidemiol Psichiatr Soc* 2003; 12(4):227–231.

133. Schlosberg A. Psychiatric stigma and mental health professionals (stigmatizers and destig-matizers). *Med Law* 1993; 12(3–5):409–416.

134. Sadow D, Ryder M, Webster D. Is education of health professionals encouraging stigma towards the mentally ill? *Journal of Mental Health* 2002; 11:657–665.

135. Crisp A. *Every Family in the Land: Understanding Prejudice and Discrimination Against People with Mental Illness.* London: Royal Society of Medicine Press; 2004.

136. Sartorius N. Stigma: what can psychiatrists do about it? *Lancet* 1998; 352(9133):1058–1059.

137. Chamberlin J. User/consumer involvement in mental health service delivery. *Epidemiol Psichiatr Soc* 2005; 14; 10–14.

138. Sutherby K, Szmukler GI, Halpern A, Alexander M, Thornicroft G, Johnson C *et al.* A study of 'crisis cards' in a community psychiatric service. *Acta Psychiatr Scand* 1999; 100(1): 56–61.

139. Henderson C, Flood C, Leese M, Thornicroft G, Sutherby K, Szmukler G. Effect of joint crisis plans on use of compulsory treatment in psychiatry: single blind randomised con-trolled trial. *BMJ* 2004; 329(7458):136–138.

140. Swanson J, Swartz M, Ferron J, Elbogen EB, Van Dom R. Psychiatric advance directives among public mental health consumers in five U.S. cities: prevalence, demand, and correl-ates. *Journal of the American Academy of Psychiatry and the Law* 2005; 34; 43–57.

141. Byng R, Jones R, Leese M, Hamilton B, McCrone P, Craig T. Exploratory cluster randomised controlled trial of shared care development for long-term mental illness. *Br J Gen Pract* 2004; 54(501):259–266.

142. Lester H, Allan T, Wilson S, Jowett S, Roberts L. A cluster randomised controlled trial of patient-held medical records for people with schizophrenia receiving shared care. *Br J Gen Pract* 2003; 53(488):197–203.

143. Allen MH, Carpenter D, Sheets JL, Miccio S, Ross R. What do consumers say they want and need during a psychiatric emergency? *J Psychiatr Pract* 2003; 9(1):39–58.

144. Repper J, Brooker C. Public attitudes towards mental health facilities in the community. *Health and Social Care in the Community* 1996; 4(5):290–299.

145. Angermeyer MC, Link BG, Majcher-Angermeyer A. Stigma perceived by patients attending modern treatment settings. Some unanticipated effects of community psychiatry reforms. *J Nerv Ment Dis* 1987; 175(1):4–11.

146. Chee CY, Ng TP, Kua EH. Comparing the stigma of mental illness in a general hospital with a state mental hospital: a Singapore study. *Soc Psychiatry Psychiatr Epidemiol* 2005; 40(8):648–653.

147. Westbrook MT, Legge V, Pennay M. Attitudes towards disabilities in a multicultural society. *Soc Sci Med* 1993; 36(5):615–623.

148. Eurobarometer. *Discrimination in Europe. For diversity, against discrimination.* Brussels: European Commission; 2003.

149. Sayce L, Curran C. Tackling social exclusion across Europe. In: Knapp M, McDaid D, Mossialos E, Thornicroft G, eds, *Mental Health Policy and Practice Across Europe. The future direction of mental health care.* Milton Keynes: Open University Press; 2006.

150. Klitzman R, Bayer R. *Mortal Secrets: Truth and lies in the age of AIDS.* Baltimore, Maryland: The Johns Hopkins University Press; 2003.

151. Sayce L. Beyond good intentions. Making anti-discrimination strategies work. *Disability and Society* 2003; 18:625–642.

152. Sayce L. *From Psychiatric Patient to Citizen. Overcoming discrimination and social exclusion.* Basingstoke: Palgrave; 2000.

153. Prince MJ. Disability. disability studies and citizenship: moving up or off the sociological agenda? *Canadian Journal of Sociology* 2004; 29:459–467.

154. Oliver M, Barnes C. *Disabled People and Social Policy.* London: Longman; 1998.

155. Degener T. Definition of Disability. *EU Network of Experts on Disability Discrimination.* Galway: National University of Ireland; 2004.

156. Perlick DA, Rosenheck RA, Clarkin JF, Sirey JA, Salahi J, Struening EL *et al.* Stigma as a barrier to recovery: adverse effects of perceived stigma on social adaptation of persons diagnosed with bipolar affective disorder. *Psychiatr Serv* 2001; 52(12):1627–1632.

157. Sapey B. From stigma to the social exclusion of disabled people. In: Mason T, Carlisle C, Watkins C, Whitehead E, eds., *Stigma and Social Exclusion in Healthcare*, pp. 270–280 London: Routledge; 2001.

158. Burchardt T, Le Grand J, Piachaud D. Social exclusion in Britain 1991–1995. *Social Psychiatry and Administration* 1999; 33:227–244.

159. Burchardt T, Le Grand J, Piachaud D. Introduction to understanding social exclusion. In: Hills D, Le Grand J, Piachaud D, eds., *Understanding Social Exclusion*, pp. Oxford: Oxford University Press; 2002, pp 1–12.

160. Evans J, Repper J. Employment, social inclusion and mental health. *J Psychiatr Ment Health Nurs* 2000; 7(1):15–24.

161. Beresford P. Developing the theoretical basis for service user/survivor-led research and equal involvement in research. *Epidemiol Psichiatr Soc* 2005; 14(1):4–9.

162. Barnes R, Auburn T, Lea S. Citizenship in practice. *Br J Soc Psychol* 2004; 43(Pt 2):187–206.

163. Poulin C, Masse R. [From deinstitutionalization to social rejection: the point of view of ex-psychiatric patients]. *Sante Ment Que* 1994; 19(1):175–194.

164. Hinshaw SP, Cicchetti D. Stigma and mental disorder: conceptions of illness, public attitudes, personal disclosure, and social policy. *Dev Psychopathol* 2000; 12(4):555–598.

165. Crisp A, Gelder MG, Goddard E, Meltzer H. Stigmatization of people with mental illnesses: a follow-up study within the Changing Minds campaign of the Royal College of Psychiatrists. *World Psychiatry* 2005; 4:106–113.

166. Zogg H, Lauber C, jdacic-Gross V, Rossler W. [Expert's and lay attitudes towards restrictions on mentally ill people]. *Psychiatr Prax* 2003; 30(7):379–383.

167. Star SA. *What the Public Thinks about Mental Health and Mental Illness.* Indianapolis, Indiana: Paper presented at the annual meeting of the National Association of Mental Health; 1952.

168. Nunnally JC. *Popular Conceptions of Mental Health.* New York: Holt, Rinehart & Winston; 1961.

169. Cumming J, Cumming E. On the stigma of mental illness. *Community Mental Health Journal* 1965; 1:135–143.

170. Phelan JC, Link BG, Stueve A, Pescosolido BA. Public conceptions of mental illness in 1950 and 1996: What is mental illness and it sit to be feared? *Journal of Health and Social Behavior* 2000; 41:188–207.

171. Regier DA, Hirschfeld RM, Goodwin FK, Burke JD, Jr., Lazar JB, Judd LL. The NIMH Depression Awareness, Recognition, and Treatment Program: structure, aims, and scientific basis. *Am J Psychiatry* 1988; 145(11):1351–1357.

172. Wells K, Miranda J, Bruce ML, Alegria M, Wallerstein N. Bridging community intervention and mental health services research. *Am J Psychiatry* 2004; 161(6):955–963.

173. Corrigan PW, Penn DL. Lessons from social psychology on discrediting psychiatric stigma. *American Psychologist* 1999; 54(9):765–776.

174. Corrigan PW, River LP, Lundin RK, Penn DL, Uphoff-Wasowski K, Campion J *et al.* Three strategies for changing attributions about severe mental illness. *Schizophr Bull* 2001; 27(2):187–195.

175. Cumming E, Cumming J. *Closed Ranks. An experiment in mental health.* Cambridge, Massachusetts: Harvard University Press; 1957.

176. Herek GM, Capitanio JP. Public reactions to AIDS in the United States: a second decade of stigma. *Am J Public Health* 1993; 83(4):574–577.

177. Herek GM, Capitanio JP, Widaman KF. HIV-related stigma and knowledge in the United States: prevalence and trends, 1991–1999. *Am J Public Health* 2002; 92(3):371–377.

178. Ellis PM, Smith DA. Treating depression: the beyondblue guidelines for treating depression in primary care. 'Not so much what you do but that you keep doing it'. *Med J Aust* 2002; 176 Suppl:S77–S83.

179. Hickie I. Can we reduce the burden of depression? The Australian experience with beyondblue: the national depression initiative. *Australas Psychiatry* 2004; 12 Suppl:S38–S46.

180. Jorm AF, Christensen H, Griffiths KM. The impact of beyondblue: the national depression initiative on the Australian public's recognition of depression and beliefs about treatments. *Aust N Z J Psychiatry* 2005; 39(4):248–254.

181. Angermeyer MC, Matschinger H. Have there been any changes in the public's attitudes towards psychiatric treatment? Results from representative population surveys in Germany in the years 1990 and 2001. *Acta Psychiatr Scand* 2005; 111(1):68–73.

182. Gaebel W, Baumann AE. Interventions to reduce the stigma associated with severe mental illness: experiences from the open the doors program in Germany. *Can J Psychiatry* 2003; 48(10):657–662.

183. Angermeyer MC, Matschinger H. Causal beliefs and attitudes to people with schizophrenia. Trend analysis based on data from two population surveys in Germany. *Br J Psychiatry* 2005; 186:331–334.

184. Priest RG, Vize C, Roberts A, Roberts M, Tylee A. Lay people's attitudes to treatment of depression: Results of opinion poll for Defeat Depression Campaign just before its launch. *BMJ* 1996; 313:858–859.

185. Paykel ES, Tylee A, Wright A, Priest RG, Rix S, Hart D. The Defeat Depression Campaign: psychiatry in the public arena. *Am J Psychiatry* 1997; 154(6 Suppl):59–65.

186. McKeon P. Defeating or preventing stigma of mental illness? *Lancet* 1998; 352(9144):1942.

187. Paykel ES, Hart D, Priest RG. Changes in public attitudes to depression during the Defeat Depression Campaign. *Br J Psychiatry* 1998; 173:519–522.

188. Rix S, Paykel ES, Lelliott P, Tylee A, Freeling P, Gask L *et al.* Impact of a national campaign on GP education: an evaluation of the Defeat Depression Campaign. *Br J Gen Pract* 1999; 49(439):99–102.

189. mcarthuresearch. *See Me Awareness.* Edinburgh: Scottish Opinion Limited; 2004.

190. Dunion L, Gordon L. Tackling the attitude problem. The achievements to date of Scotland's 'see me' anti-stigma campaign. *Ment Health Today* 2005;22–25.

191. Kotler P, Roberto EL, Lee N. *Social Marketing: improving the quality of life.* New York: Sage; 2002.

192. Thomashoff H-O, Sartorius N. *Art Against Stigma.* Stuttgart: Schattauer; 2004.

193. Scheid TL. Employment of individuals with mental disabilities: business response to the ADA's challenge. *Behav Sci Law* 1999; 17(1):73–91.

194. Scheid TL. The Americans with Disabilities Act, mental disability, and employment practices. *J Behav Health Serv Res* 1998; 25(3):312–324.

195. Sayce L, O'Brian N. The future of equality and human rights in Britain – opportunities and risks for disabled people. *Disability and Society* 2004; 19:663–667.

196. Crawford MJ, Aldridge T, Bhui K, Rutter D, Manley C, Weaver T *et al.* User involvement in the planning and delivery of mental health services: a cross-sectional survey of service users and providers. *Acta Psychiatr Scand* 2003; 107(6):410–414.

197. Entwistle VA, Sowden AJ, Watt IS. Evaluating interventions to promote patient involvement in decision-making: by what criteria should effectiveness be judged? *J Health Serv Res Policy* 1998; 3(2):100–107.

198. O'Donnell M, Entwistle V. Consumer involvement in decisions about what health-related research is funded. *Health Policy* 2004; 70(3):281–290.

199. Beresford P. Developing the theoretical basis for service user/survivor-led research and equal involvement in research. *Epidemiol Psichiatr Soc* 2005; 14(1):4–9.

200. Thornicroft G, Tansella M. Growing recognition of the importance of service user involvement in mental health service planning and evaluation. *Epidemiol Psichiatr Soc* 2005; 14(1):1–3.

201. Trivedi P, Wykes T. From passive subjects to equal partners: qualitative review of user involvement in research. *British Journal of Psychiatry* 2002; 181:468–472.

202. United Nations. *UN Standard Rules on the Equalization of Opportunities for Persons with Disabilities,* A/RES/48/96, 85th Plenary Meeting 20 December 1993. New York: United Nations; 1993.

203. European Commission. *Conclusions of the Commissioner, Seminar organized by the Council of Europe Commissioner for Human Rights and hosted by the World Health Organization Regional Office for Europe, Copenhagen, Denmark 5–7 February 2003.* Brussels: European Commission; 2003.

204. Hurstfield J, Meager N, Aston J, Davies J, Mann K, Mitchell H *et al.* Monitoring the Disability Discrimination Act (DDA) 1995: Phase 3. *London: Institute for Employment Studies; 2004.*

205. Disability Rights Commission. *Disability Equality: Making it happen - first review of the Disability Discrimination Act 1995.* London: Disability Rights Commission; 2003.

206. McDonald JJ, Jr., Kulick FB, Creighton MK. Mental disabilities under the ADA: a management rights approach. *Employee Relat Law* J 1995; 20(4):541–569.

207. Evans DC. A comparison of the other-directed stigmatization produced by legal and illegal forms of affirmative action. *J Appl Psychol* 2003; 88(1):121–130.

208. Hinkley C. *Productivity Commission Inquiry into the Disability Discrimination Act.* Canberra, ACT: Mental Health Council of Australia; 2004.

209. Heginbotham C. UK mental health policy can alter the stigma of mental illness. *Lancet* 1998; 352(9133):1052–1053.

210. Berman LE. Mental health parity. *Managed Care Interface* 2000; 13(7):63–66.

211. Read J, Baker S. *Not Just Sticks and Stones. A survey of the stigma, taboos, and discrimination experienced by people with mental health problems.* London: MIND; 1996.

212. Domenici PV. Mental health care policy in the 1990s: discrimination in health care coverage of the seriously mentally ill. *J Clin Psychiatry* 1993; 54 Suppl:5–6.

213. Rossler W, Salize HJ, Biechele U. [Social legislative and structural deficits of ambulatory management of chronic psychiatric and handicapped patients]. *Nervenarzt* 1995; 66(11):802–810.

214. Warner L. *Out of Work: A survey of experiences of people with mental health problems with the workplace.* London: Mental Health Foundation; 2002.

215. Peay J. Law and stigma: present, future and futuristic solutions. In: Crisp A, ed., *Every Family in the Land*, pp. 367–372. London: Royal Society of Medicine; 2004.

216. Thornicroft G. *Discrimination against People with Mental Illness.* Oxford: Oxford University Press; 2006.

217. Bogdan R, Biklen D, Shapiro A, Spelkoman D. The disabled: media's monster. In: Nagler M, ed., *Perspectives on Disability*, pp. 138–142. Palo Alto, California: Health Markets Research; 1990.

218. Hebl MR, Kleck RE. The social consequences of physical disability. In: Heatherton TF, Kleck RE, Hebl MR, Hull JG, eds., *The Social Psychology of Stigma*, pp. 419–439. New York: Guilford; 2000.

219. Warner R. Local projects of the world psychiatric association programme to reduce stigma and discrimination. *Psychiatr Serv* 2005; 56(5):570–575.

220. Anspach RR. From stigma to identity politics: political activism among the physically disabled and former mental patients. *Soc Sci Med* [*Med Psychol Med Sociol*] 1979; 13A(6):765–773.

221. Fine F, Asch A. Disability beyond stigma: social interaction, discrimination, and activism. *Journal of Social Issues* 1988; 44(1):3–23.

222. Raymond CA. Political campaign pinpoints 'stigma hurdle' facing nation's mental health community. *JAMA* 1988; 260(10):1338–1339.

223. Shaughnessy P. Not in my back yard. Stigma from a personal perspective. In: Mason T, Carlisle C, Watkins C, Whitehead E, eds., *Stigma and Social Exclusion in Healthcare*, pp. 181–189. London: Routledge; 2001.

224. Corrigan PW, River LP, Lundin RK, Wasowski KU, Campion J, Mathisen J *et al.* Predictors of participation in campaigns against mental illness stigma. *J Nerv Ment Dis* 1999; 187(6):378–380.

225. Sullivan M, Hamilton T, Allen H. Changing stigma through the media. In: Corrigan PW, ed., *On the Stigma of Mental Illness. Practical strategies for research and social change*, pp. 297–312. Washington, DC: American Psychological Association; 2005.

226. Sieff EF. Media frames of mental illnesses: the potential impact of negative frames. *Journal of Mental Health* 2003; 12(3):259–269.

227. Rogers A, Pilgrim D, Lacey R. *Experiencing Psychiatry. Users views of services.* London: MIND; 1993.

228. National Union of Journalists. *Guide for Journalists and Broadcasters Reporting on Schizophrenia.* Dublin: National Union of Journalists; 1999.

229. Schwitzer G. A statement of principles for health care journalists. *Am J Bioeth* 2004; 4(4):W9–13.

230. Schwitzer G, Mudur G, Henry D, Wilson A, Goozner M, Simbra M *et al.* What are the roles and responsibilities of the media in disseminating health information? *PLoS Med* 2005; 2(7):e215.

231. National Union of Journalists. *NUJ Code of Practice.* London: National Union of Journalists; 1998.

232. Norris B, Jempson M, Bygrave L. *Covering Suicide Worldwide: Media Responsibilities.* London: Presswise Trust; 2001.

233. The Samaritans. *Media Guidelines on Portrayals of Suicide.* London: The Samaritans; 2002.

234. Michel K, Frey C, Wyss K, Valach L. An exercise in improving suicide reporting in print media. *Crisis* 2000; 21(2):71–79.

235. Angermeyer MC, Dietrich S, Pott D, Matschinger H. Media consumption and desire for social distance towards people with schizophrenia. *Eur Psychiatry* 2005; 20(3):246–250.

236. Vaughan G, Hansen C. 'Like Minds, Like Mine': a New Zealand project to counter the stigma and discrimination associated with mental illness. *Australas Psychiatry* 2004; 12(2):113–117.

237. Wahl OF. Depictions of mental illness in children's media. *Journal of Mental Health* 2003; 12(3):249–258.

238. Coverdale J, Nairn R, Claasen D. Depictions of mental illness in print media: a prospective national sample. *Aust N Z J Psychiatry* 2002; 36(5):697–700.

239. Nairn R, Coverdale J, Claasen D. From source material to news story in New Zealand print media: a prospective study of the stigmatizing processes in depicting mental illness. *Aust N Z J Psychiatry* 2001; 35(5):654–659.

240. Cutcliffe JR, Hannigan B. Mass media, 'monsters' and mental health clients: the need for increased lobbying. *J Psychiatr Ment Health Nurs* 2001; 8(4):315–321.

241. Berlin FS, Malin HM. Media distortion of the public's perception of recidivism and psychiatric rehabilitation. *Am J Psychiatry* 1991; 148(11):1572–1576.

242. McKeown M, Clancy B. Media influence on societal perceptions of mental illness. *Mental Health Nursing* 1995; 15(2):10–12.

243. Penn DL, Chamberlin C, Mueser KT. The effects of a documentary film about schizophrenia on psychiatric stigma. *Schizophr Bull* 2003; 29(2):383–391.

244. Mayer A, Barry DD. Working with the media to destigmatize mental illness. *Hosp Community Psychiatry* 1992; 43(1):77–78.

245. World Psychiatric Association. *Declaration of Madrid.* Geneva: World Psychiatric Association; 1996.

246. Salter M, Byrne P. The stigma of mental illness: how you can use the media to reduce it. *Psychiatr Bull* 2004;(24):281–283.

247. Stuart H. Stigma and the daily news: evaluation of a newspaper intervention. *Can J Psychiatry* 2003; 48(10):651–656.

248. Mason T. *Stigma and Social Exclusion in Healthcare.* London: Routledge; 2001.

249. Corrigan P. *On the Stigma of Mental Illness.* Washington, DC: American Psychological Association; 2005.

250. Barchas JD, Elliott GR, Berger PA, Barchas PR, Solomon F. The ultimate stigma: inadequate funding for research on mental illness and addictive disorders. *Am J Psychiatry* 1985; 142(7):838–839.

251. Ogden J. *Health Psychology,* 3rd edn. Maidenhead: Open University Press; 2004.

252. Baum A, Newman S, Weinman J, West R, McManus C. *Cambridge Handbook of Health, Psychology and Medicine.* Cambridge: Cambridge University Press; 1997.

253. Stroebe W, Jonas K, Hewstone M. *Introduction to Social Psychology*. London: Blackwell; 2006.

254. Ajzen I, Fishbein M. *Understanding Attitudes and Predicting Social Behaviour*. New York: Prentice Hall; 1980.

255. Eagly A, Chaiken S. *The Psychology of Attitudes*. London: Thomson Learning; 1993.

256. Williams E. Patient rights: mentally disordered offenders may refuse medication. *J Law Med Ethics* 2004; 32(2):375–376.

257. Corrigan P, Thompson V, Lambert D, Sangster Y, Noel JG, Campbell J. Perceptions of discrimination among persons with serious mental illness. *Psychiatr Serv* 2003; 54(8):1105–1110.

258. Lichtenstein B. Stigma as a barrier to treatment of sexually transmitted infection in the American deep south: issues of race, gender and poverty. *Soc Sci Med* 2003; 57(12):2435–2445.

259. Harvey RD. Individual differences in the phenomenological impact of social stigma. *J Soc Psychol* 2001; 141(2):174–189.

260. Keating F, Robertson D. Fear, black people and mental illness. A vicious circle? *Health and Social Care in the Community* 2004; 12(5):439–447.

261. Pillay HM. The concepts, 'causation', 'racism' and 'mental illness'. *Int J Soc Psychiatry* 1984; 30(1–2):29–39.

262. Bailey S. Throughout Europe and North America young people at the interface of criminal justice systems and mental health services risk double jeopardy for social exclusion alienation and stigmatization. *J Adolesc* 2000; 23(3):237–241.

263. Bouras N, Szymanski L. Services for people with mental retardation and psychiatric disorders: US-UK comparative overview. *Int J Soc Psychiatry* 1997; 43(1):64–71.

264. Watkins KE, Burnam A, Kung FY, Paddock S. A national survey of care for persons with co-occurring mental and substance use disorders. *Psychiatr Serv* 2001; 52(8):1062–1068.

265. Link BG, Struening EL, Rahav M, Phelan JC, Nuttbrock L. On stigma and its consequences: evidence from a longitudinal study of men with dual diagnoses of mental illness and substance abuse. *J Health Soc Behav* 1997; 38(2):177–190.

266. Herrick CA, Pearcey LG, Ross C. Stigma and ageism: compounding influences in making an accurate mental health assessment. *Nurs Forum* 1997; 32(3):21–26.

267. Surgeon General. Surgeon General reports on mental health revolution. *Health Care Financ Rev* 1999; 21(2):293–294.

268. Cunningham R. Perspectives. Satcher Report: research is key to overcoming stigma and widespread undertreatment of mental disorders. *Med Health* 2000; 54(3):suppl-4.

269. Hegner RE. Dispelling the myths and stigma of mental illness: the Surgeon General's report on mental health. *Issue Brief Natl Health Policy Forum* 2000;(754):1–7.

270. SAMHSA. *President's New Freedom Commission on Mental Health* (SMA03–3832). Rockville, Maryland: United States Department of Health and Human Services: Substance Abuse and Mental Health Services Administration (SAMHSA); 2003.

271. Singh BS, McGorry PD. The Second National Mental Health Plan: an opportunity to take stock and move forward. *Med J Aust* 1998; 169(8):435–437.

272. Department of Health. *National Service Framework for Mental Health. Modern standards and service models*. London: Department of Health; 1999.

273. National Institute for Mental Health in England. *From Here to Equality: A strategic plan to tackle stigma and discrimination on mental health grounds*. London: Department of Health; 2004.

274. Wolff N. Risk, response, and mental health policy: learning from the experience of the United Kingdom. *Journal of Health Politics, Policy and Law* 2002; 27:801–832.

275. World Health Organisation. *WHO Resource Book on Mental Health, Human Rights and Legislation.* Geneva: World Health Organisation; 2005.

276. World Health Organisation. *Mental Health Atlas 2005.* Geneva: World Health Organisation; 2005.

277. World Health Organisation. *Mental Health Declaration for Europe.* Copenhagen: World Health Organisation; 2005.

278. World Health Organisation. *Mental Health Action Plan for Europe.* Copenhagen: World Health Organisation; 2005.

279. Thornicroft G, Rose D. Mental health in Europe. *BMJ* 2005; 330(7492):613–614.

280. Baker D. Human rights for persons with disabilities. In: Nagler M, Kemp EJ, eds., *Perspectives on Disability,* pp. 483–494. Palo Alto, California: Health Markets Research; 1993.

281. Amnesty International. *Ethical Codes and Declarations Relevant to the Health Professions.* London: Amnesty International; 2000.

282. Amnesty International. *Mental Illness, the Neglected Quarter: Summary report.* Dublin: Amnesty International; 2003.

283. United Nations. *UN Resolution 46/119 on the Protection of Persons with Mental Illness and the Improvement of Mental Health Care,* adopted by the General Assembly on 17 December 1991. New York: United Nations; 1991.

284. United Nations. *International Covenant on Civil and Political Rights.* Adopted by the UN General Assembly Resolution 2200A (XXI) of 16 December 1966. New York: United Nations (*http://www.ohchr.org/english/countries/ra 1966.*

285. United Nations. *Universal Declaration of Human Rights.* Adopted and Proclaimed by the UN General Assembly Resolution 217A (III) of 10 December 1948. New York: United Nations; 1948.

286. United Nations. *International Covenant on Economic, Social and Cultural Rights.* Adopted by UN General Assembly Resolution 2200A (XXI) of 16 December 1966. New York: United Nations; 1966.

287. United Nations. *UN Principles for the Protection of Persons with Mental Illness and for the Improvement of Mental Health Care.* Adopted by UN General Assembly Resolution 46/119 of 18 February 1992. New York: United Nations; 1992.

288. United Nations. United Nations. *Persons with Disabilities. General Comment Number 5* (Eleventh Session 1994). UN Doc E/C 12/1994/13. UN Committee on Economic, Social and Cultural Rights. New York: United Nations; 1994.

289. Kingdon D, Jones R, Lonnqvist J. Protecting the human rights of people with mental disorder: new recommendations emerging from the Council of Europe. *Br J Psychiatry* 2004; 185:277–279.

290. Bindman J, Maingay S, Szmukler G. The Human Rights Act and mental health legislation. *Br J Psychiatry* 2003; 182:91–94.

291. Thornicroft G, Szmukler G. The draft Mental Health Bill in England: without principles. *Psychiatr Bull* 2005; 29:244–247.

292. Corrigan PW. Mental illness stigma as social injustice: yet another dream to be achieved. In: Corrigan PW, ed., *On the Stigma of Mental Illness. Practical strategies for research and social change,* pp. 315–320. Washington DC: American Psychological Press; 2005.

293. Hunt P. *Economic, Cultural and Social Rights. Report of the Special Rapporteur on the right of everyone to enjoyment of the highest attainable standard of physical and mental health.*

Commission on Human Rights, 61st Session, Item 10 on the provisional agenda. New York: United Nations Economic and Social Council; 2005.

294. Allende I. *The House of the Spirits.* London: Swan Books; 1985.

295. van Oorschot W, Hvinden B. Towards convergence? Disability policies in Europe. *European Journal of Social Security* 2000; 2:293–302.

296. Magliano L, De RC, Fiorillo A, Malangone C, Maj M. Perception of patients' unpredictability and beliefs on the causes and consequences of schizophrenia – a community survey. *Soc Psychiatry Psychiatr Epidemiol* 2004; 39(5):410–416.

297. Corrigan PW, Watson AC. At issue: Stop the stigma: call mental illness a brain disease. *Schizophr Bull* 2004; 30(3):477–479.

298. Luchins DJ. At issue: will the term brain disease reduce stigma and promote parity for mental illnesses? *Schizophr Bull* 2004; 30(4):1043–1048.

299. Stuart H, Arboleda-Florez J. Community attitudes toward people with schizophrenia. *Can J Psychiatry* 2001; 46(3):245–252.

300. Baron M. Psychiatric genetics and prejudice: can the science be separated from the scientist? *Mol Psychiatry* 1998; 3(2):96–100.

301. Phelan JC. Genetic bases of mental illness – a cure for stigma? *Trends Neurosci* 2002; 25(8):430–431.

302. Read J, Harre N. The role of biological and genetic causal beliefs in the stigmatisation of 'mental patients'. *Journal of Mental Health* 2001; 10:223–235.

303. Sartorius N, Schulze H. *Reducing the Stigma of Mental Illness. A Report from the Global Programme Against Stigma of the World Psychiatric Association.* Cambridge: Cambridge University Press; 2005.

304. Jain R, Thomasma DC, Ragas R. Down syndrome: still a social stigma. *Am J Perinatol* 2002; 19(2):99–108.

305. Kim Y, Berrios GE. Impact of the term schizophrenia on the culture of ideograph: the Japanese experience. *Schizophr Bull* 2001; 27(2):181–185.

306. Penn DL, Nowlin-Drummond A. Politically correct labels and schizophrenia: a rose by any other name? *Schizophr Bull* 2001; 27(2):197–203.

307. Reaume G. Lunatic to patient to person: nomenclature in psychiatric history and the influence of patients' activism in North America. *Int J Law Psychiatry* 2002; 25(4):405–26.

308. American Psychiatric Association. *Diagnostic and Statistical Manual of Mental Disorders: DSM-IV-TR:* 4th edn Text Revision. Washington DC: American Psychiatric Publishing Inc; 2000.

309. World Health Organisation. *ICD 10: the International Classification of Mental and Behavioural Disorders: Clinical descriptions and diagnostic guidelines.* Geneva: World Health Organisation; 1992.

310. Sontag S. *AIDS and its Metaphors.* London: Penguin; 1988.

311. Nairn RG, Coverdale JH. People never see us living well: an appraisal of the personal stories about mental illness in a prospective print media sample. *Aust N Z J Psychiatry* 2005; 39(4):281–287.

312. Henderson L. Selling suffering: mental illness and media values. In: Philo G, ed., *Media and Mental Distress*, pp. 18–36. London: Longman; 1996.

313. Blaska J. The power of language: speak and write using 'person first'. In: Nagler M, Kemp EJ, eds., *Perspectives on Disability Health Markets Research*, pp. 25–32. Palo Alto, California: Health Markets Research; 1993.

314. Perkins RE, Repper JM. Exclusive language? In: Mason JM, Carlisle C, Waternaux C, Whitehead E, eds., *Stigma and Social Exclusion in Healthcare*, pp. 147–157. London: Routledge; 2001.

315. Wilson C, Nairn R, Coverdale J, Panapa A. Mental illness depictions in prime-time drama: identifying the discursive resources. *Aust N Z J Psychiatry* 1999; 33(2):232–239.

316. Wahl O. *Media Madness*. New Brunswick, New Jersey: Rutgers University Press; 1995.

317. Gilman SL. *Difference and Pathology: Stereotypes of sexuality, race and madness*. Ithaca: Cornell University Press; 1985.

318. Gilman SL. *Disease and Representation: Images of illness from madness to AIDS*. Ithaca: Cornell University Press; 1988.

319. Gilman SL. *Seeing the Insane*. Wiley: New York; 1982.

320. Rose N, Novas C. Biological citizenship. In: Ong A, Collier S, eds., *Global Assemblages. Technology, politics, and ethics as anthropological problems*, pp. London: Blackwell; 2003, pp 439–463.

321. Dunion L, Gordon L. Tackling the attitude problem. The achievements to date of Scotland's 'see me' anti-stigma campaign. *Ment Health Today* 2005; 22–25.

322. Department of Health. *Attitudes to Mental Illness 2003 Report*. London: Department of Health; 2003.

323. Estroff S. *Making it Crazy: Ethnography of psychiatric clients in an American community*. Berkeley: University of California Press; 1981.

324. Dear M, Wolch J. *Landscapes of Despair*. Princeton, New Jersey: Princeton University Press; 1992.

325. Corrigan PW, Watson AC, Gracia G, Slopen N, Rasinski K, Hall LL. Newspaper stories as measures of structural stigma. *Psychiatr Serv* 2005; 56(5):551–556.

326. Corrigan PW, Markowitz FE, Watson AC. Structural levels of mental illness stigma and discrimination. *Schizophr Bull* 2004; 30(3):481–491.

327. Corrigan PW. Towards an integrated, structural model of psychiatric rehabilitation. *Psychiatr Rehabil J* 2003; 26(4):346–358.

328. MacPherson W. *The Steven Lawrence Inquiry. Report of an Inquiry by Sir William MacPherson of Cluny*. London: Houses of Parliament, Cm 4262–1; 1999.

329. Pinfold V, Byrne P, Toulmin H. Challenging stigma and discrimination in communities: a focus group study identifying UK mental health service users' main campaign priorities. *Int J Soc Psychiatry* 2005; 51(2):128–138.

330. Goldman HH, Rachuba L, Van Tosh L. Methods of assessing mental health consumers' preferences for housing and support services. *Psychiatr Serv* 1995; 46(2):169–172.

331. March DT. Personal accounts of consumer/survivors: insights and implications. *Journal of Clinical Psychology* 2000; 56(11):1447–1457.

332. Wahl OF. Mental health consumers' experience of stigma. *Schizophr Bull* 1999; 25(3):467–478.

333. Hinshaw SP, Cicchetti D. Stigma and mental disorder: conceptions of illness, public attitudes, personal disclosure, and social policy. *Dev Psychopathol* 2000; 12(4):555–98.

334. Mercer S, Dieppe P, Chambers R, MacDonald R. Equality for people with disabilities in medicine. *BMJ* 2003; 327(7420):882–883.

335. Hanson KW. Public opinion and the mental health parity debate: lessons from the survey literature. *Psychiatr Serv* 1998; 49(8):1059–1066.

336. Thornicroft G, Rose D. Mental health in Europe. *BMJ* 2005; 330(7492):613–614.

337. Frank RG, Goldman HH, McGuire TG. Will parity in coverage result in better mental health care? *N Engl J Med* 2001; 345(23):1701–1704.

338. Kessler RC, Demler O, Frank RG, Olfson M, Pincus HA, Walters EE *et al.* Prevalence and treatment of mental disorders, 1990 to 2003. *N Engl J Med* 2005; 352(24):2515–2523.

339. Goldberg D, Goodyer I. *Genesis of Common Mental Disorders.* London: Brunner-Routledge; 2005.

340. Soanes C, Stevenson A. *Concise Oxford English Dictionary,* 11th edn. Oxford: Oxford University Press; 2003.

341. Draine J, Salzer M, Culhane D, Hadley T. Poverty, social problems, and serious mental illness. *Psychiatr Serv* 2002; 53(7):899.

342. Draine J, Salzer MS, Culhane DP, Hadley TR. Role of social disadvantage in crime, joblessness, and homelessness among persons with serious mental illness. *Psychiatr Serv* 2002; 53(5):565–573.

343. Fanon F. *The Wretched of the Earth.* New York: Grove Press; 1963.

344. Morone JA. Enemies of the people: the moral dimension to public health. *Journal of Health Politics, Policy and Law* 1997; 22(4):993–1020.

345. Kelly BD. Structural violence and schizophrenia. *Soc Sci Med* 2005; 61(3):721–730.

346. Sartorius N, Schulze H. *Reducing the Stigma of Mental Illness. A Report from a Global Programme of the World Psychiatric Association.* Cambridge: Cambridge University Press; 2005.

347. Porter R. Can the stigma of mental illness be changed? *Lancet* 1998; 352(9133):1049–1050.

348. Shorter E. *A History of Psychiatry.* New York: Wiley; 1997.

349. Goldman HH. Implementing the lessons of mental health service demonstrations: human rights issues. *Acta Psychiatr Scand* Suppl. 2000; 399:51–54.

Appendix

Internet resources

community-2.webtv.net/stigmanet/AbouttheNational/index.html
The National Stigma Clearinghouse tracks negative stereotypes of mental illnesses and provides information about fighting prejudice

stopstigma.samhsa.gov
Resource Center to Address Discrimination and Stigma of the US Department of Health and Human Services Substance Abuse and Mental Health Services Administration

www.adscenter.org
US Department of Health and Human Services Resource Center to Address Discrimination and Stigma

www.artagainststigma.org
A website dedicated to using art to fight against prejudice and stigmatisation

www.bazelon.org
The Bazelon Center for Mental Health Law aims to protect and advance the rights of adults and children who have mental disabilities

www.beyondblue.org.au
A national, independent, not-for-profit organisation to address issues associated with depression, anxiety and related substance misuse disorders in Australia, with the goal of raising community awareness about depression and reducing stigma

www.blackdoginstitute.org.au
The Black Dog Institute is a clinical, research and educational body dedicated to improving understanding, diagnosis and treatment of depression and bipolar disorder

www.drc-gb.org
The goal of the UK Disability Rights Commission is 'a society where all disabled people can participate fully as equal citizens'
www.iop.kcl.ac.uk/iopweb/departments/home/default.aspx?locator=461
Evidence of effective interventions against stigma

www.mdac.info

The Mental Disability Advocacy Center aims to promote and protect the human rights of people with mental health problems in central and eastern Europe and central Asia

www.mdri.org
Mental Disability Rights International documents conditions, publishes reports on human rights enforcement, and promotes the rights of people with mental disabilities

www.mediawise.org.uk
The MediaWise Trust promotes compliance with ethical standards of conduct and with the law by journalists, broadcasters and all others engaged in the media

www.mentalhealthcare.org.uk
A source of evidence-based information on a range of mental illnesses, provided by Rethink and the Institute of Psychiatry, King's College London

www.nami.org/Content/NavigationMenu/Take_Action/Fight_Stigma/Fight_Stigma_StigmaBusters.htm
The StigmaBusters website of the National Alliance for the Mentally Ill

www.nmha.org/newsroom/stigma/index.cfm
The Stigma Watch site of the National Mental Health Association

www.nostigma.org
The website of the National Mental Health Awareness Campaign

www.openthedoors.com
The Global Programme to Fight the Stigma and Discrimination because of Schizophrenia of the World Psychiatric Association (WPA)

www.power2u.org
The National Empowerment Center envisions a future when everyone with a mental illness will recover

www.rcpsych.ac.uk/campaigns/cminds
The Changing Minds campaign of the Royal College of Psychiatrists

www.sane.org
SANE Australia. Includes their StigmaWatch site

www.seemescotland.org
The 'See Me' campaign challenges stigma and discrimination around mental ill-health in Scotland

www.shift.org.uk
Shift is an initiative of the National Institute for Mental Health in England (NIMHE), to tackle stigma and discrimination on mental health issues

www.stigmaresearch.org
The Chicago Consortium for Stigma Research is dedicated to understanding the phenomenon of stigma, developing and testing models that explain why it occurs, and evaluating strategies that help to diminish its effects

uhaweb.hartford.edu/owahl/resources.htm
Resource page on fighting discrimination and stigma, maintained by Dr Otto Wahl

www.unhchr.ch/html/menu3/b/68.htm
Principles for the Protection of Persons with Mental Illness and the Improvement of Mental Health Care. Resolution Adopted by General Assembly of the United Nations 46/119 of 17 December 1991

Index